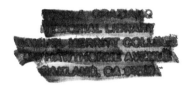

Atlas of
CARDIOVASCULAR
Monitoring

Atlas of CARDIOVASCULAR Monitoring

JONATHAN B. MARK, M.D.

Associate Professor
Department of Anesthesiology
Assistant Professor
Department of Medicine
Duke University School of Medicine
Chief, Anesthesiology Service
Veterans Affairs Medical Center
Durham, North Carolina

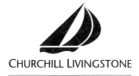

CHURCHILL LIVINGSTONE

New York, Edinburgh, London, Madrid, Melbourne, San Francisco, Tokyo

Library of Congress Cataloging-in-Publication Data

A catalog record for this book is available from the Library of Congress

ISBN: 0-443-08891-8

© **Churchill Livingstone Inc. 1998**
Medical Division of Pearson Professional Limited

 is a registered trademark of Pearson Professional Limited

Distributed in the United Kingdom by Churchill Livingstone, Robert Stevenson House, 1–3 Baxter's Place, Leith Walk, Edinburgh EH1 3AF, and by associated companies, branches, and representatives throughout the world.

Medical knowledge is constantly changing. As new information becomes available, changes in treatment, procedures, equipment and the use of drugs become necessary. The editors/authors/contributors and the publishers have, as far as it is possible, taken care to ensure that the information given in this text is accurate and up to date. However, readers are strongly advised to confirm that the information, especially with regard to drug usage, complies with the latest legislation and standards of practice.

The Publishers have made every effort to trace the copyright holders for borrowed material. If they have inadvertently overlooked any, they will be pleased to make the necessary arrangements at the first opportunity.

Acquisitions Editor: *Michael J. Houston*
Assistant Editor: *Ann Ruzycka*
Production Editor: *Elizabeth A. Plowman*
Production Supervisor: *Sharon Tuder*
Desktop Coordinator: *Barbara Ulbrich*
Cover Design: *Jeanette Jacobs*

Printed in the United States of America

To my family, Chris, Ben, Zach (and Dixie),
and to the memory of Adele Mark, who devoted her professional career to
teaching visually handicapped children.
Good eyesight is a blessing,
seeing clearly is a skill.
I hope *Atlas of Cardiovascular Monitoring* helps.

Foreword

Atlas of Cardiovascular Monitoring is a remarkable book, which is useful to anyone who wishes to maximize the information available from standard cardiovascular monitoring modalities. As such, it is a worthy supplement to the existing physiology, electrophysiology, and cardiovascular pharmacology literature. As with any atlas, it enjoys the efficiency of pictures—that is, each one is "worth a thousand words." The juxtaposition of the captions with their illustrations ties together the anatomy, physiology, pharmacology, and technology required in making proper management decisions from monitoring. In *Atlas of Cardiovascular Monitoring,* no common hemodynamic observation—real or artifact—is ignored.

One of the cardinal rules of monitoring, which is illustrated throughout this text, is the concept of *integrated monitoring.* Simply put, this means that one cannot and should not rely on a single number or tracing to make final judgments. Rather, the integration or multiple forms of information, numeric, waveform analysis, electrocardiographic, etc., are all required to enhance the probability of appropriate assessment. A good example of this is the diagnosis of junctional rhythm when P waves are difficult to discern on the electrocardiogram, but cannon a waves in the central venous pressure trace confirm the diagnosis.

Another remarkable, and now rare, aspect of *Atlas of Cardiovascular Monitoring* is that it is single-authored, giving the reader a consistent and non-duplicative presentation. Furthermore, Dr. Mark provides keen insights and attention to every detail. He is known for his "Squiggles and Wiggles" lecture at Duke University School of Medicine. The things that we all see on the screen every day are brought into exquisite and elegant translation by Dr. Mark. All of the illustrations were collected from one astute clinician's experience, not imagined or computer generated. They are *real.* Through his focus on waveform details and their relevance to the patient's condition, Dr. Mark has become legendary for his hemodynamic teaching at Duke, where he enjoys the admiration of anesthesiologists, surgeons, internists, and nurses.

Who will benefit from *Atlas of Cardiovascular Monitoring?* Patients will benefit from the more-informed care of anyone who has mastered the material. *Atlas of Cardiovascular Monitoring* was written to educate physicians, nurses, medical students, and other clinicians who make use of the bedside monitor. It will be invaluable in a wide variety of settings, including the operating room, intensive care unit, recovery room, step-down unit, and emergency room. Understanding the material which is so carefully collected and clearly presented in this book enriches the information from monitoring and provides the clinician with greater and more certain knowledge of the patient's cardiovascular condition. We are grateful to Dr. Mark for creating such a marvelous resource.

J. G. Reves, M.D.
Professor and Chairman
Department of Anesthesiology
Duke University School of Medicine
Durham, North Carolina

Preface

Atlas of Cardiovascular Monitoring actually began more than a decade ago, when I presented a Grand Rounds Lecture entitled, "Waves and Trends: Optimal Monitoring of Cardiac Filling Pressures." My talk focused on the detailed interpretation of cardiovascular waveforms, and to illustrate these teaching points, I showed real traces that I had collected from a standard bedside monitor and strip chart recorder. Over the years, as my collection of cardiovascular waveforms grew, and I continued to lecture on this subject and made it the focus of my teaching efforts in the operating room and intensive care unit, residents and other colleagues convinced me that it would be useful to reproduce these teaching materials in a more permanent form. Atlas of Cardiovascular Monitoring is the result of that request.

The critical importance of accurate waveform interpretation during cardiovascular monitoring has been emphasized in a practice guideline written by a joint task force of the American College of Physicians, the American College of Cardiology, and the American Heart Association.[4] A similar guideline sponsored by the American Society of Anesthesiologists concurs in this recommendation that "knowledge of and ability to recognize pulse waveforms for the wide array of hemodynamic conditions" be considered a prerequisite cognitive skill for safe use of hemodynamic monitoring.[10] Despite these published guidelines, a number of studies suggest that major knowledge deficits remain among physicians[5,6,7] and nurses[8] who perform hemodynamic monitoring. In fact, the ongoing clinical controversy regarding the effectiveness of pulmonary artery catheterization in reducing patient morbidity and mortality[1,2,3,9,10,12,13] may be explained in part by the improper collection and interpretation of hemodynamic data.[1,9]

In view of these concerns, I hope that Atlas of Cardiovascular Monitoring will serve as a useful educational resource for training in hemodynamic monitoring and inspire the reader to become a more astute and critical observer of monitored cardiovascular waveforms. Careful observation and detailed analysis are skills that distinguish the expert clinician, whether these skills are applied to medical history taking and physical examination or the interpretation of hemodynamic tracings.

In the pages that follow, all the standard cardiovascular waveforms from the bedside monitor are presented, beginning at the bottom of the monitor screen with central venous pressure, then moving up to pulmonary artery and wedge pressure, arterial blood pressure, and finally, the electrocardiogram (ECG). In the first half of Atlas of Cardiovascular Monitoring, normal waveforms and common artifacts are presented, as well as the technical requirements for proper ECG and pressure recording. The second half of Atlas of Cardiovascular Monitoring focuses on cardiovascular pathophysiology, including ECG and hemodynamic monitoring for myocardial ischemia, respiratory-circulatory interactions, and valvular and pericardial diseases. The final two chapters present common cardiovascular waveforms seen during cardiopulmonary bypass and intraaortic balloon counterpulsation and will prove most useful to readers who work in the same clinical environments that I inhabit as a cardiac anesthesiologist.

The waveforms contained in Atlas of Cardiovascular Monitoring have been hand-traced from the original strip chart recordings, then scanned and stored in a digital format. When a figure displays more than one type of pressure waveform, these waveforms are distinguished by lines of different intensity, in an attempt to provide the clearest possible figure for reproduction. The pressure scales are in units of millimeters of mercury (mmHg) and are labeled to allow measurement of pressure values directly from the traces. In general, standard ECG recording speed (25 mm/sec) is used, and other recording speeds are clearly noted on the figures. Most figures are reproduced at 100 percent of their original size, so that the background grid remains at a scale of 1 mm in the figure equal to 1 mm in the original tracing. Finally, the figures are segregated at the end of each chapter, accompanied by detailed legends, and presented in a horizontal format whenever possible, in order to make it easy for the reader to interpret each tracing without constantly turning pages. All of these editorial decisions were made with a single goal in mind: to present figures that would be reproduced clearly and resemble closely real strip chart tracings recorded at the bedside. I hope Atlas of Cardiovascular Monitoring will prove valuable to all clinicians who want to look beyond the numbers on the bedside monitor and learn to recognize the diagnostic clues revealed in the cardiovascular waveforms.

Jonathan B. Mark, M.D.
Durham, North Carolina

References

1. Connors AF, Speroff T, Dawson NV, et al. The effectiveness of right heart catheterization in the initial care of critically ill patients. JAMA 1996;276:889-97

2. Dalen JE, Bone RC. Is it time to pull the pulmonary artery catheter? JAMA 1996;276:916-8

3. Fink MP. The flow-directed, pulmonary artery catheter and outcome in critically ill patients: have we heard the last word? Crit Care Med 1997;25:902-3

4. Friesinger GC, Williams SV. Clinical competence in hemodynamic monitoring. JACC 1990;15:1460-4

5. Ginosar Y, Thijs LG, Sprung CL. Raising the standard of hemodynamic monitoring: targeting the practice or the practitioner? Crit Care Med 1997;25:209-11

6. Gnaegi A, Feihl F, Perret C. Intensive care physicians' insufficient knowledge of right-heart catheterization at the bedside: time to act? Crit Care Med 1997;25:213-20

7. Iberti TJ, Fischer EP, Leibowitz AB, et al. A multicenter study of physicians' knowledge of the pulmonary artery catheter. JAMA 1990;264:2928-32

8. Iberti TJ, Daily EK, Leibowitz AB, et al. Assessment of critical care nurses' knowledge of the pulmonary artery catheter. Crit Care Med 1994;22:1674-8

9. Pulmonary Artery Catheter Consensus Conference: consensus statement. Crit Care Med 1997;25:910–25

10. Rackow EC. Pulmonary Artery Catheter Consensus Conference. Crit Care Med 1997;25:901

11. Roizen MF, Berger DL, Gabel RA, et al. Practice guidelines for pulmonary artery catheterization. A report by the American Society of Anesthesiologists Task Force on Pulmonary Artery Catheterization. Anesthesiology 1993;78:380-94

12. Soni N. Swan song for the Swan-Ganz catheter? Brit Med J 1996;313:763-4

13. Tuman KJ, Roizen MF. Outcome assessment and pulmonary artery catheterization: why does the debate continue? Anesth Analg 1997;84:1-4

Acknowledgments

I would like to acknowledge the special contributions of a number of individuals who helped me along my journey as an author. In the early phases of this work, residents and colleagues in the Department of Anesthesia, Brigham and Women's Hospital, provided much needed encouragement, and the support of Chairmen, Ben Covino, and Gerry Ostheimer, was most appreciated. The single greatest influence at that time was provided by Roy Vandam, whose words of wisdom (and copious editorial red ink) helped start me on my way. The contents of *Atlas of Cardiovascular Monitoring* were enriched further through countless discussions with colleagues in the Department of Anesthesia, Duke University School of Medicine and especially the anesthesiologists at the Durham Veterans Affairs Medical Center. Not only did the VA anesthesia group offer insights to refine my own hemodynamic observations, but their dedication and hard clinical work allowed me some all-important, undisturbed writing time. Among my colleagues here in North Carolina, I want to express my special gratitude to Andrew Hilton, who reviewed the sections on electrocardiography, and my Chairman, Jerry Reves, who helped me keep my eye on the target and provided unwavering support for this project.

The technical aspects of creating the illustrations for *Atlas of Cardiovascular Monitoring* were addressed skillfully by the Duke Audiovisual Department. Jerry Schoendorf helped solve many of the initial problems of digital image creation, and Stan Coffman, the medical illustrator for this project, made it all happen. Stan's careful hand-tracings were transformed accurately into the more than 250 digitized figures contained in this book. I don't know many individuals other than Stan who would have undertaken fourth- or fifth-time figure revisions at my request in order to get the waveform, labeling and background grids just right. Although I take responsibility for any inaccuracies contained in these illustrations, Stan deserves all the credit for bringing them to the reader so clearly.

My editor at Churchill Livingstone, Michael Houston, helped keep me sane and productive during the past two years. I am grateful for the calming influence he had during the busiest and most stressful months of final writing and editing. Finally, my deepest appreciation goes to Jan Horrow, one of my first and most significant mentors in cardiac anesthesia. Jan's editorial scrutiny of the entire text resulted in innumerable improvements in both form and content.

Contents

xiii

CHAPTER ONE *Monitoring Philosophy, Displays, and Recorders*

Imagine the bedside monitor without waveform displays, no ECG or blood pressure traces, just the digital values for pressures and heart rate. So much important diagnostic information would be missing. One could not discern cardiac arrhythmias, conduction abnormalities, or ECG patterns of myocardial ischemia. Hemodynamic abnormalities such as tall v waves, cannon a waves, and pulsus alternans would be inapparent. By providing waveforms, the bedside monitor presents a wealth of cardiovascular information beyond the digital values commonly recorded on operating room or intensive care charts.[1]

Not only do waveforms provide diagnostic details, but they also corroborate the digital values displayed or warn when these values should be questioned. Flushing of a vascular pressure line is recognized immediately by the sudden disappearance and reappearance of the normal pressure trace, while the digital value may remain abnormal for an additional period (Fig. 1.1). Patient movement or electrical artifacts may distort the ECG waveform and cause an erroneous value for heart rate (Fig. 1.2). Waveform traces provide the clinician with confidence in the digital values displayed.

Monitoring is different from measuring, in that the former connotes a continuous process, while the latter implies intermittent observation. A familiar example would be the difference between direct invasive monitoring of arterial blood pressure (ABP) in contrast to periodic measurement of blood pressure with a sphygmomanometer. Similarly, central venous pressure (CVP) can be monitored continuously with a pressure transducer or measured intermittently with a water manometer. Cardiovascular waveform monitoring provides details, trends, and patterns of change over time, leading to diagnostic insights that would not be possible using intermittent measurement techniques.

In order to interpret ECG or hemodynamic tracings, the observer must have a firm appreciation of cardiac anatomy and physiology, both normal and pathologic. With sufficient knowledge and experience, the clinician will search for the expected waveforms and quickly recognize abnormal patterns, typical of many disease states. Accurate interpretation of these patterns is predicated on an understanding of underlying physiologic mechanisms. By analogy, novices of physical diagnosis may have difficulty distinguishing complicated heart sounds, while a clinician experienced in cardiac auscultation will be better able to detect and describe abnormal murmurs, snaps, clicks, and rubs.[3] Knowledge and experience improve bedside diagnostic skills, whether the clinician is using a stethoscope or the tracings on the cardiovascular monitor.

MONITOR DISPLAY

Current monitors provide a choice of scales, sweep speeds, colors, and layout configurations for the monitor display screen. When the patient has full invasive hemodynamic monitoring, the ECG, ABP, pulmonary artery pressure (PAP), and CVP should all be displayed simultaneously. In this way, patterns of change and trends in each monitored variable may be integrated together in order to arrive at the diagnosis. One might not recognize sudden disappearance of the P wave on the ECG trace, but the combination of abrupt arterial hypotension and appearance of a cannon a wave in the CVP waveform confirms that atrioventricular dissociation has developed (Fig. 1.3). (See Ch. 14 for more detail.)

In general, one or two ECG leads are displayed at the top of the monitor screen, and the ABP, PAP, and CVP are displayed beneath in that order. These waveforms can be shown in several formats. As *free waveforms*, with no adjacent scales displayed, the waveforms provide the fewest clues to the observer (Fig. 1.4). One cannot determine numeric pressure values by inspecting the traces on the monitor screen, and thus, no quantitative information can be derived. This display format is the least informative and generally should not be used.

A more common and useful display provides *separate waveforms*, each with its own scale (Fig. 1.5). The individual scales can be chosen to maximize waveform sizes, or standard default values can be chosen for each monitored pressure (e.g., 0 to 120 mmHg for ABP, 0 to 30 mmHg for PAP). Additional on-screen horizontal graticule lines aid the observer in discerning phasic pressure values like the pulmonary artery wedge pressure (Fig. 1.5). However, owing to the constraints of overall screen size, separate waveform display for individual pressure traces often makes the waveforms too small for the phasic components to be seen readily and abnormal patterns easily recognized.

The most informative display format provides *full-scale waveforms*, which occupy the entire space allotted for invasive pressure monitoring (Fig. 1.6). Temporal relations between the various invasive pressures are seen clearly, and morphologic details are observed readily, owing to the relatively large size of the display. Problems arise when the invasive pressure traces overlap, and many clinicians find this confusing. A number of solutions are available. First, many modern monitors display waveforms in different colors to provide rapid discrimination of individual traces. Monochromatic monitors may display the different pressures with lines of varying intensity or quality (e.g., dashed lines). If the clinician still objects to the overlapping traces, scales may be chosen to eliminate the problem in any individual patient. When this is done, it is best to leave the ABP scale unchanged and adjust the PAP and CVP scales to eliminate the overlap. When the clinician avoids the temptation to change the ABP scale, except under the most unusual circumstances, normal arterial pressure traces always will have the same appearance and location on the monitor screen. At a glance, the clinician can recognize important hypertension and hypotension by the location of the arterial pressure trace above or below its typical residence on the monitor screen. By analogy, a car driver rapidly recognizes the car's approximate speed by glancing at the position of the speedometer needle; if the speedometer scale changed daily, the driver could not check the speed "out of the corner of the eye," but would have to read the scale each time.

RECORDERS

Pressure waveform interpretation on the monitor screen is aided by "freeze display" or "capture screen" functions, which halt the moving traces long enough to allow time to scrutinize the waveforms. However, bedside hard copy recorders provide the best method to study pressure waveforms and document abnormalities for the medical record. Successful pressure waveform interpretation requires a multiple channel recorder, so that the ECG trace and the invasive pressure of interest can be recorded simultaneously. The ECG provides an indispensable timing marker for the cardiac cycle (Fig. 1.7), which allows unambiguous assignment of pressure waveform components as systolic or diastolic in origin. This concept is developed in detail in Chapter 2.

While a two-channel recorder is the minimum acceptable device for accurate monitoring, a four-channel recorder is preferred, since the ECG, ABP, PAP, and CVP traces can be displayed simultaneously (Fig. 1.6). Like the monitor screen, some recorders can be configured to display separate individual scale traces or full-scale traces, the latter having the potential problem of waveform overlap previously described. When waveform overlap interferes with interpretation, unneeded traces can be turned off transiently, or the PAP and CVP scales can be increased to reduce the relative size of these pressure waves and thereby obviate this problem.

Electrocardiogram and pressure waveforms generally sweep across the bedside monitor screen at a speed of 25 mm/sec. This is the same speed used in standard 12-lead ECG recordings and allows adequate resolution of temporal ECG and pressure waveform details. Similarly, 25 mm/sec is the ideal speed for routine bedside recordings; the ECG appears as it does on a standard tracing, and the pressure waveforms have sufficient temporal resolution to allow proper wave component identification (Figs. 1.6 and 1.7). Faster tracings (e.g., 50 mm/sec) are not required for most clinical work but may be preferred for research measurements. Slower speed tracings (e.g., 5 mm/sec) are chosen to display slower events, like the effect of the respiratory cycle on the pressure waveforms (Fig. 1.8). Very slow tracings (e.g., 1 or 5 mm/min) allow continuous trends of hemodynamic variables to be displayed. Although waveform detail is lost, patterns of change help elucidate transient circulatory phenomena as well as insidious patterns. In the example in Figure 1.8, a slow recording of ABP and CVP reveals sudden hypotension, lasting approximately 30 seconds and slightly preceded by an increase in CVP. Mechanical cardiac compression during mediastinal dissection produces such a pattern.

Recognizing trends of hemodynamic variables may be a valuable monitoring function, quite apart from discerning individual waveform details. From a monitoring perspective, change may be more important than absolute values, especially since patients with advanced cardiovascular diseases may have markedly abnormal baseline values when they enter the monitored environment. Inasmuch as a monitor is defined as a reminder or warning, the ability to follow trends and detect change is an important monitoring function.

INTEGRATED MONITORING

The following chapters focus on each of the major monitored waveforms, beginning at the bottom of the monitor with the CVP, and then continuing with PAP, ABP, and finally the ECG. After brief introductory discussions of each monitored variable, the text focuses on the interpretation of the various waveforms under pathologic conditions. This is considered to be *integrated monitoring*, where each waveform is interpreted in the context of other available monitored information. This approach provides the greatest clinical insight and affords the most accurate diagnostic interpretation of a given hemodynamic state. The clinician learns to look for diagnostic patterns and searches all the monitored variables for corroborative information. The goal here is to simulate the clinical monitoring environment, where clinicians have the ECG and pressure traces at their fingertips. This objective will be accomplished if the clinician can successfully answer several questions: At what am I looking? For what am I looking? Can I put all these observations together (integration!) to make a diagnosis?

Perhaps the most important element in the philosophy of integrated monitoring proposed above has been saved for last. As Marriott has opined in the introductory notes to his textbook on electrocardiography, "the electrocardiogram should always be read in the clearest light of clinical observation. All pertinent data should be in the hands of the interpreter."[2] Like electrocardiography, bedside hemodynamic monitoring is best performed when clinicians avail themselves of all pertinent medical history and physical findings, before arriving at any diagnostic decisions from the monitored hemodynamic variables. This point is illustrated in Figure 1.9, which demonstrates an elevated CVP (mean 15 mmHg) with a prominent x pressure descent and blunted y descent. Although this CVP waveform is typical for a patient with cardiac tamponade, it hardly provides a sure diagnosis as an isolated finding. However, since this patient had other *physical signs* (reduced heart sounds, distended neck veins, arterial hypotension), *symptoms* (dyspnea), and *history* (chest trauma), all consistent with the diagnosis of tamponade, the CVP trace takes on greater diagnostic value, since now it can be integrated with these other pertinent data. (See Ch. 18 for a more complete discussion of cardiac tamponade.) What follows is a guide to cardiovascular monitoring that supplements clinical information; monitoring observations never replace clinical ones.

Illustrations for Monitoring Philosophy, Displays, and Recorders

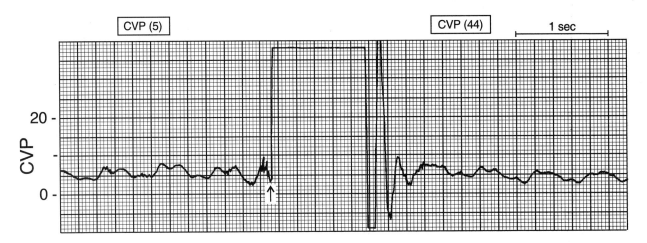

Figure 1.1 Spurious digital value for central venous pressure (CVP). The waveform is distorted by a flush artifact (*arrow*). The digital value for CVP remains abnormal after the flush (44 mmHg), even though a normal waveform trace has reappeared and confirms that the CVP is unchanged (5 mmHg).

Figure 1.2 Electrosurgical unit interference with heart rate measurement from the ECG. (*Top panel*) The ECG signal from lead V is distorted by the electrosurgical unit. As a result, the digital value for heart rate (HR) is erroneous (146 beats/min), although the pulse rate (PR) is measured accurately by the monitor from the arterial blood pressure waveform (58 beats/min). (*Lower panel*) Correct (and identical) digital values for both HR and PR are displayed by the monitor.

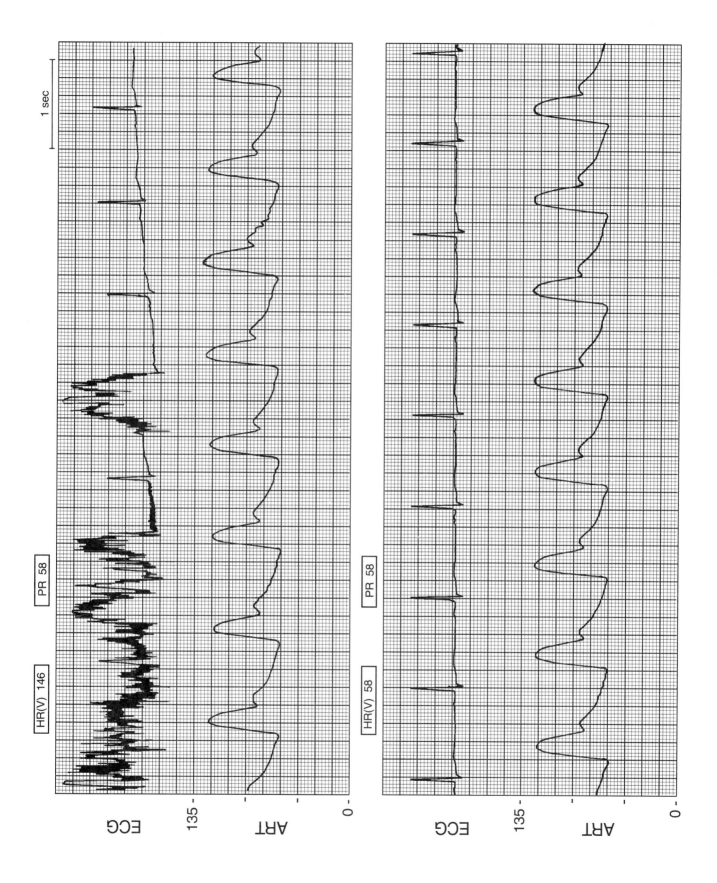

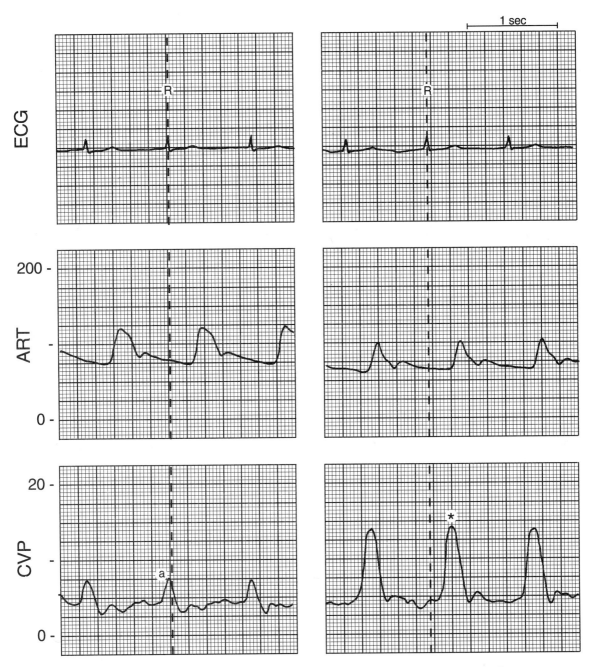

Figure 1.3 Simultaneous observation of multiple cardiovascular waveforms aids diagnosis. Compared to the left panels, those on the right show reduced arterial blood pressure (ART) associated with loss of the normal end-diastolic central venous pressure (CVP) a wave (a) and onset of a tall systolic cannon wave (°) in the CVP trace. The ECG traces do not show this change from normal sinus rhythm (*left side*) to atrioventricular dissociation (*right side*), because the ECG P waves are too small to be observed.

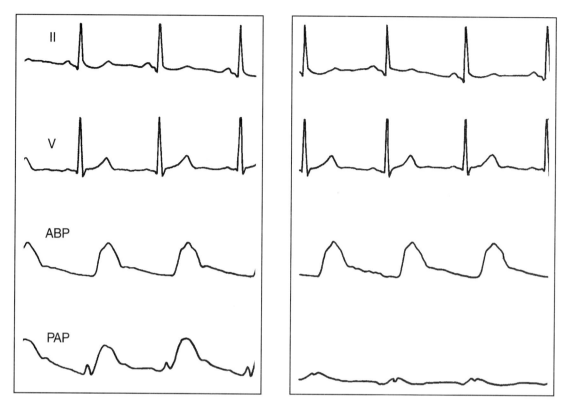

Figure 1.4 Free-waveform display. ECG leads II and V are shown in the two top traces, followed by the arterial blood pressure (ABP) and pulmonary artery pressure (PAP) traces. Waveform shape is clear, but absence of pressure scales precludes estimation of quantitative pressure values from the analog display. The PAP trace is a wedge pressure recording in the right panel.

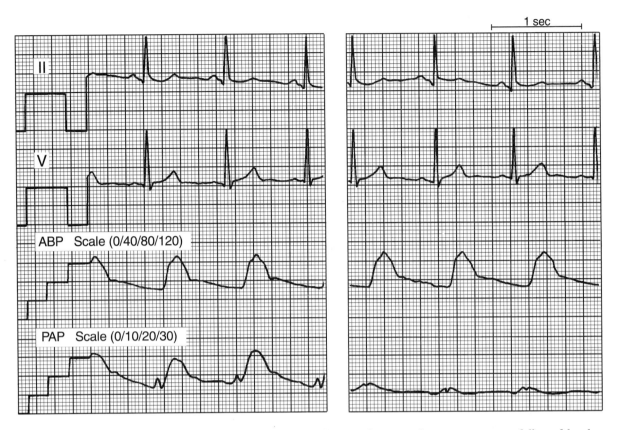

Figure 1.5 Separate waveform display. ECG leads II and V are shown in the two top traces, followed by the arterial blood pressure (ABP) and pulmonary artery pressure (PAP) traces. Individual scales are denoted by the *calibration steps* to the left of the waveforms: 10 mm/mV for ECG, 5 mm/40 mmHg for ABP, and 5 mm/10 mmHg for PAP. These scales allow reasonably accurate estimation of pressure values directly from the waveform display. The PAP trace is a wedge pressure recording in the right panel. From this trace, one can see that the wedge pressure is approximately 11 mmHg.

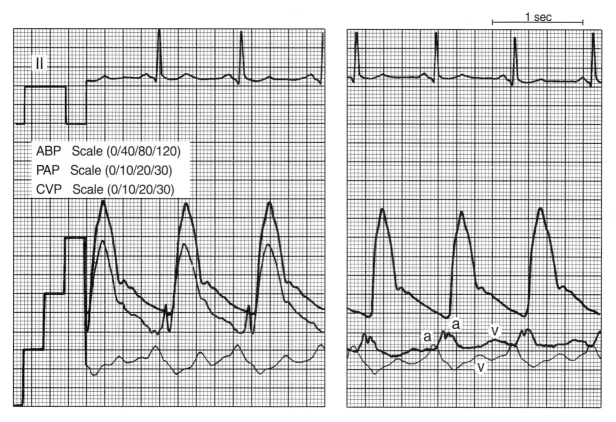

Figure 1.6 Full-scale waveform display. ECG lead II is shown in the top trace, followed by the arterial blood pressure (ABP), pulmonary artery pressure (PAP), and central venous pressure (CVP) traces from top to bottom. Lines in different colors or intensities help discriminate overlapping pressure waves on the monitor screen. Waveform details are observed easily, owing to the amplified pressure display scale: 15 mm/40 mmHg for ABP, 15 mm/10 mmHg for PAP, and 15 mm/10 mmHg for CVP. Clear a waves (a) and v waves (v) are discernible in both the CVP and PAP wedge traces in the right panel, and the temporal relation between these phasic pressure waves is easy to appreciate.

Figure 1.7 Multiple channel recording of ECG Lead II, arterial blood pressure (ABP) and central venous pressure (CVP). The pressure scales for ABP (15 mm/40 mmHg) and CVP (15 mm/10 mmHg) are noted on the left side of the panel. The ECG provides an indispensable timing marker, with the R wave denoting end of diastole and onset of systole. This helps to identify the a, c, and v waves in the CVP trace by their location in the diastolic (a wave) or systolic (c and v waves) portion of the cardiac cycle.

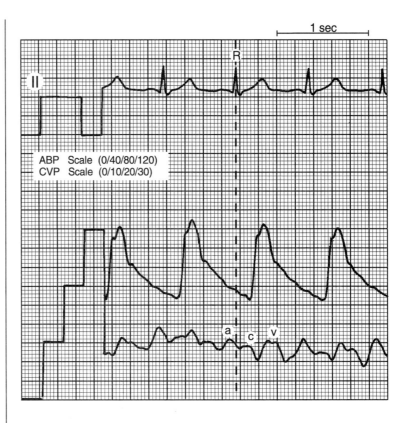

Figure 1.8 Varying sweep speeds for waveform recordings are chosen for different purposes. *Very slow speed recordings* (5 mm/min, *left panel*) elucidate the pattern and duration of cardiovascular events, like this 30-second episode of mechanical cardiac compression, which raises central venous pressure (CVP) and reduces arterial blood pressure (ART). *Slow speed recordings* (5 mm/sec, *middle panel*) are chosen to demonstrate the phasic influence of the respiratory cycle on the circulation. Inspiration during positive pressure mechanical ventilation causes the CVP to rise once on the left side of the middle panel and again 10 seconds later on the right side of the middle panel. *Standard speed recordings* (25 mm/sec, *right panel*) are those typically used for 12-lead ECGs or bedside monitors. Waveform identification is facilitated by the improved temporal resolution, so that details like the CVP a and v waves are recognized easily.

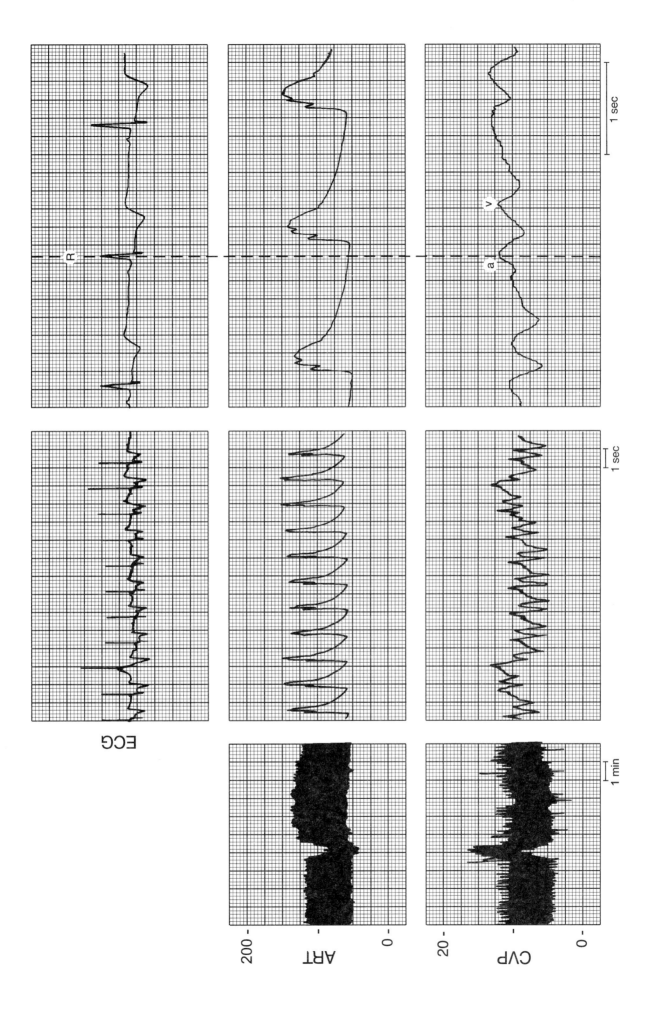

Figure 1.9 Central venous pressure (CVP) recorded from a 45-year-old trauma patient. The elevated CVP with a blunted y descent is characteristic of cardiac tamponade, but other pertinent clinical information is required to make the diagnosis.

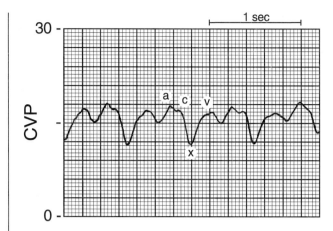

References

1. Gurushanthaiah K, Weinger MB, Englund CE. Visual display format affects the ability of anesthesiologists to detect acute physiologic changes. A laboratory study employing a clinical display simulator. Anesthesiology 1995;83:1184–93

2. Marriott HJL. Practical Electrocardiography (4th ed). Baltimore: Williams & Wilkins, 1968: xiii

3. Perloff JK. The Clinical Recognition of Congenital Heart Disease (3rd ed). Philadelphia: WB Saunders, 1987

CHAPTER TWO *Central Venous Pressure, Left Atrial Pressure*

CARDIAC CYCLE DEFINITIONS

In order to interpret invasive cardiovascular pressure waveforms, one must understand the cardiac cycle in some detail. Traditionally, the cardiac cycle is divided into two phases, systole and diastole. *Systole* connotes contraction and diastole relaxation. Although these terms are applied frequently to the action of both the atria and ventricles, confusion can develop when atrial and ventricular events do not occur in their normal sequence. During normal sinus rhythm, atrial systole occurs at the end of ventricular diastole. However, when atrioventricular dissociation develops, atrial and ventricular systole may occur at the same time.

Problems in interpretation and communication are avoided by reserving the terms *systole* and *diastole* for describing ventricular mechanics alone and always referring to atrial systole as atrial contraction. All waveform components are thus described only in reference to ventricular events and whether or not the pressure waves occur during ventricular systole or diastole. In this scheme, atrial contraction, which normally generates the atrial pressure a wave, is described as an end-diastolic pressure event.

Accurate recognition of pressure waveform components requires that the waves be properly identified as occurring in the systolic or diastolic phases of the cardiac cycle. The ECG provides the clearest reference points, and an ECG trace should always be displayed or recorded along with the pressures of interest. The ECG P wave reflects atrial depolarization, the R wave ventricular depolarization, and the T wave ventricular repolarization. Mechanical cardiac actions that result must follow these electrical signals (Fig. 2.1). Normal temporal delays between electrical and mechanical events have been identified, and it proves quite useful to keep these normal values in mind (Table 2.1 and Fig. 2.2).[1] By using the ECG as the timer and recalling that electrical-mechanical delays occur, one can identify phasic pressure waveform components accurately.

CENTRAL VENOUS PRESSURE

Central venous pressure (CVP) is recorded most commonly from a catheter with its tip in the superior vena cava or from the proximal (right atrial) lumen of a pulmonary artery catheter. Both methods yield similar pressure waveforms, and for clinical purposes, CVP and right atrial pressure (RAP) are considered to be identical, and the terms used interchangeably.

The normal CVP waveform consists of five phasic events, three peaks (a, c, v) and two descents (x, y) (Table 2.2, Figs. 2.3 and 2.4).[3] The a wave occurs at end-diastole and is the

Table 2.1 Temporal Relations of Electric and Dynamic Events in the Heart

MEASUREMENT	MEAN (MSEC)
Onset P to right atrial contraction	65
Onset P to left atrial contraction	85
Onset right to left atrial contraction	20
Onset Q to right ventricular contraction	65
Onset Q to left ventricular contraction	52
Onset left to right ventricular contraction	13
Onset Q to right ventricular ejection	80
Onset Q to left ventricular ejection	115
Onset right to left ventricular ejection	35
Duration right ventricular isovolumic contraction	16
Duration left ventricular isovolumic contraction	61

Abbreviations: P, ECG P wave; Q, ECG QRS wave.

Modified from Braunwald et al[1] with permission.

result of atrial contraction, which increases atrial pressure and provides the "atrial kick" to fill the ventricle through the tricuspid valve. The a wave follows the ECG P wave. Atrial pressure decreases following the a wave, as the atrium relaxes. This smooth decline in pressure is interrupted by the next pressure peak, the c wave. This wave is a transient increase in atrial pressure produced by isovolumic ventricular contraction, which closes the tricuspid valve and displaces it toward the atrium. The c wave always follows the ECG R wave, since it is generated by the beginning of ventricular systole.

The c wave observed in a jugular venous pressure trace may have a slightly more complex origin. This wave has

Table 2.2 Normal CVP

WAVEFORM COMPONENT	PHASE OF CARDIAC CYCLE	MECHANICAL EVENT
a wave	End diastole	Atrial contraction
c wave	Early systole	Isovolumic ventricular contraction, tricuspid motion toward right atrium
v wave	Late systole	Systolic filling of atrium
x descent	Mid-systole	Atrial relaxation, descent of the base, systolic collapse
y descent	Early diastole	Early ventricular filling, diastolic collapse

been attributed to early systolic pressure transmission from the adjacent carotid artery and may be termed a *carotid impact wave*.[4] However, since the jugular venous pressure also reflects RAP, this c wave likely represents both arterial (carotid) and venous (tricuspid motion) origins.

Atrial pressure continues its decline during ventricular systole, in part owing to continued atrial relaxation and in part owing to changes in atrial geometry produced by ventricular contraction and ejection. This is the x descent or systolic collapse in atrial pressure. The x descent can be divided into two portions, x and x′, corresponding to the segments before and after the c wave (Fig. 2.4). Although the mechanisms producing x and x′ may be distinct, the most useful clinical approach is to consider a single systolic x descent in atrial pressure.

The last atrial pressure peak is the v wave, caused by venous filling of the atrium during late systole, while the tricuspid valve remains closed. The v wave usually peaks just after the ECG T wave. Atrial pressure then decreases, inscribing the y descent or diastolic collapse, as the tricuspid valve opens and blood flows from atrium to ventricle.

This nomenclature can be remembered more easily with the following guide. The **a** wave results from *atrial* contraction, the **c** wave from atrioventricular valve *closure* and isovolumic ventricular *contraction*, and the **v** wave from *ventricular* ejection, which drives *venous* filling of the atrium.

In relation to the cardiac cycle and ventricular mechanical actions, the atrial pressure waveform can be considered to have three systolic components (c wave, x descent, v wave) and two diastolic components (y descent, a wave). By recalling the mechanical actions that generate the pressure peaks and troughs, it is easy to identify these waveform components by aligning the atrial pressure waveform and the ECG trace and marking the ECG R wave to signify the end of diastole and the onset of systole. (Although one might argue about the exact ECG reference point for end of diastole and onset of systole, the R wave has the great advantage of providing a clear, easily reproducible timing marker, thus explaining its wide acceptance in clinical practice for this purpose.) This approach has been applied to facilitate analysis of many of the tracings in this book. Furthermore, this is a simple, reliable technique to use for interpreting pressure tracings at the bedside: Find the ECG R wave, and analyze the pressure waveform in reference to this timing marker.

Attempts to identify the phasic components of the CVP trace are more difficult when the arterial blood pressure trace is used for timing, rather than the ECG. The problems encountered are highlighted in the example in Figure 2.5, where the radial arterial pressure upstroke is seen to be delayed for approximately 200 msec following the ECG R wave. Four events contribute to this apparent delay: (1) spread of electrical depolarization through the ventricle, producing an electrical-mechanical delay (approximately 60 msec), (2) isovolumic left ventricular contraction (approximately 60 msec), (3) transmission of aortic pressure rise to the radial artery (approximately 50 msec), and (4) transmission of radial artery pressure rise through fluid-filled tubing to the transducer (approximately 10 msec) (Table 2.1).[1,5] As a consequence of these events, the radial artery systolic upstroke appears delayed relative to the RAP systolic c wave, since the latter is produced by isovolumic right ventricular contraction, and the former by left ventricular ejection (Figs. 2.2 and 2.5).

The normal atrial pressure peaks have been designated systolic (c, v) or diastolic (a), according to the phase of the cardiac cycle in which the wave begins. However, one generally identifies these atrial pressure waves not by their onset or upstroke, but rather by the location of the pressure peaks. For instance, the a wave generally begins and peaks in end-diastole, but the peak may appear delayed to coincide with the ECG R wave, especially in a patient with short PR interval. In this instance, a and c waves merge, and this composite wave is termed an a-c wave (Fig. 2.6). Despite their close temporal association, the a and c waves arise from different phases of the cardiac cycle. The a wave reflects atrial contraction at end-*diastole*, while the c wave is produced by early *systolic* isovolumic ventricular contraction.

Designation of an atrial pressure wave as systolic or diastolic in origin can be even more confusing for the v wave. Recall that the v wave is caused by venous filling of the atrium in late systole, while the atrioventricular valve is closed. Clearly, the v wave ascent commences during late systole. However, the v wave peak is achieved during isovolumic ventricular relaxation, immediately prior to atrioventricular valve opening and the y descent of diastole (Fig. 2.1). Consequently, the most precise description would be that the v wave begins in late systole but peaks during isovolumic ventricular relaxation, the earliest portion of diastole. For clinical purposes, it is simplest to consider the v wave to be a systolic wave, and most authors have adopted this approach.[2,4]

Although three individual atrial pressure peaks (a, c, v) and two distinct troughs (x, y) are usually identified in the atrial pressure trace, heart rate abnormalities may alter this pattern. With sinus bradycardia, which prolongs diastole, an additional mid-late diastolic plateau pressure, termed an h wave, may be inscribed (Fig. 2.7).[4] Furthermore, separate x and x′ descents are more evident with prolonged PR intervals or when bradycardia causes all phasic waveform components to become more temporally distinct. In contrast, tachycardia causes the atrial pressure waves to fuse, just as S3 and S4 heart sounds may merge to form a summation gallup.[4] In this situation, the a-c wave appears more monophasic and x and y descents are shortened (Fig. 2.6), making waveform analysis more difficult.

RIGHT vs. LEFT ATRIAL PRESSURE

Direct left atrial pressure (LAP) measurement is far less common than RAP measurement. It is usually restricted to the cardiac catheterization laboratory or cardiac surgical operating rooms and intensive care units, where patients may have transthoracic left atrial catheters remaining in place following heart surgery (Fig. 2.8). Despite the infrequent clinical measurement of LAP, it is important to understand similarities and differences between LAP and RAP waveforms and their temporal relationships. (The value of understanding LAP waveforms will become clearer in Ch. 4, when pulmonary artery wedge pressure measurements are discussed.)

Although mean LAP exceeds mean RAP in normal subjects, transient reversal of this pressure gradient occurs during the cardiac cycle in many individuals, particularly during the a wave of atrial contraction (Fig. 2.9).[1] This serves as a reminder of the ever-present risk of paradoxic embolization of gaseous or solid material through a patent foramen ovale.

Normal RAP and LAP waveforms have typical temporal relations and subtle morphologic distinctions. Since atrial depolarization originates in the sinoatrial node located at the junction of the superior vena cava and the right atrium, the right-sided a wave appears prior to the left-sided a wave (Table 2.1 and Fig. 2.9). Furthermore, the a wave is the most prominent pressure wave in a normal RAP trace, while the v wave is often taller than the a wave in a normal LAP trace. These observations suggest that end-diastolic right atrial contraction may be more vigorous than left atrial contraction and that the left atrium is less distensible than the right atrium during passive systolic filling.[1] Finally, the interval between right atrial contraction and right ventricular contraction exceeds the interval between left atrial contraction and left ventricular contraction by approximately 40 msec (Table 2.1 and Fig. 2.2). Consequently, a and c waves are seen more often as separate waves in an RAP trace than in an LAP trace.

Although examples of abnormal CVP, LAP, and pulmonary artery wedge pressure traces can be found throughout the ensuing chapters of the book, most of these are presented in Chapters 12, 14, 17, and 18.

Illustrations for
Central Venous Pressure,
Left Atrial Pressure

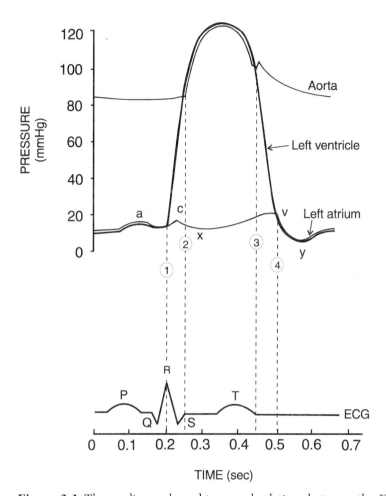

Figure 2.1 The cardiac cycle and temporal relations between the ECG and pressures in the aorta, left ventricle, and left atrium. Normal left atrial pressure (LAP) waves (a, c, and v) and descents (x and y) and components of the ECG (P, Q, R, S, and T waves) are noted. Actions of the left-sided cardiac valves are (1) mitral closure, (2) aortic opening, (3) aortic closure, and (4) mitral opening. Phases of the cardiac cycle are (1) to (2) isovolumic ventricular contraction, (2) to (3) ventricular ejection, (3) to (4) isovolumic ventricular relaxation, and (4) to (1) ventricular filling. In general, ventricular *systole* is considered to include phases 1 to 3 and ventricular *diastole* includes phases 3 to 1. Similarly, the LAP waves can be designated as systolic (c, x, and v) or diastolic (y and a) events in relation to the phase of the cardiac cycle in which they begin. (See text for details.) Note that the ECG records electrical events, which always precede mechanical events seen in the pressure waveforms. The ECG P wave precedes the LAP a wave, the ECG R wave precedes the LAP c wave and the increase in left ventricular and aortic pressures, and the ECG T wave precedes the decline in left ventricular and aortic pressures and the y descent in left atrial pressure. For simplicity, only left-sided cardiac chamber pressures are illustrated, but analogous temporal relations exist for the ECG and right-sided chamber pressures and valvular events, except that the isovolumic phases are shorter and the ejection and filling phases are longer on the right side of the heart. (See Fig. 2.2 for more detail.)

Figure 2.2 Temporal relations between electrical and mechanical events in the heart. Normal ECG waves (P, Q, R, S, and T) precede their mechanical counterparts. (1) Onset right atrial contraction, (2) onset left atrial contraction, (3) onset left ventricular contraction, (4) onset right ventricular contraction, (5) onset right ventricular ejection, (6) onset left ventricular ejection, (7) end left ventricular ejection, and (8) end right ventricular ejection. (Modified from Braunwald et al,[1] with permission.)

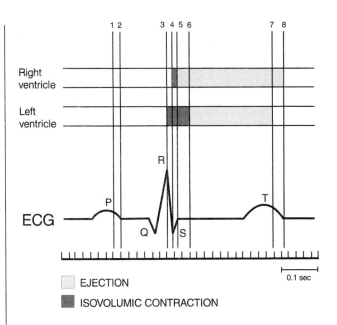

Figure 2.3 A normal central venous pressure (CVP) waveform has three systolic components (c wave, x descent, v wave) and two diastolic components (y descent, a wave). (From Mark,[3] with permission.)

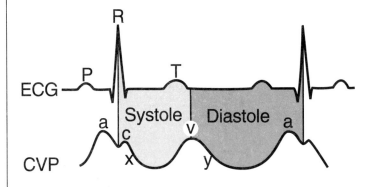

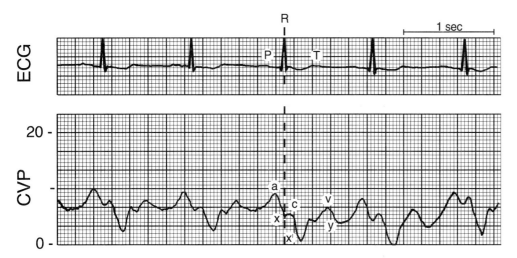

Figure 2.4 Normal central venous pressure (CVP) waveform showing the systolic descent divided into x and x′ components, corresponding to the segments before and after the c wave. (Modified from Mark,[3] with permission.)

Figure *2.5* The arterial pressure (ART) upstroke follows the ECG R wave by approximately 200 msec. This apparent delay in the onset of systole must be considered when using the ART waveform to identify venous waveform components. (See text for more detail.) (Modified from Mark,[3] with permission.)

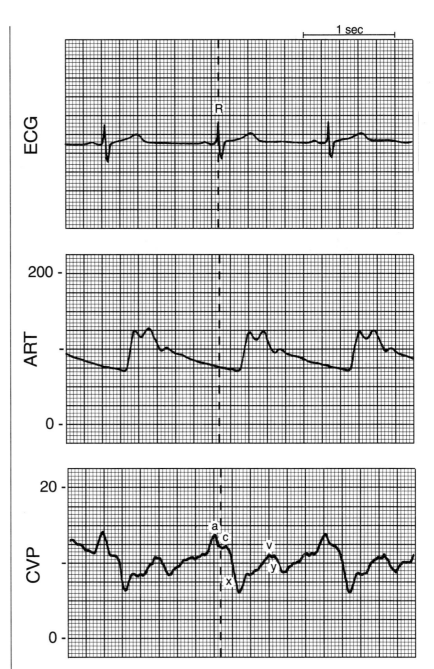

Figure 2.6 Tachycardia and short PR intervals produce fusion of individual central venous pressure (CVP) waveform components, particularly the a and c waves. (Modified from Mark,[3] with permission.)

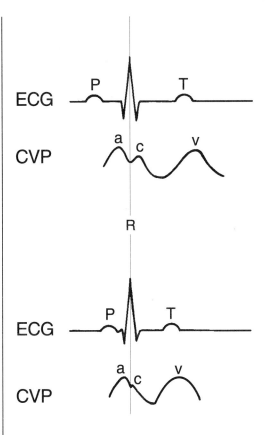

Figure 2.7 A mid-diastolic plateau pressure wave (h) becomes evident in the central venous pressure (CVP) trace when the heart rate is slow. (Modified from Mark,[3] with permission.)

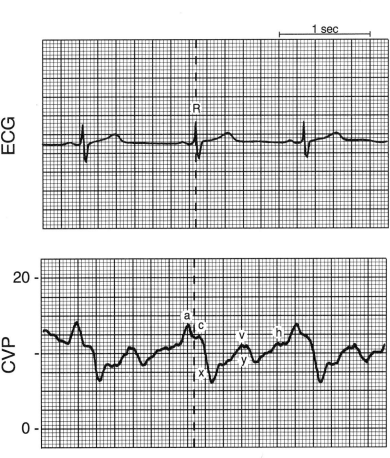

***Figure* 2.8** A normal left atrial pressure (LAP) waveform resembles a central venous pressure waveform and displays a clear end-diastolic a wave and end-systolic v wave. Mean LAP is 13 mmHg. (Modified from Mark,[3] with permission.)

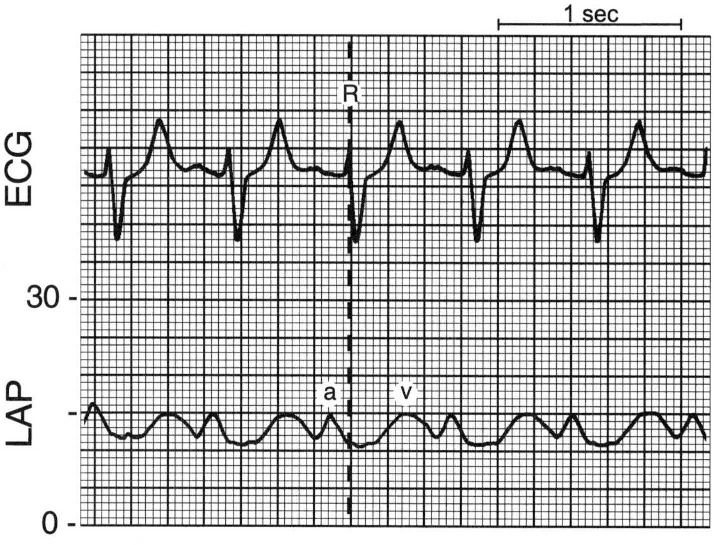

***Figure* 2.9** Temporal relation between the ECG and normal central venous pressure (CVP) and left atrial pressure (LAP) waveforms. Note that the CVP a wave slightly precedes the LAP a wave because the sinoatrial node is located in the right atrium. (Modified from Mark,[3] with permission.)

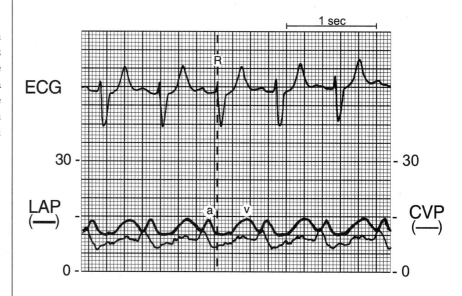

References

1. Braunwald E, Fishman AP, Cournand A. Time relationship of dynamic events in the cardiac chambers, pulmonary artery and aorta in man. Circ Res 1956;4:100–7

2. Mark JB. The cardiac cycle. Response. J Cardiothorac Vasc Anesth 1991;5:651

3. Mark JB. Getting the most from your central venous pressure catheter, 157–75. In: Barash PG, ed: ASA Refresher Courses in Anesthesiology (vol 23). Philadelphia: Lippincott-Raven, 1995

4. O'Rourke RA, Silverman ME, Schlant RC. General examination of the patient. In: Schlant RC, Alexander RW, eds. The Heart Arteries and Veins. New York: McGraw-Hill, 1994:238–41

5. Shinozaki T, Deane RS, Mazuzan JE. The dynamic responses of liquid-filled catheter systems for direct measurements of blood pressure. Anesthesiology 1980;53:498–504

CHAPTER THREE Pulmonary Artery Pressure

FLOATING THE PULMONARY ARTERY CATHETER: WAVEFORM MORPHOLOGIES

As the flow-directed, balloon-tipped pulmonary artery catheter is floated from a central vein to its proper position in the pulmonary artery, characteristic pressure waveforms are recorded (Fig. 3.1). Initially, the pulmonary artery catheter is passed through the introducer sheath until its tip is located in the right atrium. This central venous or right atrial pressure (RAP) is recognized by the characteristic a, c, and v waves and the low mean pressure value. Once the catheter tip is positioned in the right atrium, the pulmonary artery catheter balloon is inflated fully with 1.5 ml of air, and the catheter is advanced until it crosses the tricuspid valve.

Right ventricular pressure is now recorded. This waveform is recognized by the marked increase in systolic pressure and by the low diastolic pressure, which approximates RAP. In early diastole, right ventricular pressure falls to its nadir, then increases during diastole as right ventricular filling proceeds. Right ventricular end-diastolic pressure (RVEDP) is measured at the ECG R wave. Although right ventricular diastolic pressure approximates mean RAP, right ventricular end-diastolic pressure is influenced by right atrial end-diastolic contraction and is best estimated by the peak of the right atrial a wave pressure (Fig. 3.1, shaded boxes).

The pulmonary artery catheter next enters the right ventricular outflow tract and floats across the pulmonic valve into the main pulmonary artery Fig. 3.1. Often, this passage is heralded by arrhythmias, especially premature ventricular beats, as the balloon-tipped catheter strikes the right ventricular infundibulum. Pulmonary artery systolic pressure should closely approximate right ventricular systolic pressure, but pulmonary artery diastolic pressure generally exceeds right ventricular diastolic pressure. This *diastolic pressure step-up* is generally considered to be evidence that the catheter has crossed from right ventricle to pulmonary artery successfully.

On occasion, it may be difficult to distinguish right ventricular pressure from pulmonary artery pressure (PAP), particularly if only the digital values for these pressures are examined. In the example in Figure 3.1, a pressure of 30/10 mmHg could be recorded from either the pulmonary artery or the right ventricle. However, examination of the diastolic pressure contours clarifies the distinction between right ventricular pressure and pulmonary artery pressure. Pulmonary artery pressure *decreases* steadily with time in diastole as blood flows from the pulmonary artery toward the left atrium. In contrast, right ventricular pressure *increases* steadily with time in diastole as blood flows into the right ventricle through the open tricuspid valve (Fig. 3.2).

The pulmonary artery catheter, with balloon inflated, finally reaches the wedge position (Figs. 3.1 and 3.3). The waveform again changes, and the pulmonary artery wedge pressure (PAWP) resembles left atrial pressure, with typical a, c, and v waves. Mean PAWP will always be less than mean PAP, otherwise blood would not flow in an antegrade direction.

GUIDELINES FOR CATHETER PLACEMENT

From a right internal jugular vein puncture site, the right atrium should be reached when the catheter is inserted 20 cm, the right ventricle at 30 to 35 cm, the pulmonary artery at 40 to 45 cm, and the wedge position at 50 cm. When

Table 3.1 Typical Distances for Placing a Pulmonary Artery Catheter

PUNCTURE SITE	DESTINATION	DISTANCE (CM)
Right internal jugular vein		
	Right atrium	20
	Right ventricle	30–35
	Pulmonary artery	40–45
	Pulmonary artery wedge	50
Right or left subclavian vein		No change
Left internal jugular vein		Add 5
Right external jugular vein		Add 5
Left external jugular vein		Add 10
Right or left femoral vein		Add 15
Right antecubital vein		Add 30
Left antecubital vein		Add 35

other vascular puncture sites are chosen for catheter placement, additional distance is required (Table 3.1). Keeping in mind typical distances from the skin to right atrium, right ventricle, and pulmonary artery will aid proper waveform identification and help avoid complications caused by unintended catheter loops and knots. These distances serve as a rough guide: Waveform morphology must be verified from the continuous display on the bedside monitor, and catheter position should be confirmed with a chest x-ray.

Prior to pulmonary artery catheter flotation, proper assembly and functioning of the catheter and pressure monitoring system must be confirmed. Each vascular lumen should be flushed and the balloon checked to confirm symmetric inflation, with the balloon surrounding the tip of the catheter without obstructing the distal lumen. A simple maneuver can now be performed to check assembly of the catheter monitoring system (Fig. 3.4).[3] First, the pressure monitoring transducer is adjusted to the level of the patient's heart. Next, the pulmonary artery catheter tip is held at the level of the heart, and the monitor screen checked to ensure that a pressure of 0 mmHg is recorded. Finally, the catheter is held at the 30-cm mark, and the tip is elevated to create a vertical fluid column approximately 30 cm in height, which should produce a pressure equivalent to 22 mmHg (Fig. 3.4). (Recall that the density of mercury is 13.6 times that of water. Thus, a "water column" created by the distal 30 cm of the fluid-filled pulmonary artery catheter will produce a calibrating pressure signal equal to approximately 22 mmHg. See Ch. 9 for more detail.)

A few additional points might be considered to aid successful positioning of the pulmonary artery catheter. It is important to recognize that the air-filled balloon tends to float to nondependent regions as it passes through the heart into the pulmonary artery vasculature. Consequently, positioning a patient head-down will aid flotation past the tricuspid valve, and tilting the patient onto the right side or placing the head up will aid flotation out of the right ventricle. Furthermore, the head-up position may reduce the frequency of arrhythmias during catheterization.[4] Owing to gravitational and anatomic factors, most catheters float to the right pulmonary artery.[2] Thus, in order to selectively catheterize the left pulmonary artery, the patient should be positioned with the right side down.[6] Deep inspiration during spontaneous ventilation will increase venous return and right ventricular output transiently. This may facilitate catheter flotation in a patient with low cardiac output. On occasion, a catheter may be floated to proper position when stiffened by injecting, through the distal lumen, 10 to 20 ml of the iced solution prepared for cardiac output measurement. Finally, a catheter that is difficult to place initially may be positioned easily when hemodynamic conditions change, as commonly occurs after induction of general anesthesia and initiation of positive pressure ventilation.

TEMPORAL RELATIONS: PULMONARY ARTERY PRESSURE

Under normal conditions, the PAP upstroke slightly precedes the radial artery pressure upstroke (Figs. 3.3 and 3.5). This reflects the longer duration of left ventricular isovolumic contraction[1] (see Ch. 2, Fig. 2.2 and Table 2.1) as well as the transmission time of the central aortic pressure upstroke to the downstream radial artery recording site. Although the PAP upstroke precedes the radial artery pressure upstroke by 50 msec, peak PAP precedes peak radial artery pressure by only 10 msec.[5] As a practical matter, PAP and systemic arterial pressure contours appear to overlap on the bedside monitor, with these pressures rising, peaking, and falling at approximately the same points (Figs. 3.3 and 3.5).

Cardiac conduction abnormalities alter these normal temporal relations between PAP and systemic artery pressures. Left bundle branch block delays left ventricular systole, and thus, radial artery pressure appears even more delayed relative to the PAP (Fig. 3.6). Right bundle branch block has the opposite effect (Fig. 3.7). These timing observations are important to bear in mind when attempting to distinguish a PAP waveform from a PAWP waveform that displays a tall v wave. A PAP trace will coincide temporally with the systemic arterial pressure trace (Figs. 3.3 and 3.5) or will peak slightly before (Fig. 3.6) or after (Fig. 3.7) systemic arterial pressure. In contrast, the systolic pressure peak generated by a tall regurgitant v wave in a PAWP trace will appear much later in the cardiac cycle (Fig. 3.8) (see Ch. 17, Figs. 17.5 through 17.13).

Illustrations for Pulmonary Artery Pressure

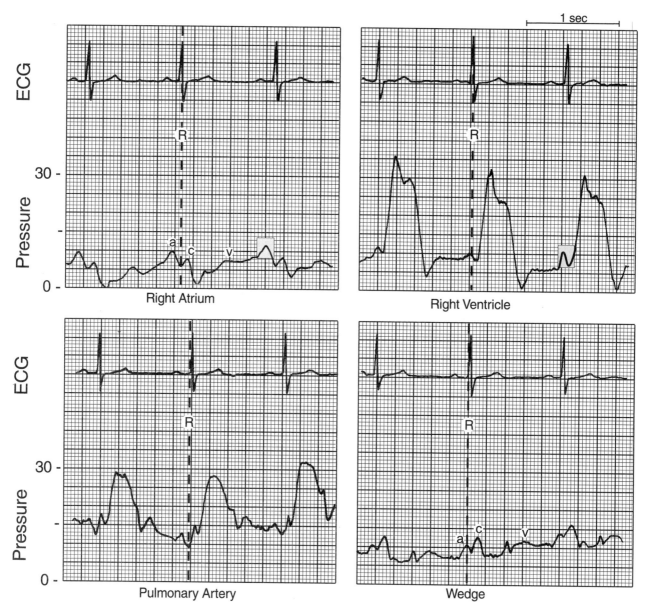

Figure 3.1 Pressure waveforms recorded from a pulmonary artery catheter as it passes through the right atrium and right ventricle to the pulmonary artery and wedge positions. Right ventricular end-diastolic pressure is measured at the time of the ECG R wave and is estimated best by the right atrial a wave pressure peak (*shaded boxes*). A, c, and v waves are recorded from both the right atrium and pulmonary artery wedge positions. (See text for more detail.)

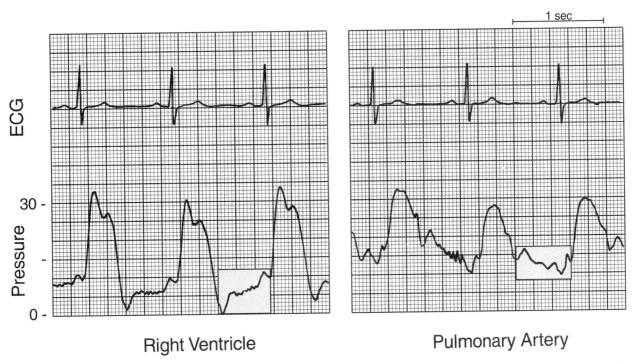

Figure 3.2 The diastolic contour helps distinguish right ventricular from pulmonary artery pressure (*shaded boxes*). During diastole, right ventricular pressure increases as the ventricle fills, while pulmonary artery pressure decreases as blood flows toward the left atrium.

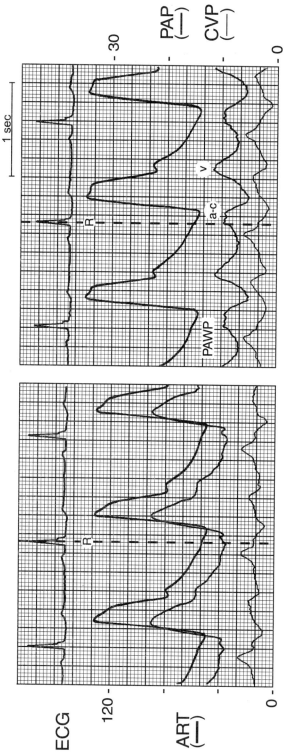

Figure 3.3 (*Left panel*) Normal ECG, arterial blood pressure (ART), pulmonary artery pressure (PAP), and central venous pressure (CVP) waveforms are displayed from top to bottom. (*Right panel*) The pulmonary artery wedge pressure (PAWP) is recorded, with typical a-c and v waves. The morphologic features of these waveforms and their temporal relationships are clearly illustrated. Mean PAWP is less than mean PAP. The PAWP waveform closely resembles the CVP waveform except that the a-c and v waves appear later in the PAWP trace than in the CVP trace. (See Ch. 4 for more detail.)

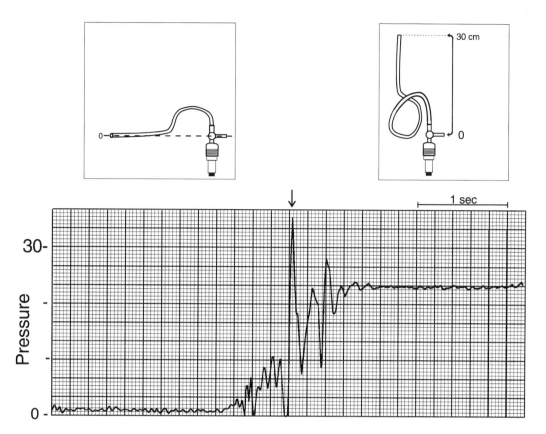

Figure 3.4 Proper assembly and function of the pulmonary artery catheter–pressure transducer system is confirmed by recording the pressure at the level of the heart, which should read 0 mmHg (*left side*), and then raising the catheter tip to create a 30-cm vertical water column, which should read 22 mmHg (*right side*). Catheter motion (*arrow*) produces the pressure artifacts in the middle of the trace. (See text for details.)

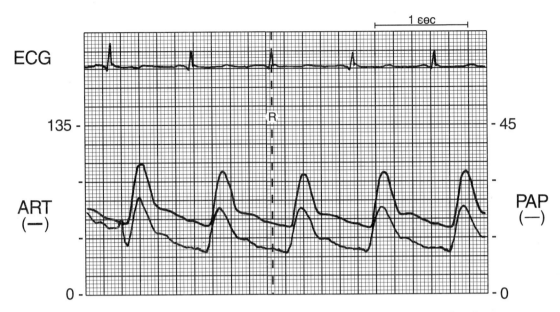

***Figure* 3.5** The pulmonary artery pressure (PAP) upstroke precedes the arterial blood pressure (ART) upstroke by 40 msec. As a first approximation, however, these two pressure waveforms appear to have the same temporal relationship to the ECG under normal conditions.

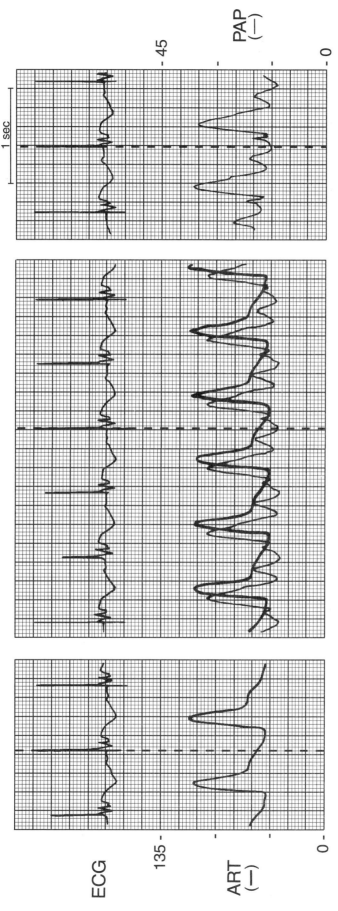

Figure 3.6 Left bundle branch block produces further delay in the arterial blood pressure (ART) upstroke relative to the pulmonary artery pressure (PAP) upstroke. The vertical dashed lines mark ECG pacing spikes resulting from right ventricular endocardial pacing. (*Left panel*) ART. (*Right panel*) PAP. (*Center panel*) Both pressures are superimposed. Compare with Fig. 3.5.

Figure 3.7 Right bundle branch block delays onset of right ventricular systole and causes the arterial blood pressure (ART) upstroke to precede the pulmonary artery pressure (PAP) upstroke. Left ventricular epicardial pacing produces a pacing spike and a wide S wave in ECG lead V_5. Compare with Figs. 3.5 and 3.6.

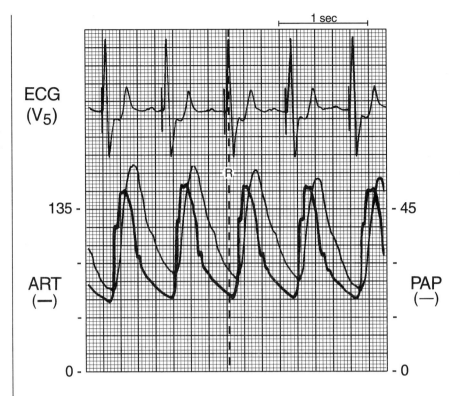

Figure 3.8 A tall systolic v wave in the pulmonary artery wedge pressure (PAWP) trace appears later in the cardiac cycle than the pulmonary artery pressure peak. Contrast this PAWP peak with the pulmonary artery pressure peaks in Figs. 3.5 to 3.7. Note the timing of the PAWP peak relative to the ECG and arterial blood pressure (ART) waveforms.

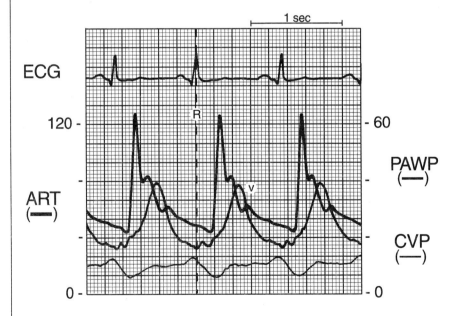

References

1. Braunwald E, Fishman AP, Cournand A. Time relationship of dynamic events in the cardiac chambers, pulmonary artery and aorta in man. Circ Res 1956;4:100–7

2. Benumof JL, Saidman LJ, Arkin DB, Diamant M. Where pulmonary arterial catheters go: intrathoracic distribution. Anesthesiology 1977;46:336–8

3. Donahue PJ, Satwicz PR. A method for ensuring proper function of multiorifice catheters. Anesthesiology 1992;76:148–9

4. Keusch DJ, Winters S, Thys DM. The patient's position influences the incidence of dysrhythmias during pulmonary artery catheterization. Anesthesiology 1989;70:582–4

5. Moore RA, Neary MJ, Gallagher JD, Clark DL. Determination of the pulmonary capillary wedge position in patients with giant left atrial V waves. J Cardiothorac Anesth 1987;1:108–13

6. Parlow JL, Milne B, Cervenko FW. Balloon flotation is more important than flow direction in determining the position of flow-directed pulmonary artery catheters. J Cardiothorac Vasc Anesth 1992;6:20–3

CHAPTER FOUR *Pulmonary Artery Wedge Pressure*

WHAT IS WEDGE PRESSURE?

When the pulmonary artery catheter floats to the wedge position, the balloon occludes anterograde blood flow to a portion of the pulmonary vasculature. Blood flow ceases between the pulmonary artery catheter tip and a junction point where pulmonary veins draining the occluded pulmonary vascular region join other veins in which blood still flows toward the left atrium (Fig. 4.1). A continuous static column of blood now connects the wedged pulmonary artery catheter tip to this junction point in the pulmonary veins near the left atrium. Inasmuch as resistance to flow in these large pulmonary veins is negligible, pulmonary artery wedge pressure (PAWP) reflects pulmonary venous pressure and thus left atrial pressure (LAP).[16] Put more succinctly, PAWP measures the pressure where blood flow resumes on the venous side of the pulmonary circuit.[20]

Provided that the fluid column between catheter tip and left atrium remains patent, narrowing of the static portion of this column does not alter the close agreement between wedge pressure and LAP. This must be the case, since there is no pressure drop across the zero flow segment. However, a similar narrowing of the flowing column distal to the junction point will cause wedge pressure to overestimate LAP (Fig. 4.2). Fortunately, this latter condition, pulmonary venoocclusive disease, is rare.[2,3] (See Ch. 6 for more detail.)

WEDGE PRESSURE vs. LEFT ATRIAL PRESSURE

As a surrogate for LAP, the PAWP waveform shares many morphologic features. Phasic a and v waves and x and y descents are usually identifiable in the wedge pressure trace. However, owing to the pulmonary vascular bed interposed between pulmonary artery catheter tip and left atrium, PAWP is a *delayed* representation of LAP[13] (Fig. 4.3). On average, 160 msec are required for the LAP pulse to traverse the pulmonary veins, pulmonary capillaries, and pulmonary arterioles and arteries. As a consequence of this delay, the wedge pressure a wave appears to follow the ECG R wave in early ventricular systole (Fig. 4.3). However, the a wave is an end-diastolic pressure event, produced by left atrial contraction. This time delay in phasic wedge pressure waves must be appreciated for proper waveform interpretation.

Not only is PAWP a delayed representation of LAP, but it is also a *damped* reflection of phasic atrial pressure waves (Figs. 4.3 and 4.4). The amount of damping is variable, but when the LAP waves are prominent, the pressure peaks may be significantly underestimated and the pressure nadirs measured as spuriously high in the wedge trace. Figure 4.4 shows LAP and PAWP traces recorded from a patient with severe mitral regurgitation. Tall systolic regurgitant c-v waves are inscribed in both pressure traces. Although mean pressure values are similar (22 mmHg), the c-v wave pressure peak is lower in the PAWP trace than in the LAP trace (30 vs. 42 mmHg), and the wedge pressure waveform appears to be a damped, delayed version of LAP.[15]

Instead of recording PAWP by balloon inflation, a wedge pressure can be obtained by advancing the pulmonary artery catheter into a distal, smaller branch of the pulmonary artery without prior balloon inflation. This distal wedge pressure measurement by catheter tip impaction may allow indirect LAP measurement with less intervening pulmonary vasculature and consequently less damping and delay of the LAP trace.[17] Patients with chronic lung diseases or other conditions that produce regional disturbances in the pulmonary circulation may have more marked differences between wedge pressures obtained proximally (by balloon inflation) versus those obtained distally (by catheter tip impaction).[11] This makes sense, considering the previously developed notion of what the wedge pressure measures. By occluding a smaller pulmonary artery, the wedged catheter is now measuring pressure where flow resumes in a smaller vein more proximally (Fig. 4.5). Hence, increased resistance to flow in diseased smaller veins distal to the junction point will be detected and will cause the distal impaction wedge pressure to exceed the proximal balloon wedge pressure.[20] Since the clinical safety of repeated short balloon inflation to measure PAWP is well accepted, whereas wedge measurement by tip impaction is not widely practiced and may carry considerably greater risk of pulmonary vascular trauma, these distal catheter impaction wedge pressures are not recorded in routine clinical practice.

In summary, PAWP measured with a balloon-tipped pulmonary artery catheter provides a delayed, damped estimate of LAP, by measuring the pressure where flow resumes at a pulmonary venous junction point near the left atrium. The PAWP waveform should display small a and v waves like the LAP waveform, and these phasic components should be identifiable if the pressure trace is displayed with sufficient gain and resolution on the monitor screen.

WEDGE PRESSURE vs. RIGHT ATRIAL PRESSURE

The PAWP waveform generally has two prominent pressure peaks, the a and v waves, in contrast to the three peaks commonly seen in the central venous pressure trace (Fig. 4.6).[15] The c wave is difficult to discern in a normal wedge pressure trace for several reasons. First, a and c waves are normally less prominent in the left atrium than in the right atrium.[1] Second, the interval between onset of atrial and ventricular contraction (and thus a and c waves) is shorter on the left side of the heart than on the right side. Consequently, left atrial a and c waves appear more superimposed, and this composite wave is sometimes termed an a-c wave (Fig. 4.7). Third, the PAWP trace is a damped reflection of LAP. This further obscures distinct a and c waves in the wedge pressure trace. For all of these reasons, the PAWP trace usually shows only two pressure peaks, a and v.

REPORTING WEDGE PRESSURE

When a and v waves are trivial in magnitude, the PAWP is reported as one value, the mean pressure. On the other hand, when the waves are prominent, it is best to note three values: a, v, and mean pressures. Each pressure value may have particular significance. The wedge a wave peak pressure reflects end-diastolic atrial contraction and is the most accurate predictor of left ventricular end-diastolic pressure in patients with left ventricular dysfunction (Fig. 4.8).[7,13] The magnitude of the wedge pressure v wave is often used to estimate severity of mitral valve regurgitation.[9] Finally, mean PAWP estimates mean LAP and, thus, the average hydrostatic back-pressure exerted upon the pulmonary vasculature. Consequently, mean wedge pressure would be expected to predict a patient's risk for developing hydrostatic (high filling pressure) pulmonary edema, better than the a or v wave peak pressure values. (These concepts are developed in much greater detail in Ch. 6.)

WEDGE PRESSURE, OCCLUSION PRESSURE, AND CAPILLARY PRESSURE

The terms *pulmonary artery wedge pressure* and *pulmonary artery occlusion pressure* can be used interchangeably. Both refer to the measurement obtained from the tip of a pulmonary artery catheter following balloon inflation and flotation to the wedged position. For the reasons described above, this wedge pressure measurement is generally a close approximation of LAP.

In contrast, the hydrostatic pressure in the pulmonary capillaries is a different pressure, which must exceed LAP to maintain anterograde blood flow through the lungs.[18] Pulmonary capillary pressure should not be confused with wedge pressure or LAP. However, this misconception has been perpetuated by frequent use of the phrase *pulmonary capillary wedge pressure*, when pulmonary artery wedge or occlusion pressure was intended. The magnitude of the difference between pulmonary capillary pressure and PAWP is generally small but can increase markedly when resistance to flow in the pulmonary veins is elevated (Fig. 4.5). This may occur in rare conditions like pulmonary veno-occlusive disease (see Ch. 6) or more common causes of elevated pulmonary venous resistance, such as central ner-

vous system injury, acute lung injury, hypovolemic shock, endotoxemia, and norepinephrine infusion.[18] Under these conditions, measurement of PAWP will underestimate pulmonary capillary pressure substantially and thereby underestimate the risk of hydrostatic pulmonary edema.

Pulmonary capillary pressure may be measured at the bedside by analyzing the pulmonary artery pressure decay following balloon inflation,[4,5,8,10,12,19] but these techniques have not been adopted widely in clinical practice. In summary, it is important to recognize that in patients with pulmonary hypertension caused by abnormally high resistance to flow in the *small* pulmonary veins, measurement of a normal wedge pressure accurately indicates normal LAP (Fig. 4.5, top) but underestimates true pulmonary capillary pressure (Fig. 4.5, bottom). Under these conditions, high pulmonary capillary pressure may coexist with normal LAP and hydrostatic pulmonary edema may be misdiagnosed as low-pressure, capillary leak, or noncardiogenic in origin.[4-6] To avoid confusion, the phrase *pulmonary capillary wedge pressure* should be abandoned.[18]

IDENTIFYING WEDGE PRESSURE IN THE UNWEDGED PULMONARY ARTERY PRESSURE TRACE

In order to recognize prominent a or v waves in the wedge pressure trace, it is not always necessary to inflate the pulmonary artery catheter balloon and obtain wedge position (Fig. 4.9). Since the wedge pressure records LAP waves transmitted in retrograde fashion from the left atrium, these waves will normally sum with the anterograde pulmonary artery pressure (PAP) waves produced by right ventricular ejection. The PAP trace then becomes a composite wave, reflecting both retrograde and anterograde components. Consequently, tall left atrial a and v waves distort the normal PAP contour: the a wave is inscribed at the onset of the systolic upstroke, and the v wave can be seen distorting the dicrotic notch (Figs. 4.9 and 4.10).[14] When the PAWP v wave is unusually prominent, the unwedged PAP trace takes on a bifid appearance, with the second peak being caused by the large v wave (Fig. 4.11).

Once these waves are recognized by observing the wedge pressure and comparing it with the PAP trace, it is convenient, and perhaps more prudent, to follow the wedge pressure a and v waves in the PAP trace, without repeatedly inflating the balloon to measure wedge pressure. However, marked changes in PAP values or wave morphology should initiate balloon inflation and wedge pressure measurement, since artifacts occasionally mimic these observations. Some of these artifacts are considered in Chapter 5.

Illustrations for Pulmonary Artery Wedge Pressure

Figure 4.1 Pulmonary artery wedge pressure measurement. The wedged catheter creates a static column of blood connecting the catheter tip to a junction point where flow resumes in the pulmonary veins (PV) near the left atrium (LA). Right atrium, RA, right ventricle, RV, pulmonary artery, PA, and left ventricle, LV.

Figure 4.2 Pulmonary veno-occlusive disease. *(Top)* Obstruction to flow is confined to the static column of blood in the small pulmonary veins (PV), and pulmonary artery wedge (PAW) pressure (10 mmHg) closely approximates left atrial (LA) pressure (10 mmHg). *(Bottom)* Obstruction to flow beyond the static column of blood in the larger PV creates a pressure gradient beyond the junction point and causes the PAW and PV pressures (15 mmHg) to exceed LA pressure (10 mmHg) and overestimate diastolic pressure in the left ventricle (LV). See text for more detail.

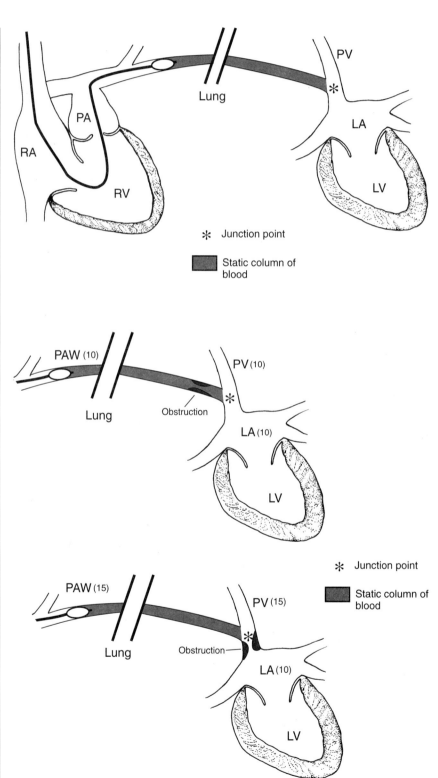

Figure 4.3 Pulmonary artery wedge pressure (PAWP) is a delayed reflection of left atrial pressure (LAP). Note the PAWP a and v waves (square boxes) are delayed relative to the corresponding LAP a and v waves (circles). The a wave in the PAWP trace usually appears after the ECG QRS, even though this pressure wave results from end-diastolic left atrial contraction. The rhythm is sinus bradycardia, although the ECG P waves are not well seen. (Modified from Kern and Deligonul,[13] with permission.)

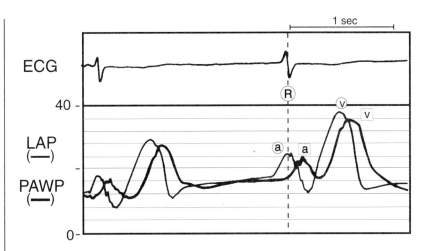

Figure 4.4 Pulmonary artery wedge pressure (PAWP) is a damped reflection of left atrial pressure (LAP). Recorded from a patient with severe mitral regurgitation, the tall v wave in the PAWP trace is smaller in magnitude than the v wave simultaneously recorded from the LAP trace (30 vs. 42 mmHg), and the y pressure descent and nadir are steeper and lower in the LAP trace compared to the PAWP trace. This recording also illustrates the delayed arrival of LAP waves in the PAWP trace. (Modified from Mark,[15] with permission.)

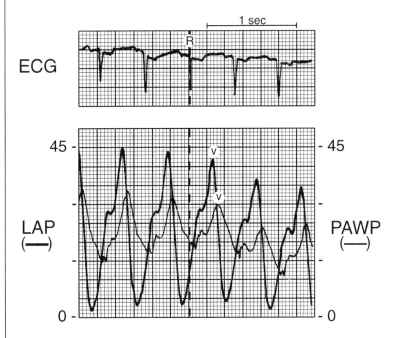

Figure 4.5 Pulmonary artery wedge (PAW) pressure recorded by balloon flotation (*top figure*) occludes flow in a larger vessel than PAW pressure recorded by catheter tip impaction (*bottom figure*). Obstruction to flow confined to small pulmonary veins (PV) would not be detected in the former instance, and PAW pressure (10 mmHg) would equal the pressure in the large PV (10 mmHg) and left atrium (LA) (10 mmHg) (*top figure*). In contrast, PAW pressure measurement by catheter impaction moves the PV junction point upstream to smaller veins, and this PAW pressure (15 mmHg) would exceed large PV pressure (10 mmHg) and LAP (10 mmHg) (*bottom figure*). See text for more detail.

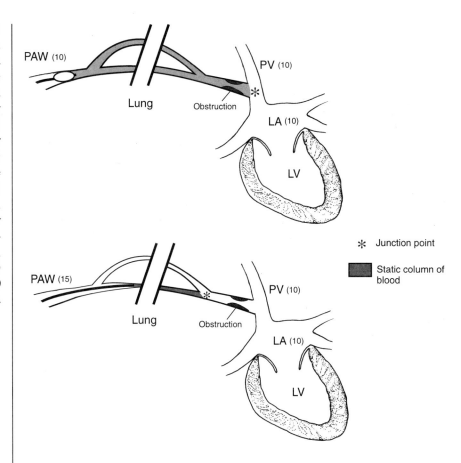

✳ Junction point

▨ Static column of blood

Figure 4.6 The pulmonary artery wedge pressure (PAWP) waveform generally displays two pressure peaks (a and v waves) compared to the three pressure peaks (a, c, and v waves) seen in the central venous pressure (CVP) trace. The ECG P, R, and T waves are labeled to aid identification of pressure waveforms. Note that both the mean PAWP (28 mmHg) and the mean CVP (12 mmHg) are abnormally elevated in this example. See text for more detail. (Modified from Mark,[15] with permission.)

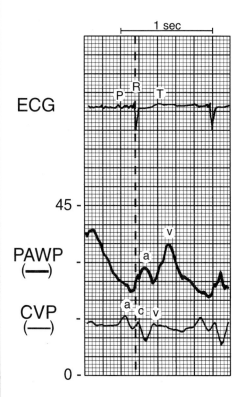

Figure 4.7 Normal pulmonary artery wedge pressure (PAWP) displays two small pressure peaks. The first wave inscribed after the ECG R wave is the a wave and is described as a composite a-c wave (9 mmHg) when the a and c components can be discerned individually, as in this example. The second wave is the v wave (7 mmHg) and is inscribed after the ECG T wave. Arterial blood pressure (ART) and ECG traces are shown to emphasize timing of PAWP a-c and v waves.

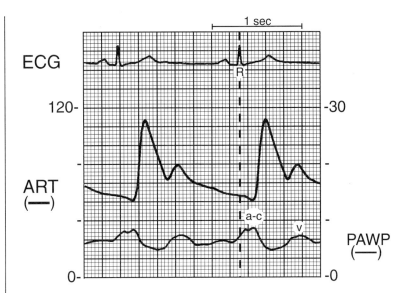

Figure 4.8 Pulmonary artery wedge pressure (PAWP) recorded at the peak of the a wave (18 mmHg) provides the best estimate of left ventricular end-diastolic pressure (*arrow*, 23 mmHg) in patients with left ventricular dysfunction because the a wave peak pressure reflects the booster pump effect of left atrial contraction at end-diastole. (Modified from Kern and Deligonul,[13] with permission.)

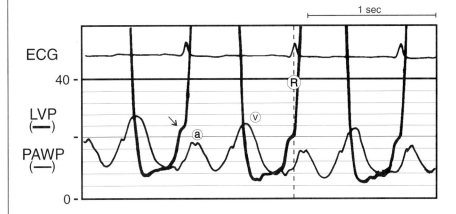

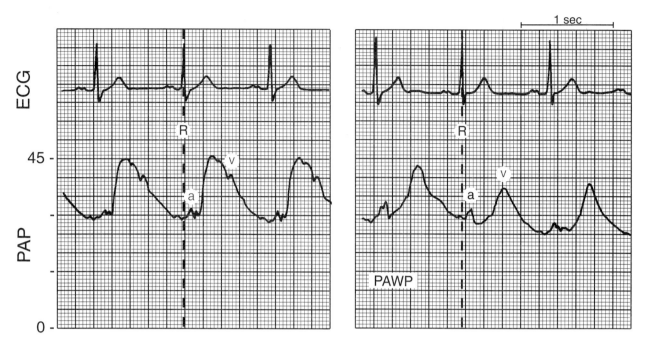

Figure 4.9 Prominent a and v waves in the pulmonary artery wedge pressure (PAWP) trace can be detected in the unwedged pulmonary artery pressure (PAP) trace. Note that the timing of the a and v waves relative to the ECG R wave is similar in both panels.

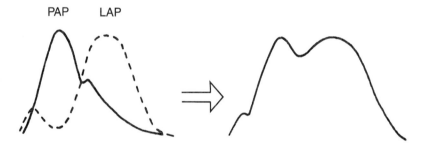

Figure 4.10 Left atrial pressure (LAP) a and v waves are transmitted in a retrograde manner through the lung vasculature to sum with anterograde pulmonary artery pressure (PAP) waves, thus creating a composite wave. The LAP a wave distorts the systolic upstroke, and the v wave distorts the dicrotic notch. (Modified from Mark,[14] with permission.)

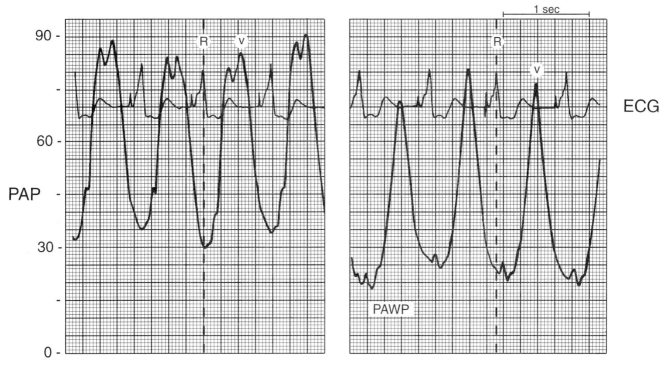

Figure 4.11 Giant pulmonary artery wedge pressure (PAWP) v waves recorded from a patient with severe mitral regurgitation (*right panel*) will distort the unwedged pulmonary artery pressure (PAP) trace and give it a bifid appearance (*left panel*), with the giant v wave producing the second pressure peak.

References

1. Braunwald E, Fishman AP, Cournand A. Time relationship of dynamic events in the cardiac chambers, pulmonary artery and aorta in man. Circ Res 1956;4:100–7

2. Case records of the Massachusetts General Hospital (Case 21-1986). N Engl J Med 1986;314:1435–45

3. Case records of the Massachusetts General Hospital (Case 48-1993). N Engl J Med 1993;329:1720–8

4. Collee GG, Lynch KE, Hill RD, Zapol WM. Bedside measurement of pulmonary capillary pressure in patients with acute respiratory failure. Anethesiology 1987;66:614–20

5. Cope DK, Allison RC, Parmentier JL, et al. Measurement of effective pulmonary capillary pressure using the pressure profile after pulmonary artery occlusion. Crit Care Med 1986;14:16–22

6. Cope DK, Allison RC, Dumond ME, Taylor AE. Changes in the pulmonary capillary pressure after cardiac surgery. J Cardiothorac Anesth 1988;2:182–7

7. Falicov RE, Resnekov L. Relationship of the pulmonary artery end-diastolic pressure to the left ventricular end-diastolic and mean filling pressures in patients with and without left ventricular dysfunction. Circulation 1970;42:65–73

8. Gilbert E, Hakim TS. Derivation of pulmonary capillary pressure from arterial occlusion in intact conditions. Crit Care Med 1994;22:986–93

9. Grossman W. Profiles in valvular heart disease, 557–81. In: Grossman W, Baim DS, eds: Cardiac Catheterization, Angiography, and Intervention. Philadelphia: Lea & Febiger, 1991

10. Hakim TS, Maarek JI, Chang HK. Estimation of pulmonary capillary pressure in intact dog lungs using the arterial occlusion technique. Am Rev Respir Dis 1989;140:217–24

11. Henriquez AH, Schrijen FV, Redondo J, Delorme N. Local variations of pulmonary arterial wedge pressure and wedge angiograms in patients with chronic lung disease. Chest 1988;94:491–5

12. Holloway H, Perry M, Downey J, et al. Estimation of effective pulmonary capillary pressure in intact lungs. J Appl Physiol 1983;54:846–51

13. Kern MJ, Deligonul U. The left-sided V wave, 49–56. In: Kern MJ, ed: Hemodynamic Rounds. Interpretation of Cardiac Pathophysiology from Pressure Waveform Analysis. New York: Wiley-Liss, 1993

14. Mark JB, Chetham PM. Ventricular pacing can induce hemodynamically significant mitral valve regurgitation. Anesthesiology 1991;74:375–7

15. Mark JB. Getting the most from your central venous pressure catheter, 157–75. In: Barash PG, ed: ASA Refresher Courses in Anesthesiology (vol 23). Philadelphia: Lippincott-Raven, 1995

16. O'Quin R, Marini JJ. Pulmonary artery occlusion pressure: clinical physiology, measurement, and interpretation. Am Rev Respir Dis 1983;128:319–26

17. Royster RL, Johnson JC, Prough DS, et al. Differences in pulmonary artery wedge pressures obtained by balloon inflation versus impaction techniques. Anesthesiology 1984;61:339–41

18. Wiedemann HP. Wedge pressure in pulmonary veno-occlusive disease. N Engl J Med 1986;315:1233

19. Yamada Y, Komatsu K, Suzukawa M, et al. Pulmonary capillary pressure measured with a pulmonary arterial double port catheter in surgical patients. Anesth Analg 1993;77:1130–4

20. Zidulka A, Hakim TS. Wedge pressure in large vs. small pulmonary arteries to detect pulmonary venoconstriction. J Appl Physiol 1985;59:1329–32

CHAPTER FIVE Pulmonary Artery and Wedge Pressure Artifacts

Intravascular pressure monitoring systems that use fluid-filled catheters and tubing connected to mechanical transducers are subject to artifactual distortion of the waveforms and pressure values. Blood clots, air bubbles, and soft, compliant tubing all tend to dampen the transmitted waveform, obscuring the pulsatile details. On the other hand, monitored pressure signals may contain high-frequency components that are amplified artifactually because of the mechanical limitations of the recording system. This artifact is commonly referred to by the terms *resonance, ringing,* or *overshoot*. These technical aspects of pressure recording are covered in much greater detail in Chapter 9. Here, we consider two somewhat unique pressure monitoring artifacts that are seen commonly during pulmonary artery pressure (PAP) monitoring.[2,4,5]

Since the pulmonary artery catheter is longer than other intravascular catheters, even greater attention must be paid to ensure that the lumens are free of clot or air, thereby obviating the waveform distortion that would result. Furthermore, the pulmonary artery catheter passes through the heart and therefore is subject to pressure recording artifacts resulting from cardiac-induced catheter motion. In order to discern whether or not artifactual pressure waves have been generated, the displayed waveform is examined with one specific question in mind: *what are the anticipated physiologic waveform components?* For example, the PAP trace should have a steep systolic upstroke, systolic peak, dicrotic notch, and diastolic trough, while wedge or atrial pressure waveforms should display a and v waves, even if these waves are small in magnitude (Fig. 5.1). Commonly, other bumps are superimposed on these expected physiologic waves that do not conform to normal physiologic patterns and that cannot be ascribed readily to known pathophysiologic states (Fig. 5.2). These additional bumps are generated when the pulmonary artery catheter is set in motion during the cardiac cycle by the actions of the heart and heart valves. Fluid contained within the moving catheter accelerates and generates artifactual pressure waves when the catheter moves or strikes the walls of the heart and pulmonary artery. These artifactual pressure waves appear as sharp spikes in contrast to the smoother, more rounded physiologic pressure waves. These high-frequency spikes result from the inertia of the fluid contained within the lumen when the catheter is moved by the beating heart.

The most prominent spike pressure artifact is observed commonly in a pulmonary artery or wedge pressure trace following the ECG R wave at the onset of systole.[1] At this time, tricuspid valve closure and right ventricular contraction and ejection may set the pulmonary artery catheter in motion and inscribe a spurious, nonphysiologic pressure wave (Figs. 5.2 and 5.3). Note that this artifactual PAP wave occurs at the same time as the right atrial pressure c wave, the latter resulting from isovolumic right ventricular contraction (Fig. 5.3).

Catheter motion artifacts may inscribe artifactual pressure troughs, as well as artifactual pressure peaks (Figs. 5.4 to 5.6). These nadir pressures may produce erroneous digital values on the bedside monitor if the trough pressure is detected and recorded as diastolic pressure. Repositioning the catheter by advancing or withdrawing it a few centimeters may produce a different position in the right side of the heart, ameliorate the artifact, and allow the digital value on the monitor to be a more accurate estimate of pulmonary artery diastolic pressure (Figs. 5.4 and 5.5).

Another common artifact in PAP measurement occurs when attempts to inflate the balloon cause the catheter tip to become obstructed and no longer measure intravascular pressure, a phenomenon generally termed *overwedging*. This is usually caused by distal catheter migration, with subsequent eccentric balloon inflation that forces the catheter tip against the pulmonary artery wall. Rather than recording intravascular pressure, the catheter now records the gradually rising pressure produced by the pressurized continuous flush system as it builds up against the obstructed distal opening until it frees the orifice from the vessel wall (Fig. 5.7). Note that the overwedged pressure is devoid of pulsatile detail, much higher than pulmonary artery diastolic pressure, and continuously rising until the balloon is deflated. All of these observations suggest that this cannot be an accurate measurement of pulmonary artery wedge pressure.

With each balloon inflation to measure wedge pressure, the pulmonary artery catheter tip floats several centimeters to its wedged position. This flotation process generally occurs over one or two cardiac cycles. Instant wedge pressure occurring before full balloon inflation suggests the pulmonary artery catheter is located inappropriately in a smaller, distal branch of the pulmonary artery. The catheter should be withdrawn before overwedging occurs and results in pulmonary arterial trauma or tissue infarction downstream. A distally positioned catheter may overwedge itself without balloon inflation as the inspiratory phase of mechanical ventilation displaces the catheter tip into the wall of the pulmonary artery (Fig. 5.8). Withdrawing the catheter several centimeters will eliminate this problem. An alternative explanation of this artifactual pressure recording is that the pulmonary artery catheter is positioned in lung zones 1 or 2, resulting in airway pressures rather than vascular pressures being measured during positive pressure inspiration.[3] In Chapter 16, these respiratory–circulatory interactions are discussed in more detail.

Illustrations for Pulmonary Artery and Wedge Pressure Artifacts

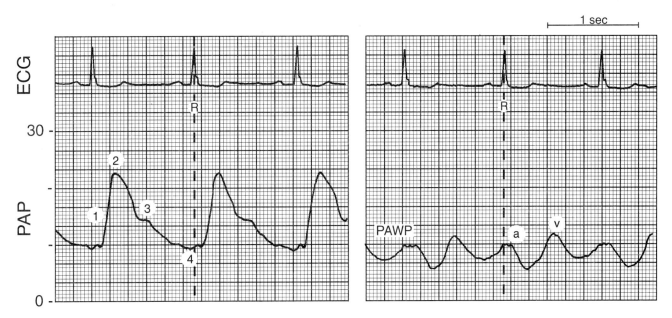

Figure 5.1 Normal pulmonary artery pressure (PAP) and pulmonary artery wedge pressure (PAWP) waveforms. The PAP waveform consists of (1) a steep systolic upstroke, (2) systolic peak, (3) dicrotic notch, and (4) diastolic trough pressures, the latter commonly termed the *pulmonary artery diastolic pressure*. The PAWP waveform displays small a and v waves. In this example, PAP is 22/9 mmHg, and mean PAWP is 9 mmHg (a 10 mmHg, v 12 mmHg).

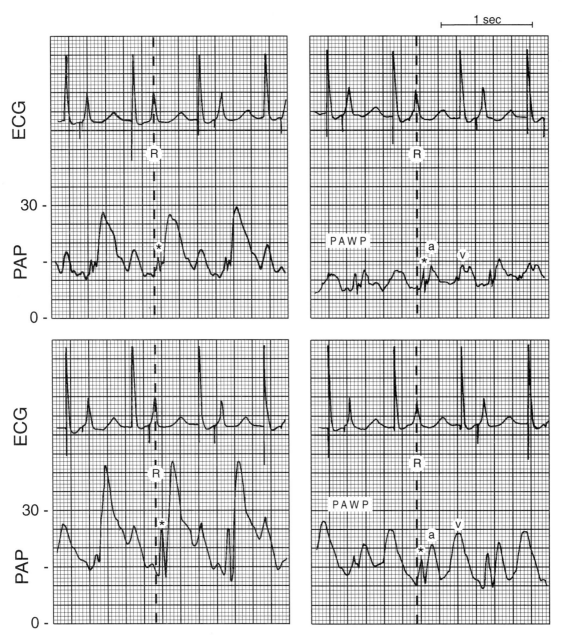

Figure 5.2 Pressure artifacts in pulmonary artery pressure (PAP) and pulmonary artery wedge pressure (PAWP) traces. A sharp pressure spike (*) inscribed immediately after the ECG R wave distorts both the PAP and PAWP waveforms. This artifact is more noticeable at higher pressure (*bottom panels*). Note that the ECG shows atrioventricular sequential pacing. See text for more detail.

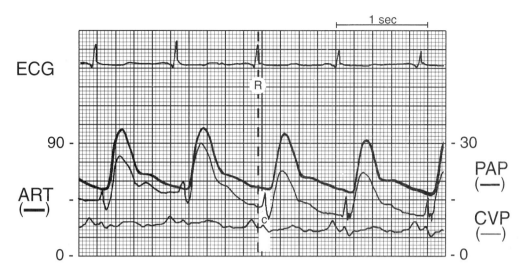

Figure 5.3 Pressure artifact in the pulmonary artery pressure (PAP) trace. This common artifact is inscribed immediately following the ECG R wave and occurs at the time of tricuspid valve closure and onset of right ventricular systole. Note that the PAP artifact also coincides with the central venous pressure (CVP) c wave, which results from right ventricular isovolumic contraction. Arterial blood pressure (ART).

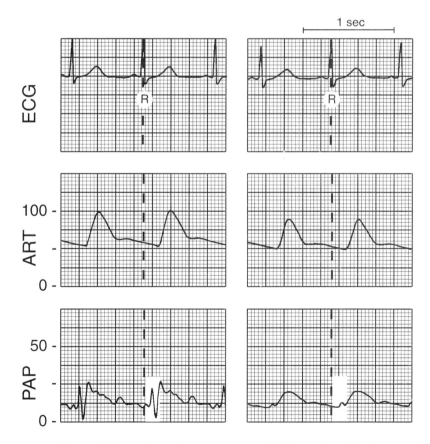

Figure 5.4 Artifactual pressure trough (*left panels, white box*) in the pulmonary artery pressure (PAP) trace. Displayed digital value for PAP (27/2 mmHg) provides a spuriously low value for pulmonary artery diastolic pressure because of this artifact. After the pulmonary artery catheter is repositioned, the pressure artifact is no longer evident (*right panels, white box*), and the digital value displayed by the monitor for PAP (20/10 mmHg) is now accurate.

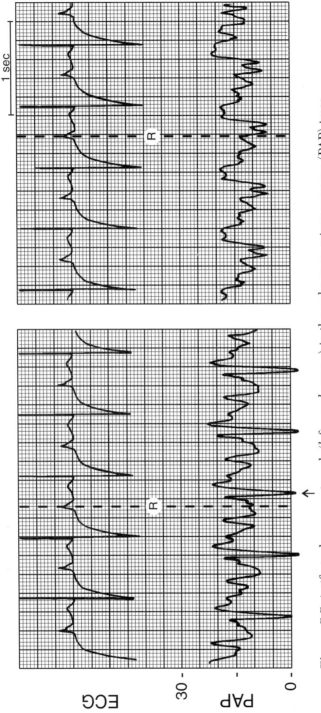

Figure 5.5 Artifactual pressure trough (*left panel, arrow*) in the pulmonary artery pressure (PAP) trace. Displayed digital value for PAP (22/0 mmHg) provides a spuriously low value for pulmonary artery diastolic pressure because of this artifact. The pressure artifact disappears after the pulmonary artery catheter is repositioned (*right panel*). Note that the ECG shows atrial pacing with first-degree atrioventricular block.

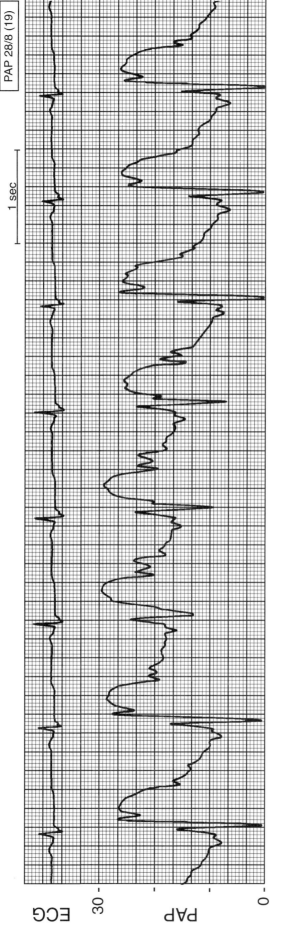

Figure 5.6 Artifactual pressure trough in the pulmonary artery pressure (PAP) trace. In this instance, the displayed digital value for PAP (28/8 mmHg, mean PAP 19 mmHg) provides a reasonable estimate for pulmonary artery diastolic pressure (8 mmHg). More often, this common PAP artifact produces a falsely low displayed digital value for pulmonary artery diastolic pressure of 0 mmHg. Note the cyclic variation in PAP resulting from positive pressure ventilation and elevated intrathoracic pressure during inspiration, which increases pulmonary artery diastolic pressure to approximately 15 mmHg on the second, third, and fourth beats.

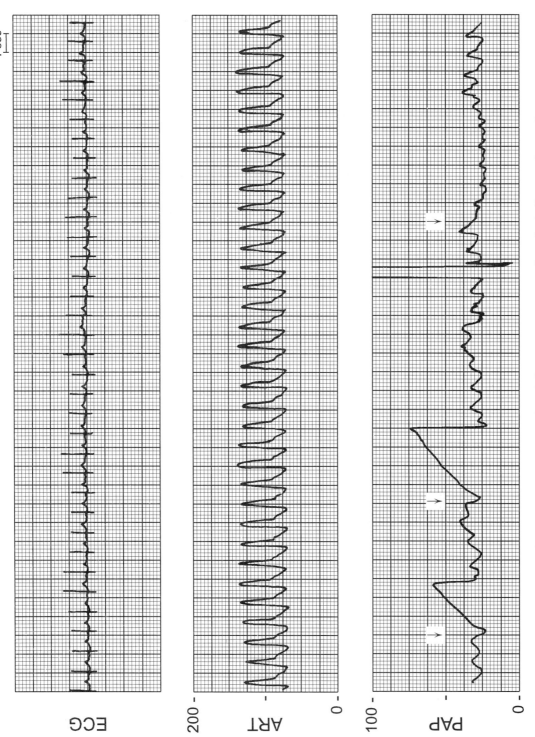

Figure 5.7 Artifactual pulmonary artery pressure (PAP) during attempts to inflate the balloon and record wedge pressure. As the balloon is partially inflated (*first two arrows*), a nonpulsatile increasing pressure is seen as a result of an occluded catheter tip. This pressure artifact is commonly termed *overwedging*. The pulmonary artery catheter should be withdrawn slightly in order to allow complete balloon inflation and pulmonary artery wedge pressure measurement (*third arrow*). Note that mean wedge pressure is always less than mean PAP. See text for more detail.

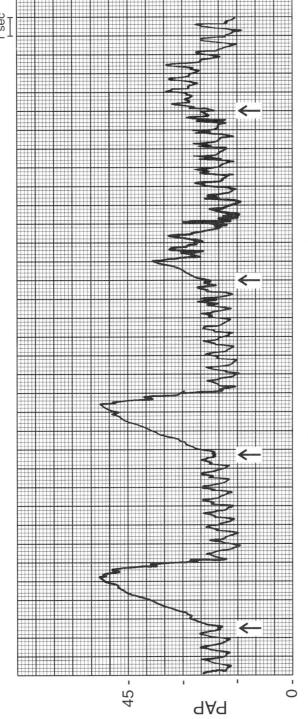

Figure 5.8 Artifactual pressure recording from a pulmonary artery catheter. The pulmonary artery pressure (PAP) trace appears to be overwedged even though the balloon has not been inflated. In this example, the inspiratory phase of positive pressure mechanical ventilation causes the catheter tip to be displaced into the vessel wall (*first three arrows*) until the catheter is withdrawn several centimeters (*last arrow*). This phasic pressure disturbance occurs approximately every 9 seconds, corresponding to a respiratory rate of seven breaths per minute.

References

1. Bashein G. Another source of artifact in the pulmonary artery pressure waveform. Anesthesiology 1988;68:310

2. Morris AH, Chapman RH, Gardner RM. Frequency of technical problems encountered in the measurement of pulmonary artery wedge pressure. Crit Care Med 1984;12:164–70

3. O'Quin R, Marini JJ. Pulmonary artery occlusion pressure: clinical physiology, measurement, and interpretation. Am Rev Respir Dis 1983;128:319–26

4. Schmitt EA, Brantigan CO. Common artifacts of pulmonary artery and pulmonary artery wedge pressures: recognition and interpretation. J Clin Monit 1986;2:44–52

5. Shin B, Ayella RJ, McAslan TC. Pitfalls of Swan-Ganz catheterization. Crit Care Med 1977;5:125–7

CHAPTER SIX Predicting Left Ventricular End-Diastolic Pressure

ON THE DISTINCTION BETWEEN MEAN AND PHASIC PRESSURE

Pulmonary artery catheter monitoring is performed to measure a number of hemodynamic variables in critically ill patients, including cardiac output, mixed venous oxygen saturation, and most importantly, pulmonary artery diastolic and wedge pressures. These pressure measurements are used to estimate left ventricular filling pressure and to help guide fluid and vasoactive drug administration when clinical signs, symptoms, or other monitored variables are felt to be inadequate or unreliable.[24]

Accurate measurement of the left ventricular filling pressure has two somewhat distinct purposes. First, knowledge of the filling pressure provides an estimate of the hydrostatic pressure within the pulmonary capillaries, which is a major determinant of the vascular back-pressure favoring the formation of pulmonary edema. For this purpose, the *mean* pulmonary artery wedge pressure (PAWP) averaged over the cardiac cycle is the pressure of interest. Note that wedge pressure and capillary pressure are not identical, but in general, increases in wedge pressure lead to increases in capillary pressure. (See Ch. 4 for details.)

The second purpose for measuring left ventricular filling pressure is to estimate the preload of the left ventricle. In this instance, the *end-diastolic* wedge pressure resulting from atrial contraction best predicts the end-diastolic filling pressure or preload of the left ventricle.[28] Measurement of left ventricular end-diastolic pressure (LVEDP) is performed at the Z-point, which is identified on the left ventricular pressure trace as the point at which the slope of the ventricular pressure upstroke changes, approximately 50 msec after the ECG Q wave, and generally coinciding with the ECG R wave (Fig. 6.1).[5] Most importantly, this is a phasic pressure point measured at end-diastole, not a mean diastolic pressure in the left ventricle.

Although PAWP is generally reported as mean pressure, an end-diastolic component of wedge pressure can be identified in its phasic pressure trace as well. In the presence of normal sinus rhythm, atrial contraction provides this end-diastolic mechanical event. Thus, measurement of the PAWP a wave pressure peak provides a more accurate estimate of LVEDP than that provided by mean PAWP (Fig. 6.1).

The distinction here is subtle: *average* or *mean* wedge pressure as an estimate of hydrostatic pressure on the lungs vs. *phasic* or *end-diastolic* wedge pressure, the pressure recorded after the a wave, as a predictor of LVEDP. Perhaps a more eloquent description of this point is offered by others:

While the ventricular end diastolic pressure may be considered to be the hemodynamic "stimulus" which determines the force of ventricular contraction, the mean atrial pressure may be considered the hemodynamic "price" which the organism must pay for this stimulus to be provided.[19]

The pressure tracings from two patients in Figure 6.2, one with aortic stenosis and one with mitral regurgitation, help illustrate this point. The LVEDP in both patients is elevated (25 mmHg) and well approximated by the left atrial (or wedge) pressure a wave peak, the phasic pressure produced by end-diastolic atrial contraction. In both patients, this pressure (25 mmHg) provides the best single pressure estimate of left ventricular preload, that is, the *stimulus* for left ventricular contraction. (One should recognize, however, that a filling pressure is at best only an estimate of filling volume. These pressure–volume relations are discussed in greater detail in Ch. 15). Although both patients have the same end-diastolic pressure, mean left atrial (or wedge) pressure is much higher in the patient with mitral regurgitation (30 mmHg) than in the patient with aortic stenosis (15 mmHg). The patient with aortic stenosis produces an LVEDP of 25 mmHg with a strong left atrial contraction, as evidenced by the tall left atrial a wave. This effective booster pump mechanism provides adequate left ventricular preload or end-diastolic pressure (the *stimulus*) with a reasonable mean left atrial pressure (LAP) (the *price*), which does not place the patient at risk for developing hydrostatic pulmonary edema. In contrast, the patient with mitral regurgitation and an LVEDP of 25 mmHg has a very high mean LAP (30 mmHg) caused by the tall regurgitant c-v wave inscribed during systole. In order to provide a similar LVEDP (the *stimulus*), mean LAP (the *price*) is excessive and would likely result in pulmonary edema.

The distinction between *mean* and *phasic* filling pressures should now be evident. Clearly, the mean wedge pressure is not always equal to the end-diastolic pressure value, and the taller the pulsatile a and v wave components, the greater the discrepancy may be. This distinction is important and has been obscured in daily clinical practice by our emphasis on single digital values for *the* PAWP.

In this chapter, we focus on how we can use the pulmonary artery diastolic pressure (PADP) or PAWP to predict LVEDP most accurately. Although these routinely monitored pressures may provide a reasonable estimate of left ventricular filling pressure under many circumstances, under some clinical conditions, like the one just illustrated, these measurements from the left atrium or pulmonary artery may either underestimate or overestimate LVEDP. The following sections highlight conditions where there is lack of agreement between these measurements. Table 6.1 lists conditions where LVEDP is underestimated, and Table 6.2 lists conditions where it is overestimated.

Underestimation of Left Ventricular End-Diastolic Pressure

DECREASED LEFT VENTRICULAR COMPLIANCE

Under normal circumstances, the atrial contribution to left ventricular end-diastolic volume and pressure is less than 20 percent.[23] However, when there is left ventricular diastolic dysfunction causing delayed relaxation or abnormal ventricular compliance, the atrial contribution to left ventricular filling volume and pressure can be as much as 40 to 50 percent.[23,26] Atrial contraction into an incompletely relaxed or stiff left ventricle inscribes a prominent end-diastolic a wave in the PAWP trace (Figs. 6.2 to 6.4). Under these conditions, the peak of the wedge pressure a wave provides a close estimate of LVEDP[12] while mean wedge pressure will underestimate LVEDP (Figs. 6.2 and 6.5). Conditions in which left ventricular compliance is reduced or ventricular relaxation is impaired include myocardial ischemia and infarction (Figs. 6.4 and 6.6), left ventricular hypertrophy caused by systemic hypertension, aortic stenosis (Figs. 6.2, 6.3, and 6.5), hypertrophic cardiomyopathy, and other primary myocardial diseases.

AORTIC VALVE REGURGITATION

Normal left ventricular filling commences after isovolumic ventricular relaxation, when ventricular pressure falls below atrial pressure and the mitral valve opens. Ventricular filling proceeds until the onset of isovolumic ventricular contraction and mitral valve closure. When there is aortic valve regurgitation, the duration and sources for left ventricular filling change. In this condition, abnormal diastolic filling occurs from the aorta as soon as left ventricular pressure falls below aortic pressure, thus eliminating isovolumic ventricular relaxation. Diastolic ventricular filling precedes mitral valve opening and continues after left atrial contraction and closure of the mitral valve. Left ventricular diastolic pressure continues to rise until LVEDP is reached at the onset of mechanical systole and the re-establishment of anterograde flow from left ventricle to aorta. Since mitral valve closure occurs prior to end-diastole, mean PAWP as well as the wedge a wave pressure both underestimate LVEDP (Fig. 6.7).[12] Despite the very high LVEDP so generated, mean wedge pressure may remain low, thereby protecting the pulmonary vasculature from elevated luminal hydrostatic pressure and reducing the risk of pulmonary edema.

PULMONIC VALVE REGURGITATION

In the presence of pulmonic valve regurgitation, diastolic flow from the proximal pulmonary artery becomes bidirectional, anterograde into the left atrium and retrograde into the right ventricle. When the right ventricular diastolic pressure is lower than LAP, and coexists with a significant degree of pulmonic regurgitation, pulmonary artery diastolic flow will seek the lower pressure pathway, in this instance, that of the right ventricle (Fig. 6.8). As a consequence, PADP will underestimate wedge pressure, LAP, and LVEDP.

RIGHT BUNDLE BRANCH BLOCK

When pulmonary vascular resistance is normal, there is no pressure gradient across the pulmonary vascular bed at end of diastole, and PADP equilibrates with its downstream pressure, LAP. When right ventricular systole is delayed because of right bundle branch block, pulmonary artery pressure continues to fall with the x or systolic descent of downstream LAP. Under such conditions, PADP will underestimate LVEDP (Fig. 6.9).[17]

Not only does right bundle branch block cause a delayed onset of right ventricular contraction, the aberrant conduction pathway through the right ventricle also causes a loss of synchronous contraction, reducing right ventricular dp/dt and further contributing to the delayed opening of the pulmonic valve. Herbert[17] found that PADP underestimated LVEDP by 4 mmHg in these circumstances. Note that the PADP underestimates LVEDP because the left atrial a wave pressure peak best estimates LVEDP. Since the PADP continues to decline after the left atrial a wave during the systolic x descent, underestimation of LVEDP results. How-

Table 6.1 Underestimation of LVEDP

CONDITION	DISCREPANCY	CAUSE
Decreased left ventricular compliance	Mean LAP<LVEDP	Increased end-diastolic a wave
Aortic valve regurgitation	LAP a wave<LVEDP	Mitral valve closure prior to end-diastole
Pulmonic valve regurgitation	PADP<LVEDP	Bidirectional runoff for pulmonary artery flow
Right bundle branch block	PADP<LVEDP	Delayed pulmonic valve opening
Decreased pulmonary vascular bed	PAWP<LVEDP	Obstruction of pulmonary blood flow

Abbreviations: LVEDP, left ventricular end-diastolic pressure; PADP, pulmonary artery diastolic pressure; PAWP, pulmonary artery wedge pressure; LAP, left atrial pressure.

Table 6.2 Overestimation of LVEDP

CONDITION	DISCREPANCY	CAUSE
Positive end-expiratory pressure	Mean PAWP>mean LAP	Creation of lung zone 1 or 2 or pericardial pressure changes
Pulmonary arterial hypertension	PADP>mean PAWP	Increased pulmonary vascular resistance
Pulmonary veno-occlusive disease	Mean PAWP>mean LAP	Obstruction to flow in large pulmonary veins
Mitral valve stenosis	Mean LAP>LVEDP	Obstruction to flow across mitral valve
Mitral valve regurgitation	Mean LAP>LVEDP	Systolic v wave raises mean atrial pressure
Tachycardia	PADP>mean LAP>LVEDP	Short diastole creates pulmonary vascular and mitral valve gradients
Ventricular septal defect	Mean LAP>LVEDP	Systolic v wave raises mean atrial pressure

Abbreviations: LVEDP, left ventricular end-diastolic pressure; PADP, pulmonary artery diastolic pressure; PAWP, pulmonary artery wedge pressure; LAP, left atrial pressure.

ever, the pulmonary artery wedge a wave peak pressure will remain a close estimate of LVEDP in this circumstance.

REDUCED PULMONARY VASCULAR BED

Inflation of the pulmonary artery catheter balloon to measure PAWP interrupts anterograde blood flow through a small section of the lung. Normally, this minor reduction in the pulmonary vascular tree has no measurable effect upon total pulmonary blood flow or left atrial filling. However, after pneumonectomy, and possibly other conditions that markedly reduce the pulmonary vascular bed, pulmonary artery catheter balloon inflation may occlude a significant portion of the remaining pulmonary vascular cross-sectional area. Mechanical obstruction of pulmonary blood flow results, causing increased central venous pressure and decreased left ventricular filling, cardiac output, and systemic blood pressure. This phenomenon has been reported in patients after pneumonectomy[1,32] and confirmed in dog experiments.[32] By obstructing pulmonary blood flow, balloon inflation reduces left atrial and wedge pressures. Consequently, this falsely low value for PAWP underestimates the LVEDP that existed prior to balloon inflation. This artifact should be suspected in the appropriate clinical setting, when a sudden reduction in systemic arterial pressure occurs coincident with pulmonary artery catheter balloon inflation.

Note that this condition is quite different from the other causes of pulmonary artery diastolic or wedge pressure underestimation of LVEDP. In the setting of a reduced pulmonary vascular bed, the balloon inflation procedure itself reduces pulmonary blood flow and left ventricular filling. The resulting wedge pressure measurement correctly reflects LVEDP at the time of the measurement. However, this left ventricular filling pressure has been reduced by the measurement procedure itself, analogous to the Heisenberg Uncertainty Principle in physics, where the act of measurement changes the quantity you wish to measure.

Overestimation of Left Ventricular End-Diastolic Pressure

POSITIVE END-EXPIRATORY PRESSURE

In order for PAWP to be a valid estimate of LVEDP, a continuous, static column of blood must exist between the tip of the wedged catheter and the draining pulmonary venous radicle. At the microcirculatory level, this connecting channel consists of thin pulmonary capillaries, which are subject to extramural compressive forces exerted by surrounding alveoli. In lung physiologic zones 1 and 2,[30] alveolar pressure can exceed pulmonary venous pressure (zone 2) or both pulmonary arterial and pulmonary venous pressure (zone 1) (Fig. 6.10). When this occurs, the pressure sensed by the pulmonary artery catheter will be influenced by alveolar pressure and may bear little relationship to pulmonary venous pressure, LAP, or LVEDP. Under these circumstances, alveolar or airway pressures are being monitored, rather than the intended downstream vascular pressure in the left atrium or ventricle. In other words, zone 3 lung conditions must apply for PAWP to reflect LAP accurately. In most clinical settings in which pulmonary artery catheters are used, patients are supine, which favors the creation of zone 3 conditions. However, patients nursed in the lateral or semi-sitting position may have considerable nondependent portions of their lungs behave like zone 2.

Catheters that are wedged outside zone 3 may be suspected when the normal phasic a and v waves are absent and wedge pressure varies markedly with the respiratory cycle.[21] In addition, mean wedge pressure should not exceed PADP unless tall a or v waves are present in the wedge pressure trace. Otherwise, the clinician should suspect that the wedged catheter is no longer in zone 3 and that alveolar pressures are being measured unintentionally.

Several factors conspire to make these respiratory effects more or less of a problem.[2,14,25] In general, zones 1 and 2 become more extensive when LAP is low, when the pulmonary artery catheter tip is located vertically above the left atrium, or when alveolar pressure is high. This last condition is particularly common when positive end-expiratory pressure (PEEP) is applied to improve arterial blood oxygenation. How should PAWP be interpreted when PEEP is being used, and alveolar pressure may exceed pulmonary venous or pulmonary arterial pressures?

Formulae have been derived to adjust for the effects of PEEP on wedge pressure measurement. In general, mechanical ventilation with PEEP raises wedge pressure by an amount less than one-half the value of PEEP applied (i.e., 10 cm H_2O PEEP will raise wedge pressure less than 5 cm H_2O or 4 mmHg).[16,21] The mathematical basis for this relation depends on the ratio of chest wall to lung compliance, and details of its derivation may be found in several reviews.[20,21,29] Unfortunately, simple quantitative corrections such as these are not entirely reliable.[22]

Alternative methods to correct for PEEP are problematic also. Measurement of pleural pressure as an estimate of pericardial or juxtacardiac pressure is possible using an esophageal balloon,[21] but this technique has not found widespread clinical application. Prolonged discontinuation of PEEP before measuring wedge pressure is to be discouraged. Not only will circulatory dynamics change dramatically owing to rebound central hypervolemia caused by translocation of blood from the periphery, but respiratory gas exchange may deteriorate and be slow to recover.[21]

On the other hand, Pinsky et al[22] found that transient airway disconnection for 2 to 3 seconds in patients receiving mechanical ventilation with PEEP allowed measurement of *nadir wedge pressure*, which proved to be a better estimate of left ventricular filling pressure at higher levels of PEEP. This transient airway disconnection should not produce sustained alteration of circulatory or respiratory function. When wedge pressure measurement did not change after abrupt airway disconnection, the on-PEEP wedge pressure measurement accurately reflected left ventricular filling pressure. However, when wedge pressure decreased after airway disconnection, the nadir wedge pressure reached within 3 seconds provided a better estimate of ventricular filling pressure.

Fortunately, most patients who require high levels of PEEP may not manifest these artifactual wedge pressure measurement problems. In patients with the adult respiratory distress syndrome, PAWP closely estimates LVEDP at all levels of PEEP up to 20 cm H_2O.[27] While transmission of alveolar pressures to the wedged pulmonary artery catheter was seen in previous dog experiments,[2,25] measurements in critically ill patients who require pulmonary ventilation with PEEP confirm that alveolar pressures do not interrupt the continuous vascular channel connecting the wedged pulmonary artery catheter tip to the left atrium, producing relative microvascular protection from the effects of PEEP.[27] Consequently, PAWP remains a close estimate for LVEDP in most patients requiring PEEP ventilation for advanced respiratory failure, as a result of increased intrapulmonary shunting and low pulmonary compliance, which are the hallmarks of this disease.[27]

In summary, mechanical ventilation with PEEP may cause PAWP to overestimate LAP. However, higher levels of PEEP, more than 10 cm H_2O, should only be required in patients with severe pulmonary dysfunction, and in these patients, wedge pressure remains a close estimate for LAP and LVEDP.[27]

PULMONARY ARTERIAL HYPERTENSION

When the pulmonary vasculature is normal, pulmonary blood flow ceases at end-diastole,[10] and PADP equals LAP. However, if pulmonary vascular resistance is increased, pulmonary artery pressure equilibration with downstream pressure does not occur. Under these conditions, the pulmonary vascular bed begins to resemble the systemic vasculature, where a large pressure gradient exists at end-diastole, with systemic arterial diastolic pressure markedly exceeding downstream right artrial pressure. Therefore, in the presence of pulmonary hypertension caused by elevated pulmonary vascular resistance, PADP overestimates PAWP, LAP, and LVEDP (Fig. 6.11). Although the PADP may be misleading, the wedge pressure should provide an accurate estimate of the left ventricular filling pressure.

Owing to an anatomic distortion of the pulmonary vasculature that develops in this condition, it may be very difficult to wedge the pulmonary artery catheter. Instead of the normal gradual tapering of the pulmonary arteries, enlarged proximal arteries rapidly taper to small distal vessels. A balloon-tipped catheter often will coil in these proximal ectatic arteries and return to the right ventricle, rather than wedge and occlude the pulmonary artery (Fig. 6.12). Consequently, the fact that PADP exceeds LAP in this condition becomes even more important to remember, since the wedge pressure may be unobtainable.

Pulmonary hypertension can develop in a variety of clinical conditions: pulmonary embolism,[10] mitral valve stenosis and regurgitation, left ventricular dysfunction, primary pulmonary hypertension, and left to right shunts. When remodeling of the pulmonary vasculature occurs as these diseases become chronic, pulmonary vascular resistance rises and a pressure gradient develops across the pulmonary vasculature at end-diastole. In general, a greater pressure gradient across the lung at end-diastole (defined as PADP minus PAWP) is associated with a greater calculated pulmonary vascular resistance.[10] In this example (Fig. 6.13), severe pulmonary hypertension is present, and PADP markedly exceeds LAP and LVEDP. Note that the long R-R interval on the fourth beat allows the PADP to decline from 41 mmHg to 27 mmHg and thus provide a much better estimate of left ventricular filling pressure because of the increased time for downstream diastolic runoff.

PULMONARY VENO-OCCLUSIVE DISEASE

In contrast to the precapillary pulmonary vascular constriction that exists in patients with pulmonary arterial hypertension, postcapillary obstruction to flow in the pulmonary veins may occur in the rare condition, pulmonary veno-occlusive disease. Patients with this condition have normal LAP, but some disagreement exists as to whether these patients have normal or elevated PAWP.[7,8,21,31] In part, these different observations may relate to whether the pulmonary artery catheter has been wedged successfully, since the wedge position may be difficult to obtain in these patients. For example, the wedge pressure may be obtained in a lung vascular channel that is already totally occluded. This no-flow region would not communicate with downstream venous pressure or LAP, and a factitious wedge pressure value would be recorded.

However, as explained in detail in Chapter 4, one would expect that a normal wedge pressure would be recorded when the patient has small vessel veno-occlusive disease, but an elevated wedge pressure would be recorded in large vessel disease.[7,8,21,31] Small vein obstruction (Fig. 6.14) narrows the *static* column of blood connecting the wedged pulmonary artery catheter tip with the flowing column in the larger pulmonary veins. Since the partial obstruction only involves the static column, wedge pressure will measure normal pulmonary venous pressures and LAPs because there is no pressure drop across the stenotic segment in the absence of flow. On the other hand, large vein obstruction (Fig. 6.14) creates a gradient in the column of blood *flowing* from these veins toward the left atrium. In this instance, wedge pressure will detect an increased pulmonary venous pressure and overestimate LAP.

This model is consistent with the observations of Zidulka and Hakim,[33] who measured PAWPs from both large and small pulmonary arteries (see Ch. 4, Fig. 4.5). Large artery wedge pressure measurement, similar to clinical wedge pressure measurement with a balloon-tipped catheter, closely estimated the pressure in large pulmonary veins near their entrance to the left atrium. In contrast, small artery wedge pressure estimated the pressure in small pulmonary veins. This upstream venous pressure detected obstruction to flow in small pulmonary veins, and the difference between large artery and small artery wedge pressure values aided detection of elevated pulmonary venous resistance. These observations help explain why the PAWP, as commonly recorded in clinical practice, can either accurately estimate *or* falsely overestimate LAP, depending upon the site of venous obstruction and the site of wedge pressure measurement. Other conditions that mimic pulmonary veno-occlusive disease in this regard include mediastinal fibrosis and intrathoracic or atrial tumors, which obstruct pulmonary venous flow near the left atrium.

MITRAL VALVE STENOSIS

Mitral valve stenosis causes obstruction to blood flow from left atrium to left ventricle during diastole, thereby creating a pressure gradient. Consequently, LAP will exceed left ventricular pressure throughout diastole. Furthermore, all upstream pressures (PADP, PAWP, and LAP) will overestimate LVEDP, owing to the valvular obstruction (Fig. 6.15).[18]

The pressure gradient across the stenotic mitral valve increases as the flow across the valve increases with changes in cardiac output and heart rate. In particular, tachycardia shortens the duration of diastole and can produce a dramatic increase in the mitral valve gradient because the same total flow across the mitral valve must now occur during a reduced period for diastolic filling. Consequently, pulmonary artery diastolic or wedge pressures will overestimate left ventricular filling pressures, and the magnitude of this overestimation will change during altered hemodynamic states.

Other conditions can mimic mitral stenosis by causing obstruction to diastolic filling of the left ventricle. Cardiac tumors, especially left atrial myxoma, can produce a diastolic atrial to ventricular pressure gradient.

MITRAL VALVE REGURGITATION

LAP is elevated in mitral valve regurgitation, owing to the abnormal leakage of blood across the incompetent valve, which inscribes a prominent c-v wave during systole and raises mean LAP and PAWP. In this instance, LVEDP is better approximated by measuring wedge pressure prior to the onset of this regurgitant wave (Figs. 6.16 and 6.17).[15] This presystolic pressure can be estimated accurately from examining the wedge pressure trace (Fig. 6.17), but the digital display of the bedside monitor will report mean wedge pressure and thereby overestimate LVEDP.

In contrast to the patient with mitral stenosis where LAP exceeds left ventricular pressure throughout diastole, the patient with mitral regurgitation has appropriate diastolic equilibration of atrial and ventricular pressures. The problem in mitral regurgitation is choosing the appropriate end-diastolic, pre-v wave pressure to use as an estimate of LVEDP. (See Ch. 17 for more detail about mitral regurgitation and other valvular heart disease.)

TACHYCARDIA

As heart rate increases, the duration of diastole is shortened, and the time available for egress of blood from the pulmonary vasculature to the left atrium and from left atrium to left ventricle is reduced.[4,11,19] At both mitral valve and pulmonary vascular levels, pressure gradients develop as the duration of diastole progressively decreases during tachycardia. As tachycardia worsens, left atrial contraction may occur during the previous ventricular systole, prior to full mitral valve opening. Like cannon a waves inscribed during atrioventricular dissociation, these prominent pre-diastolic left atrial a waves raise mean atrial pressure at a time when ventricular end-diastolic pressure is falling.[19]

In addition to this atrial–ventricular pressure gradient during tachycardia, a gradient may also develop between PADP and LAP. As the duration of diastole is progressively reduced, egress of blood from the pulmonary vasculature into the left atrium is incomplete, and a PADP–LAP gradient develops, similar to that seen in patients with pulmonary arterial hypertension. Consequently, PADP overestimates mean wedge pressure, which in turn overestimates LVEDP[4,11] (Fig. 6.18). Note that progressive increase in heart rate may accentuate these gradients, as PADP continues to rise, while LVEDP continues to fall. Patients with irregular heart rates, such as those with atrial fibrillation, will have more complete equilibration of PADP and LVEDP during longer R-R intervals. Consequently, these beats should be chosen to provide the best estimate of LVEDP (Fig. 6.19)

VENTRICULAR SEPTAL DEFECT

Tall systolic v waves of any cause will raise mean left atrial and wedge pressures and drive these mean pressures above LVEDP. It cannot be overemphasized that LVEDP is a phasic pressure measurement at end-diastole, whereas clinical reporting of wedge pressure or LAP focuses on the mean pressure only. As in mitral regurgitation, selecting wedge pressure before the onset of the v wave will identify end-diastole and provide a reasonable estimate for LVEDP.

Ventricular septal defect with intact atrial septum may cause large v waves in the wedge pressure trace.[3] The increased pulmonary blood flow caused by the left to right shunt increases pulmonary venous inflow to the left atrium. The systolic component of this venous inflow generates a tall atrial v wave, raising mean wedge pressure above LVEDP. Other conditions that produce left to right shunting,[9] left ventricular failure, volume overload, and elevated mean wedge pressure can be associated with prominent v waves in the absence of mitral regurgitation.[13] In all these cases, mean wedge pressure overestimates LVEDP.

SUMMARY: PREDICTING LEFT VENTRICULAR END-DIASTOLIC PRESSURE

This chapter has highlighted conditions where the PADP or PAWP either underestimate or overestimate LVEDP. Some conditions are relatively common, such as diastolic dysfunction or mitral regurgitation, while others are extremely rare, such as pulmonary veno-occlusive disease or decreased pulmonary vascular bed. Often, several conditions coexist, further compounding the magnitude of the measurement problem. For example, a patient with mitral stenosis resulting in pulmonary hypertension who develops tachycardia now has three reasons for PADP to overestimate LVEDP. Major clinical errors would result if the high PADP were presumed to indicate increased left ventricular preload in this patient.

Although the magnitude of the discrepancy between PADP or PAWP and LVEDP may be slight, such as a 4-mmHg underestimation in the case of right bundle branch block,[17] in some cases, these differences can be very great, particularly in the presence of pulmonary arterial hypertension.[6] Most importantly, an awareness of these confounding circumstances will allow the clinician to interpret more critically the data available from the pulmonary artery catheter.

Illustrations for Predicting Left Ventricular End-Diastolic Pressure

Figure 6.1 Simultaneous left ventricular pressure (LVP) and left atrial pressure (LAP) a, c, and v waves. Left ventricular end-diastolic pressure (LVEDP) is recorded at the Z-point where the slope of the LVP upstroke increases, approximately 50 msec after the ECG Q wave, near the peak of the ECG R wave. Note that LVEDP is a phasic pressure, measured at end-diastole, and best approximated by the LAP a wave pressure (15 mmHg), rather than mean LAP ($\overline{\text{LAP}}$ 9 mmHg).

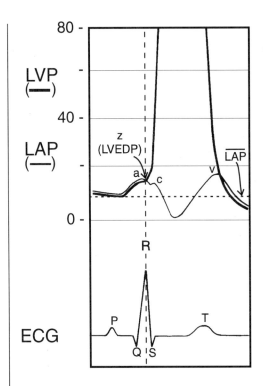

Figure 6.2 Simultaneous left ventricular pressure (LVP) and left atrial pressure (LAP) traces comparing these pressure relations in aortic stenosis with mitral regurgitation. Left ventricular end-diastolic pressure (LVEDP) is elevated in both conditions (25 mmHg). Mean LAP remains low in aortic stenosis ($\overline{LAP}$ 15 mmHg) but is high in mitral regurgitation ($\overline{LAP}$ 30 mmHg), owing to the regurgitant c-v wave inscribed during systole. LAP a, c, and v waves are identified. See text for more detail.

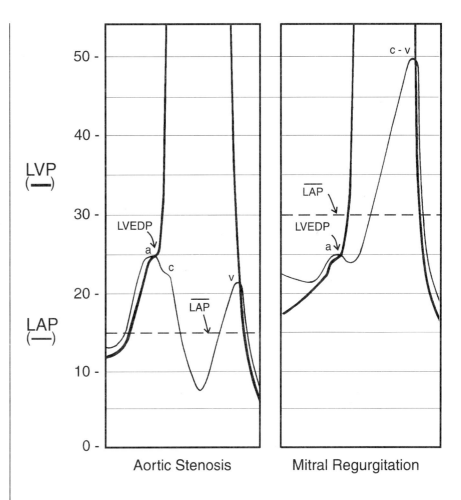

Aortic Stenosis   Mitral Regurgitation

Figure 6.3 Pulmonary artery wedge pressure (PAWP) a, c, and v waves recorded from a patient with reduced left ventricular compliance caused by aortic stenosis and coronary artery disease. The PAWP a wave peak pressure (26 mmHg) is greater than the mean wedge pressure and provides the best estimate of left ventricular end-diastolic pressure (LVEDP). At the time of cardiac catheterization in this patient, mean wedge pressure was 18 mmHg and LVEDP was 28 mmHg.

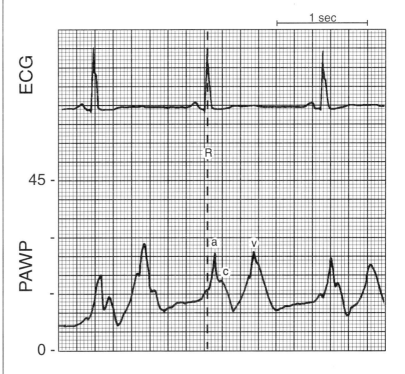

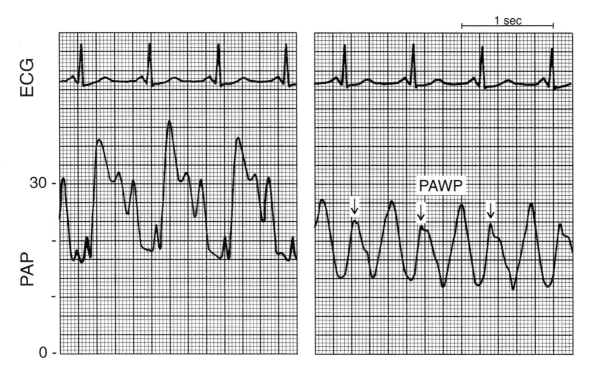

Figure 6.4 Pulmonary artery pressure (PAP) and pulmonary artery wedge pressure (PAWP) recorded from a patient with reduced left ventricular compliance caused by myocardial ischemia following induction of anesthesia and tracheal intubation. Mean PAWP is well approximated by the pulmonary artery diastolic pressure (approximately 17 mmHg), but both these pressures likely underestimate left ventricular end-diastolic pressure (LVEDP). The prominent wedge pressure *a* wave (*arrows*, 23 mmHg) provides a better estimate of LVEDP.

Figure 6.5 Simultaneous left ventricular pressure (LVP) and pulmonary artery wedge pressure (PAWP) recorded from a patient with moderately severe aortic stenosis. Left ventricular end-diastolic pressure (LVEDP, 15 mmHg) is closely approximated by PAWP a wave peak pressure (14 mmHg), while mean wedge pressure is significantly lower (PAWP 11 mmHg). Note that the PAWP a and v waves appear delayed relative to the LVP trace. Compare with Figs. 6.1 and 6.2, which illustrate the temporal relation of LVP and direct left atrial pressure measurement. (Modified from Falicov and Resnekov,[12] with permission.)

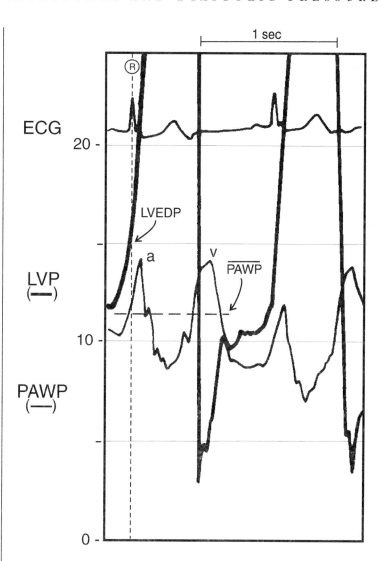

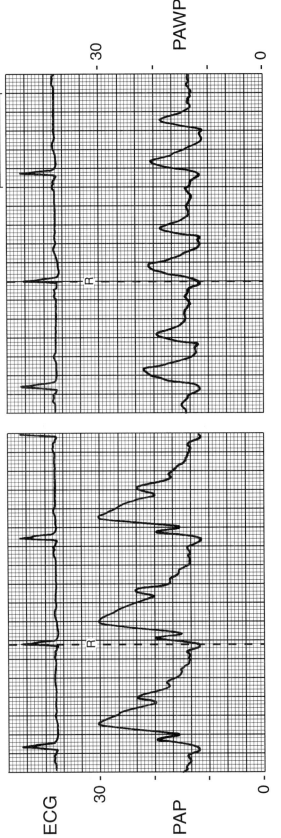

Figure 6.6 Pulmonary artery pressure (PAP) and pulmonary artery wedge pressure (PAWP) recorded from a patient undergoing coronary artery revascularization. The tall PAWP a wave (21 mmHg) inscribed after the ECG R wave suggests impaired left ventricular relaxation, a sign of myocardial ischemia. The tall wedge pressure waves are evident in the unwedged PAP trace.

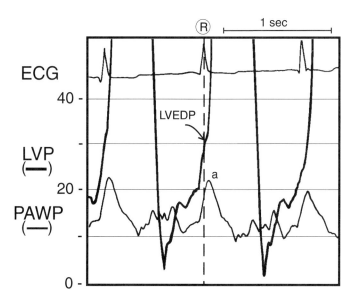

Figure 6.7 Simultaneous left ventricular pressure (LVP) and pulmonary artery wedge pressure (PAWP) recorded from a patient with severe aortic regurgitation. Abnormal diastolic filling of the left ventricle through the incompetent aortic valve proceeds throughout diastole, even after closure of the mitral valve. Consequently, left ventricular end-diastolic pressure (LVEDP, 30 mmHg) exceeds both the mean PAWP (15 mmHg) as well as the PAWP a wave peak pressure (22 mmHg). (Modified from Falicov and Resnekov,[12] with permission.)

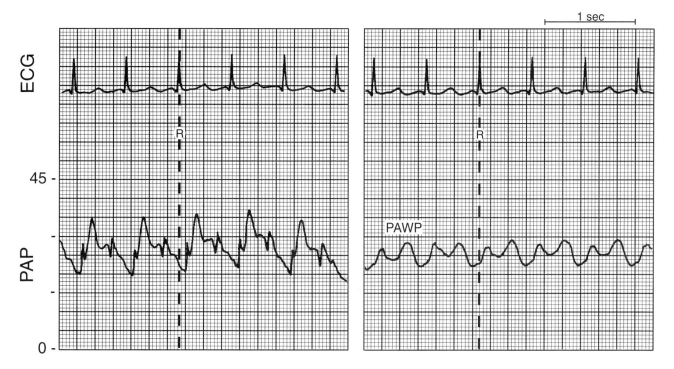

Figure 6.8 Pulmonary artery pressure (PAP) and pulmonary artery wedge pressure (PAWP) recorded from a patient with pulmonic valve regurgitation. Abnormal pulmonary artery diastolic flow back into the right ventricle causes the pulmonary artery diastolic pressure (20 mmHg) to underestimate mean PAWP (26 mmHg) and thereby also underestimate left ventricular filling pressure.

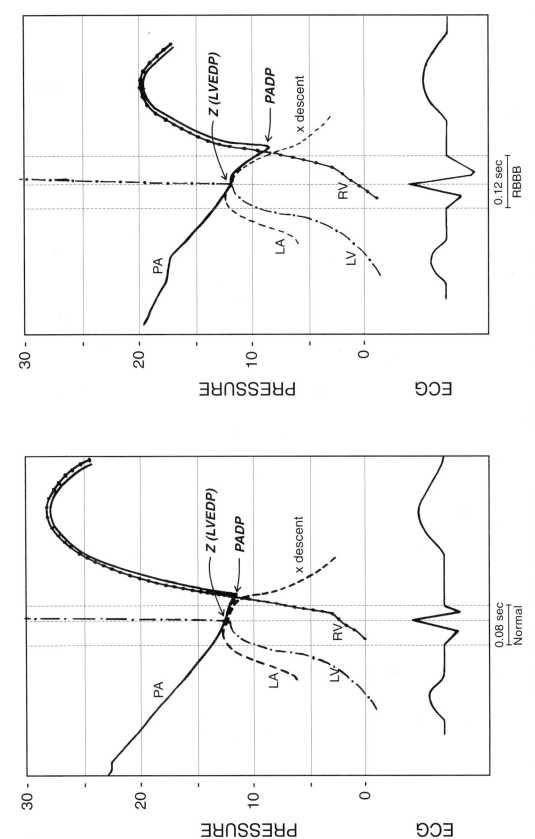

Figure 6.9 Right bundle branch block (RBBB) delays onset of right ventricular (RV) systole. As a result, pulmonary artery (PA) pressure falls with the x descent in left atrial (LA) pressure, and PA diastolic pressure (PADP) underestimates left ventricular (LV) end-diastolic pressure (LVEDP). LVEDP is measured at the Z-point corresponding to the ECG R wave. Under normal conditions (*left panel*), PADP and LVEDP are approximately equal (12 mmHg), while RBBB (*right panel*) causes PADP (8 mmHg) to underestimate LVEDP (12 mmHg). See text for more detail. (Modified from Herbert,[17] with permission.)

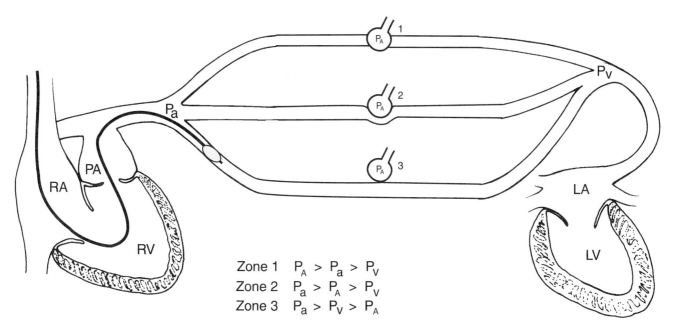

Zone 1 $P_A > P_a > P_v$
Zone 2 $P_a > P_A > P_v$
Zone 3 $P_a > P_v > P_A$

Figure 6.10 A pulmonary artery catheter is shown traversing the right atrium (RA), right ventricle (RV), and pulmonary artery (PA), with its tip wedged in lung zone 3, where pulmonary artery pressure (P_a) exceeds both pulmonary vein pressure (P_v) and alveolar pressure (P_A). Under these conditions, the pulmonary artery wedge pressure will provide an accurate estimate for downstream left atrial (LA) and left ventricular (LV) pressures. When P_A rises above P_v (zone 2) or P_a (zone 1), the continuous, static column of blood between the tip of the wedged catheter and the LA no longer exists, and the wedge pressure will reflect alveolar rather than intravascular pressure. See text for more detail.

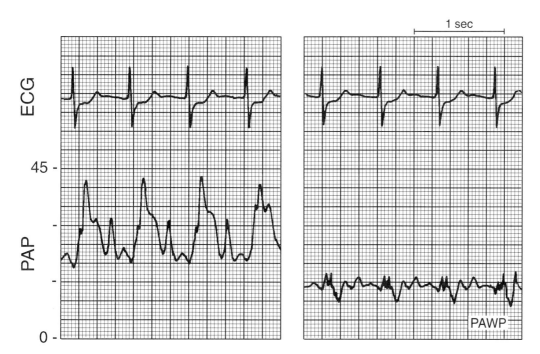

Figure 6.11 Pulmonary artery pressure (PAP) and pulmonary artery wedge pressure (PAWP) recorded from a patient with pulmonary artery hypertension. PAP is 42/20 mmHg, and mean PAWP is 13 mmHg. Abnormal pulmonary vascular resistance causes pulmonary artery diastolic pressure to overestimate wedge pressure. See text for more detail.

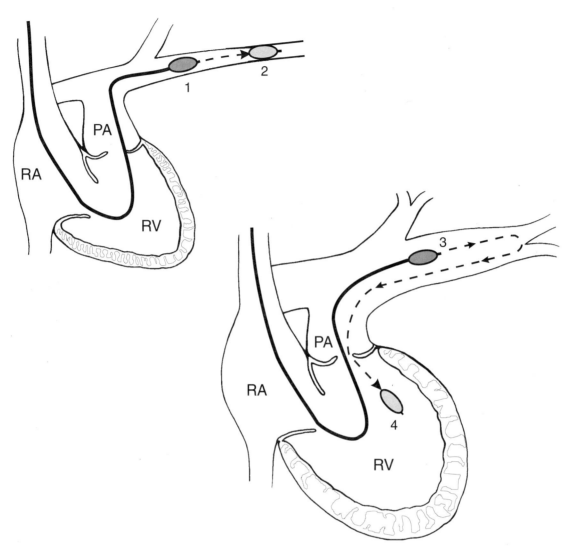

Figure 6.12 A pulmonary artery catheter is shown traversing the right atrium (RA) and right ventricle (RV). (*Top figure*) Under normal conditions balloon inflation causes the catheter to float out into the pulmonary artery (PA) (*position 1*) and achieve the wedge position (*position 2*). (*Bottom figure*) In patients with severe pulmonary hypertension, enlarged, rapidly tapering pulmonary arteries make it difficult for the balloon-tipped catheter to wedge in the PA, and attempts to measure wedge pressure (*position 3*) often result in the catheter coiling and returning to the RV (*position 4*). See text for more detail.

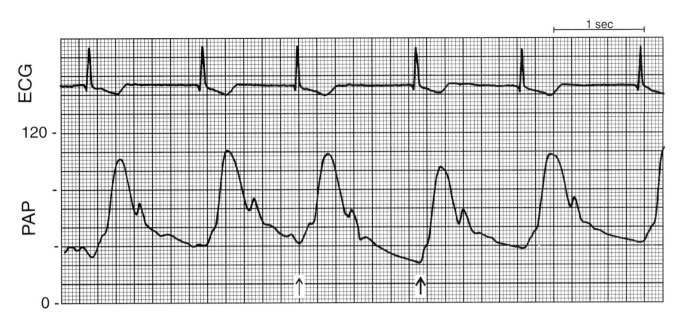

Figure 6.13 Pulmonary artery pressure (PAP) recorded from a patient with severe pulmonary hypertension and atrial fibrillation caused by chronic mitral valve regurgitation. The lower pulmonary artery diastolic pressure recorded after a long ECG R-R interval (*dark arrow*, 27 mmHg) provides a better estimate of left ventricular filling pressure than the pulmonary artery diastolic pressure recorded after a shorter R-R interval (*light arrow*, 41 mmHg). See text for more detail.

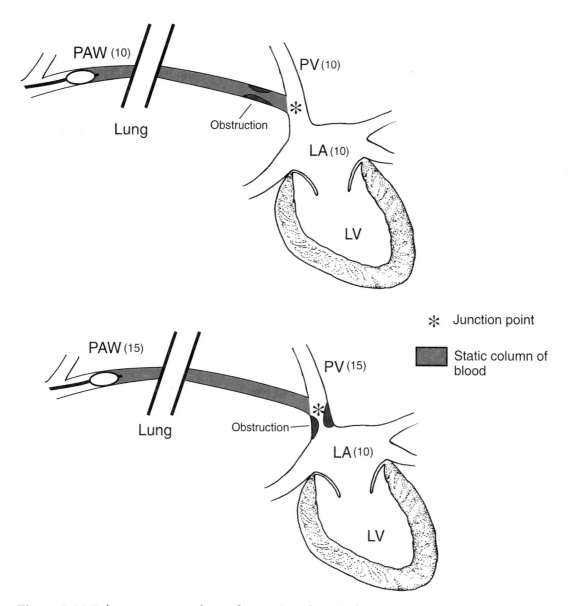

✳ Junction point

▇ Static column of blood

Figure 6.14 Pulmonary veno-occlusive disease. (*Top figure*) Obstruction to flow is confined to the static column of blood in the small pulmonary veins (PV), and pulmonary artery wedge (PAW) pressure (10 mmHg) closely approximates left atrial (LA) pressure (10 mmHg). (*Bottom figure*) Obstruction to flow beyond the static column of blood in the larger PV creates a pressure gradient beyond the junction point and causes the PAW and PV pressures (15 mmHg) to exceed LA pressure (10 mmHg) and overestimate diastolic pressure in the left ventricle (LV). See text for more detail.

Figure 6.15 Simultaneous left ventricular pressure (LVP) and left atrial pressure (LAP) recorded from a patient with severe mitral stenosis. The pressure gradient across the mitral valve during diastole causes all upstream pressures (pulmonary artery diastolic pressure, wedge pressure, and LAP) to overestimate LVP. The rhythm is atrial fibrillation, and consequently, the LAP trace displays a v wave but no a wave. (Modified from Kern and Aguirre,[18] with permission.)

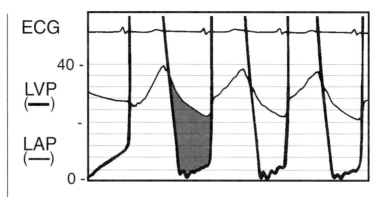

Figure 6.16 Simultaneous left ventricular pressure (LVP) and pulmonary artery wedge pressure (PAWP) recorded from a patient with severe mitral regurgitation. Mean PAWP seriously overestimates left ventricular end-diastolic pressure (LVEDP), owing to the huge regurgitant c-v wave inscribed during systole in the PAWP trace. The best estimate of LVEDP (*dark arrow*) is provided by the end-diastolic PAWP (*light arrow*) prior to inscription of the regurgitant c-v wave. (Modified from Grossman,[15] with permission.)

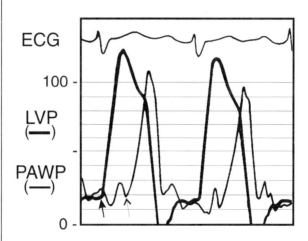

Figure 6.17 Arterial blood pressure (ART), pulmonary artery wedge pressure (PAWP), and central venous pressure (CVP) recorded from a patient with mitral regurgitation. Mean PAWP overestimates left ventricular filling pressure because the regurgitant c-v wave raises mean PAWP during systole. Left ventricular end-diastolic pressure is best estimated by choosing the wedge pressure value prior to onset of the regurgitant wave (*arrow*).

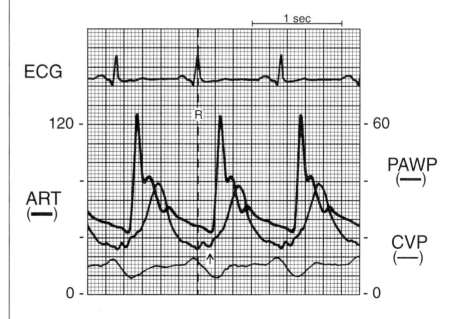

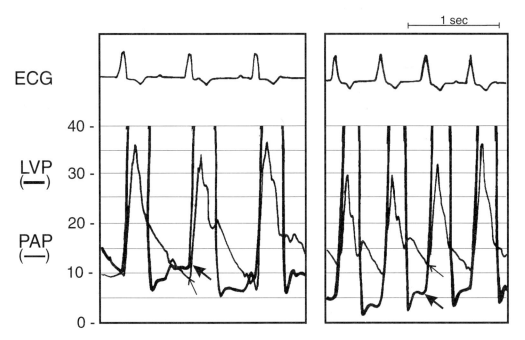

Figure 6.18 Simultaneous left ventricular pressure (LVP) and pulmonary artery pressure (PAP) recorded during artificial pacing at a heart rate of 80 beats/min (*left panel*) and 120 beats/min (*right panel*). At the slower heart rate (*left panel*), pulmonary artery diastolic pressure (PADP, *thin arrow*) closely approximates left ventricular end-diastolic pressure (LVEDP, *thick arrow*). During tachycardia (*right panel*), a pressure gradient develops, and PADP (*thin arrow*, 12 mmHg) significantly overestimates LVEDP (*thick arrow*, 6 mmHg). See text for more detail. (Modified from Enson et al,[11] with permission.)

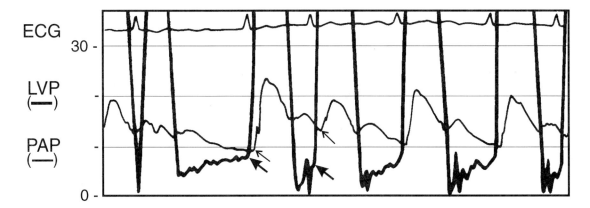

Figure 6.19 Simultaneous left ventricular pressure (LVP) and pulmonary artery pressure (PAP) traces illustrate the effect of cardiac cycle length on the relation between pulmonary artery diastolic pressure (PADP) and left ventricular end-diastolic pressure (LVEDP). During the second cardiac cycle, the long preceding ECG R-R interval provides sufficient time for equilibration between PADP (*thin arrow*, 9 mmHg) and LVEDP (*thick arrow*, 8 mmHg). The next beat follows a shorter cycle length and produces a gradient between PADP (*thin arrow*, 13 mmHg) and LVEDP (*thick arrow*, 6 mmHg). See text for more detail. (Modified from Bouchard et al[4] with permission.)

References

1. Berry AJ, Geer RT, Marshall BE. Alteration of pulmonary blood flow by pulmonary-artery occluded pressure measurement. Anesthesiology 1979;51:164–6

2. Berryhill RE, Benumof JL. PEEP-induced discrepancy between pulmonary arterial wedge pressure and left atrial pressure: the effects of controlled vs. spontaneous ventilation and compliant vs. noncompliant lungs in the dog. Anesthesiology 1979;51:303–8

3. Bethea CF, Peter RH, Behar VS, et al. The hemodynamic simulation of mitral regurgitation in ventricular septal defect after myocardial infarction. Cathet Cardiovasc Diagn 1976;2: 97–104

4. Bouchard RJ, Gault JH, Ross J. Evaluation of pulmonary arterial end-diastolic pressure as an estimate of left ventricular end-diastolic pressure in patients with normal and abnormal left ventricular performance. Circulation 1971;44:1072–9

5. Braunwald E, Fishman AP, Cournand A. Time relationship of dynamic events in the cardiac chambers, pulmonary artery and aorta in man. Circ Res 1956;4:100–7

6. Buchbinder N, Ganz W. Hemodynamic monitoring: invasive techniques. Anesthesiology 1976;45:146–55

7. Case records of the Massachusetts General Hospital (Case 21–1986). N Engl J Med 1986;314:1435–45

8. Case records of the Massachusetts General Hospital (Case 48-1993). N Engl J Med 1993;329:1720–8

9. Case records of the Massachusetts General Hospital (Case 1-1996). N Engl J Med 1996;334:105–11

10. Cozzi PJ, Hall JB, Schmidt GA. Pulmonary artery diastolic-occlusion pressure gradient is increased in acute pulmonary embolism. Crit Care Med 1995;23:1481–4

11. Enson Y, Wood JA, Mantaras NB, Harvey RM. The influence of heart rate on pulmonary arterial-left ventricular pressure relationships at end-diastole. Circulation 1977;56:533–9

12. Falicov RE, Resnekov L. Relationship of the pulmonary artery end-diastolic pressure to the left ventricular end-diastolic and mean filling pressures in patients with and without left ventricular dysfunction. Circulation 1970;42:65–73

13. Fuchs RM, Heuser RR, Yin FCP, Brinker JA. Limitations of pulmonary wedge V waves in diagnosing mitral regurgitation. Am J Cardiol 1982;49:849–54

14. Geer RT. Interpretation of pulmonary-artery wedge pressure when PEEP is used. Anesthesiology 1977;46:383–4

15. Grossman W. Profiles in valvular heart disease, 557–81. In: Grossman W, Baim DS, eds: Cardiac Catheterization, Angiography, and Intervention. Philadelphia: Lea & Febiger, 1991

16. Guyton RA, Chiavarelli M, Padgett CA, et al. The influence of positive end-expiratory pressure on intrapericardial pressure and cardiac function after coronary artery bypass surgery. J Cardiothorac Anesth 1987;1:98–107

17. Herbert WH. Pulmonary artery and left heart end-diastolic pressure relations. Br Heart J 1970;32:774–8

18. Kern MJ, Aguirre FV. Mitral valve gradients: part I, 35–42. In: Kern MJ, ed: Hemodynamic Rounds. Interpretation of Cardiac Pathophysiology From Pressure Waveform Analysis. New York: Wiley-Liss, 1993

19. Mitchell JH, Gilmore JP, Sarnoff SJ. The transport function of the atrium. Factors influencing the relation between mean left atrial pressure and left ventricular end diastolic pressure. Am J Cardiol 1962;9:237–47

20. Nadeau S, Noble WH. Misinterpretation of pressure measurements from the pulmonary artery catheter. Can Anaesth Soc J 1986;33:352–63

21. O'Quin R, Marini JJ. Pulmonary artery occlusion pressure: clinical physiology, measurement, and interpretation. Am Rev Respir Dis 1983;128:319–26

22. Pinsky M, Vincent J-L, De Smet J-M. Estimating left ventricular filling pressure during positive end-expiratory pressure in humans. Am Rev Respir Dis 1991;143:25–31

23. Rahimtoola SH, Loeb HS, Ehsani A, et al. Relationship of pulmonary artery to left ventricular diastolic pressures in acute myocardial infarction. Circulation 1972;46:283–90

24. Roizen MF, Berger DL, Gabel RA, et al. Practice guidelines for pulmonary artery catheterization. A report by the American Society of Anesthesiologists task force on pulmonary artery catheterization. Anesthesiology 1993;78:380–94

25. Roy R, Powers SR, Feustel PJ, Dutton RE. Pulmonary wedge catheterization during positive end-expiratory pressure ventilation in the dog. Anesthesiology 1977;46:385–90

26. Stott DK, Marpole DGF, Bristow JD, et al. The role of left atrial transport in aortic and mitral stenosis. Circulation 1970; 41:1031–41

27. Teboul JL, Zapol WM, Brun-Buisson C, et al. A comparison of pulmonary artery occlusion pressure and left ventricular end-diastolic pressure during mechanical ventilation with PEEP in patients with severe ARDS. Anesthesiology 1989;70:261–6

28. Teplick RS. Measuring central vascular pressures a surprisingly complex problem. Anesthesiology 1987;67:289–91

29. Tuman KJ, Carroll GC, Ivankovich AD. Pitfalls in interpretation of pulmonary artery catheter data. J Cardiothorac Anesth 1989;3:625–41

30. West JB, Dollery CT, Naimark A. Distribution of blood flow in isolated lung: relation to vascular and alveolar pressures. J Appl Physiol 1964;19:713–24

31. Wiedemann HP. Wedge pressure in pulmonary veno-occlusive disease. N Engl J Med 1986;315:1233

32. Wittnich C, Trudel J, Zidulka A, Chiu RC. Misleading "pulmonary wedge pressure" after pneumonectomy: its importance in postoperative fluid therapy. Ann Thorac Surg 1986;42:192–6

33. Zidulka A, Hakim TS. Wedge pressure in large vs. small pulmonary arteries to detect pulmonary venoconstriction. J Appl Physiol 1985;59:1329–32

CHAPTER SEVEN Arterial Blood Pressure

DIRECT VS. INDIRECT MEASUREMENT

WHY MEASURE BLOOD PRESSURE DIRECTLY?

Unlike pulmonary artery pressure, systemic arterial blood pressure (ABP) can be monitored by both direct invasive techniques or indirect noninvasive ones. Although direct blood pressure measurement is more costly, has the potential for more complications, and requires more technical expertise to initiate and maintain, this technique is selected in many critically ill patients. Furthermore, direct ABP monitoring is chosen frequently for patients undergoing anesthesia and operation for the following reasons:

ACCURACY   When the operative procedure demands that the blood pressure be known with greatest accuracy, direct ABP measurement is considered to be the reference standard. A typical example might be its use for a patient undergoing clipping of a cerebral aneurysm with controlled hypotension. In order for direct ABP monitoring to achieve this standard for accuracy, many technical requirements must be met. These are discussed in detail in Chapter 9.

CONTINUOUS REAL-TIME MONITORING   Noninvasive techniques, both manual and automated, provide only intermittent measurement of blood pressure. Although a number of devices have been developed that provide both continuous and noninvasive measurement of blood pressure, their widespread clinical application has been limited, owing to a variety of technical problems in their application.[9,16,38] Continuous invasive monitoring of blood pressure is chosen when acute, moment to moment pressure changes are anticipated, and their immediate detection is considered to be a high priority. These changes in blood pressure might be expected when the patient has circulatory instability caused by the underlying medical condition, or when the planned operative procedure will cause dramatic cardiovascular changes (e.g., thoracic aortic cross-clamping).

It should be noted that even direct ABP monitoring is not truely continuous, since valid blood pressure waveforms from invasive arterial cannulae are not always present on the monitor display. Wesseling and Smith[35] have shown that ABP waveforms are not usable up to 15 percent of the time during anesthesia and operation, owing to artifacts, blood sampling, and line flushing. However, intermittent noninvasive techniques clearly provide less data, particularly if manual methods are employed instead of automated techniques.[11,28]

ARTERIAL BLOOD SAMPLING   When repeated sampling of arterial blood is required, an arterial catheter provides reliable vascular access and obviates the need for multiple arterial punctures. New clinical devices allow continuous monitoring of arterial blood gas values using fiberoptic sensors placed directly into the artery through the vascular catheter.[21,34]

UNMEASURABLE BLOOD PRESSURE   Under some clinical circumstances, the blood pressure cannot be detected or measured by indirect methods, and direct arterial catheterization is the only reliable method available. During cardiopulmonary bypass (Fig. 7.1), nonpulsatile perfusion precludes indirect measurement of blood pressure because the pulse pressure is not sufficient to allow measurement by noninvasive means. On occasion, patients with cardiogenic shock or severe systemic vasoconstriction may have no auscultatory blood pressure or palpable peripheral pulses, yet direct arterial cannulation may reveal a normal or even elevated blood pressure.[7] Furthermore, severely burned or morbidly obese patients may not have a suitable extremity on which to place a blood pressure cuff.

DIAGNOSTIC CLUES   Although not emphasized by most clinicians as an important reason to select direct ABP monitoring, many diagnostic clues about the patient's condition may be derived from a *critical analysis of the arterial pressure waveform*. More than 40 years ago, Eather et al[10] emphasized these diagnostic insights in a paper in which they introduced and promoted the use of direct monitoring of "arterial pressure and pressure pulse contours" in anesthetized patients. Some of these diagnostic insights are readily apparent and commonly sought, such as the identification of the ABP dicrotic notch to guide proper timing of inflation of an intraaortic balloon pump. However, careful analysis of the ABP waveform can provide many additional subtle pathophysiologic insights. These are explored in much greater detail in later chapters (see Chs. 17, 19, and 20).

DIRECT vs. INDIRECT ARTERIAL BLOOD PRESSURE

Direct measurement of ABP requires cannulation of a major artery. Radial artery pressure monitoring is most common, because it is technically easy to perform and rarely associated with complications. Slogoff et al.[30] studied 1,700 cardiovascular surgical patients who underwent radial artery cannulation without any ischemic complications, despite evidence of arterial occlusion after decannulation in more than 25 percent of patients. Major complications are extremely rare in the absence of other contributing factors,[22] such as previous arterial injury, protracted shock, high-dose vasopressor administration, prolonged cannulation, or infection.

In contrast to direct pressure measurement, indirect measurement of blood pressure can be performed by a number of different techniques, in addition to the standard auscultatory method. Virtually all these techniques are noninvasive except for the return-to-flow method, in which both an occluding cuff and indwelling arterial catheter are employed. Consequently, noninvasive indirect measurement of blood pressure is widely applied, even when direct ABP measurement is in place. This makes good clinical sense, since the noninvasive technique serves to corroborate the direct method and occasionally may elucidate major technical problems with the latter.[23] When noninvasive indirect blood pressure measurement is used in combination with direct ABP monitoring, frequent noninvasive pressure measurement should not be necessary. One must remember that repeated cuff inflation at short intervals, especially common with automated devices, has been associated with clinical complications such as venostasis, limb edema, and neuropathy.[2,14]

When both direct and indirect methods of blood pressure measurement are employed simultaneously, clinical caregivers are confronted with a common problem. When the blood pressure measurements produce different numbers, which should be relied upon as *the true blood pressure*? It is not surprising, really, that direct and indirect measurements of blood pressure yield different values in routine clinical practice. Direct techniques measure pressure, while indirect techniques measure flow beneath or beyond an occluding cuff. Since the energy package differs in these two forms of measurement, one should not expect a priori that the different methods will provide identical results.[4,5]

Under controlled clinical conditions, some investigators have shown that noninvasive blood pressure measurements closely approximate directly measured ABP values.[3,27,36] However, other studies underscore the fact that marked disagreement occurs when direct and indirect pressure measurements are compared,[33] particularly when radial artery pressure is used as the direct measurement standard[4,24] or when the techniques are compared under changing clinical conditions.[18] Gravlee and Brockschmidt[18] compared direct brachial artery pressure with a variety of indirect methods, including manual auscultation, automated oscillometry, aneroid manometer visual "flicker" (onset of needle oscillations), and return-to-flow. These authors found that the relation between these indirect pressure values and directly measured pressures varied between patients, within patients over time, and with changing hemodynamic conditions.[18] In view of the uncertain relation between direct and indirect measurements of ABP, one needs some general principles to guide clinical practice. These will become clearer as we examine these pressure relations in more detail and consider some of the potential problems that complicate monitoring practice.

SYSTOLIC, DIASTOLIC, OR MEAN ARTERIAL PRESSURE: WHICH TO MEASURE? REAL OR ARTIFACT?

Epidemiologic studies examining long-term cardiac risk have focused on measurement of diastolic pressure and more recently pulse pressure as a measure of vascular overload or stress.[13] However, short-term clinical monitoring of critically patients and those undergoing operations has focused on either the systolic or the mean arterial pressure (MAP). Ream[29] has argued that MAP is the most useful single measurement on theoretical grounds and is less subject to some of the technical problems inherent in invasive ABP measurement. (See Ch. 9 for more detail.) Other investigators have pointed out that measurement of diastolic or pulse pressure adds little useful information about acute changes in the circulation during anesthesia to that available from measurement of systolic pressure alone.[8,26] Consequently, in both the operating room and intensive care unit, monitoring of the MAP or systolic arterial pressure has been the central focus for most clinicians.

In view of the fact that different blood pressure values can be measured using either invasive or noninvasive techniques, how can one use all of this arterial pressure information to guide clinical decisions most effectively? In order to answer this question, the clinician must understand the usual relationship between invasive and noninvasive measurements of systolic, mean, and diastolic arterial pressure. In addition, an appreciation for some of the technical limitations of all measurement techniques will help avoid misinterpreting the monitored values.

As a general rule, indirect measurements of *systolic arterial pressure* equal or slightly underestimate direct systolic pressure values in normotensive patients. In hypertensive patients, indirect noninvasive methods generally underestimate direct systolic pressure values, while under conditions of hypotension, indirect methods generally overestimate direct systolic pressure (Fig. 7.2).[3,4,18]

Interpretation of *mean arterial pressure* values is a bit more complicated. Oscillometric techniques for indirect measurement of blood pressure actually measure three separate variables to determine systolic, diastolic, and mean pressures,[27] while auscultatory or Doppler ultrasound methods determine systolic and diastolic pressures, then calculate the mean. Consequently, most studies comparing direct and indirect measurement of MAP have used oscillometric measurement for the noninvasive method to be compared with direct invasive blood pressure.[3,4,18,36] Most investigations demonstrate that indirect measurements of MAP equal or slightly overestimate direct MAP values.

Diastolic arterial pressure is an important determinant of coronary blood flow, yet its perioperative monitoring has received less attention than the measurement of systolic or mean pressure. In general, when diastolic blood pressure is measured by noninvasive indirect techniques, the values obtained slightly overestimate directly measured values.

Despite the fact that perfect agreement between direct and indirect blood pressure measurements is rarely seen in practice, the preceding generalizations provide some clinical guidelines. However, marked differences greater than 40 mmHg between direct and indirect measurements of blood pressure do not occur normally and demand an explanation. The inaccuracy may lie in either the direct or indirect values or both. When major disagreements occur, it is difficult to know which method is closer to the truth and where to search for problems and explanations. Always check the patient first, since other signs and symptoms of the adequacy of circulation will dictate which blood pressure values are to be believed initially, while the cause of the discrepancy between invasive and noninvasive pressure measurements is sought.

The sources of disagreement between direct and indirect measurements of blood pressure may be categorized as those related to the patient's condition and those resulting from technical problems related to either the direct or indirect measurement technique. A variety of patient factors may produce true pressure differences when the blood pressure is measured at different sites in the body (Table 7.1). These real differences may be interpreted erroneously as problems inherent in the measurement techniques. For example, patients undergoing vascular surgery are known to have marked differences in blood pressure between right and left arms as a result of their underlying peripheral vascular disease.[12] In such patients, direct blood pressure measurement in one arm and indirect measurement from the contralateral arm might yield different values because of these patient factors rather than technical methodologic factors. Regional ABP gradients may result from atherosclerosis, arterial dissection or embolism, placement of surgical retractors (Fig. 7.3),[6,20] and unusual patient positions resulting in vascular compression. Furthermore, more widespread arterial pressure gradients are seen in patients in shock with peripheral vasoconstriction[7] and in those rapidly rewarmed[32] at the termination of cardiopulmonary bypass.[17,25,31] Finally, one must recognize that even under normal circumstances, the ABP waveform changes its morphology as it is transmitted through the vascular tree, resulting in a wider pulse pressure recorded from a peripheral artery than from a more central location.[1] In Chapter 8, these characteristic morphologic features of the arterial waveform and their physiologic basis are examined in greater detail.

Technical factors influence both the direct and indirect measurement of blood pressure. The technical factors governing direct measurement of pressure are discussed in Chapter 9. While it seems self-evident that direct invasive blood pressure measurement requires careful attention to technical detail, the same attention to detail is required for the accurate measurement of blood pressure using any of the indirect methods. These technical details are reviewed at length by Geddes[15] and Ramsey,[27] but a few must be emphasized here (Table 7.2). Blood pressure cuff width should be 20 percent greater than arm diameter, and the cuff should be applied snugly after any residual air has been squeezed out. While too large a cuff generally will work well, cuffs that are too small yield erroneously high values for blood pressure.[19,27] Overly rapid cuff deflation rates (greater than 3 mmHg/sec) may cause underestimation of blood pressure, especially at slow heart rates.[37] Oscillometric techniques for blood pressure measurement are influenced by patient movement or shivering and by extrinsic cuff compression, as when a surgeon leans against the arm. Finally, all indirect techniques have limitations in providing accurate pressure values under certain pathophysiologic conditions, including rapid pressure changes, dysrhythmias, and shock.

Table 7.1 Patient Factors: Causes of Disagreement Between Direct and Indirect Blood Pressure Measurement

Regional arterial pressure gradients
 Atherosclerosis
 Peripheral vascular disease
 Aortic dissection
 Arterial embolism
 Surgical retractors
 Patient position
Generalized arterial pressure gradients
 Severe vasoconstriction and shock
 Peripheral vasodilation with rewarming after
  cardiopulmonary bypass
 Normal peripheral pulse pressure widening

Table 7.2 Technical Factors in Indirect Blood Pressure Measurement: Causes of Disagreement Between Direct and Indirect Blood Pressure Measurement

Cuff problems
 Size too small leads to overestimation
 Fit in a conical-shaped arm
 Extrinsic cuff compression
 Limb position relative to heart
Rapid deflation leads to underestimation
Physiologic problems and method limitations
 Rapid pressure changes
 Dysrhythmias
 Severe vasoconstriction and shock
 Shivering and patient movement
 Beat-to-beat variation (e.g., pulsus alternans)

Illustrations for
Arterial Blood Pressure

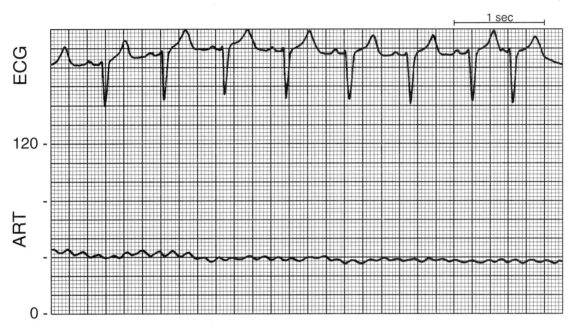

Figure 7.1 Arterial blood pressure (ART) during cardiopulmonary bypass. Direct invasive blood pressure measurement is required because of the nonpulsatile perfusion technique. Mean arterial pressure is approximately 38 mmHg. The small oscillations in the ART trace result from the mechanical action of the extracorporeal pump. (See Ch. 19 for more detail.)

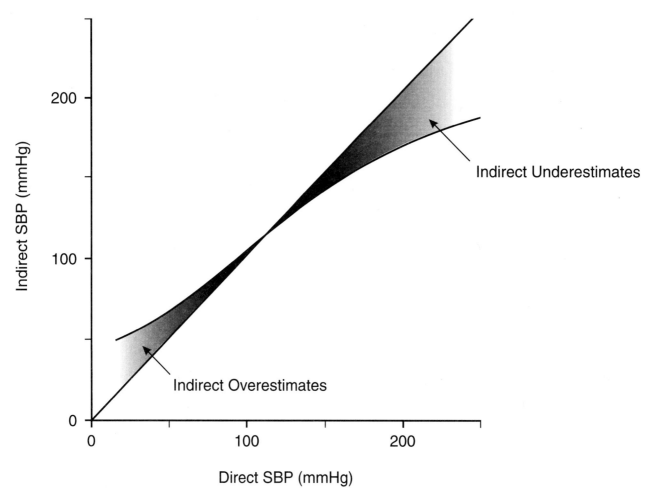

Figure 7.2 Relationship between direct invasive and indirect noninvasive measurement of systolic blood pressure (SBP). In the normotensive range, SBP 120 mmHg, the two methods provide a similar measurement. In the hypertensive range, indirect methods underestimate direct measurements, while in the hypotensive range, indirect methods overestimate direct measurements.

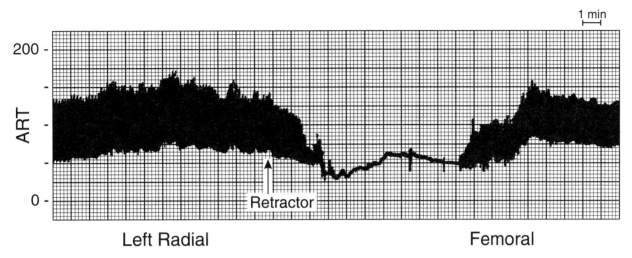

Figure 7.3 Left radial arterial blood pressure (ART) trace is severely damped after placement of a surgical chest retractor used to aid dissection of the internal mammary artery from the chest wall. Femoral ART monitoring is established several minutes later on the right side of the tracing, suggesting that the hypotension resulted from a regional pressure gradient produced by the retractor. (Modified from Camann et al[6] with permission.)

References

1. Abrams JH, Cerra F, Holcroft JW. Cardiopulmonary monitoring, 1–27. In: Wilmore DW, Brennan MF, Harken AH, et al, eds: Care of the Surgical Patient. Volume 1. Critical Care. New York: Scientific American Medicine, 1989

2. Bickler PE, Schapera A, Bainton CR. Acute radial nerve injury from use of an automatic blood pressure monitor. Anesthesiology 1990;73:186–8

3. Borow KM, Newburger JW. Noninvasive estimation of central aortic pressure using the oscillometric method for analyzing systemic artery pulsatile blood flow: comparative study of indirect systolic, diastolic, and mean brachial artery pressure with simultaneous direct ascending aortic pressure measurements. Am Heart J 1982;103:879–86

4. Bruner JMR, Krenis LJ, Kunsman JM, Sherman AP. Comparison of direct and indirect methods of measuring arterial blood pressure. Med Instrument 1981;15:11–21, 97–101, 182–8

5. Bruner JMR. On the calibration of artifacts. J Clin Monit 1994; 10:143–6

6. Camann WR, Wojtowicz SR, Mark JB. Reoperation for coronary artery bypass grafting: anesthetic challenge. J Cardiothorac Anesth 1987;1:458–67

7. Cohn JN. Blood pressure measurement in shock. Mechanism of inaccuracy in auscultatory and palpatory methods. JAMA 1967;199:972–6

8. Cullen DJ. Interpretation of blood-pressure measurements in anesthesia. Anesthesiology 1974;40:6–12

9. de Jong JR, Tepaske R, Scheffer G-J, et al. Noninvasive continuous blood pressure measurement: a clinical evaluation of the Cortronic APM 770. J Clin Monit 1993;9:18–24

10. Eather KF, Peterson LH, Dripps RD. Studies of the circulation of anesthetized patients by a new method for recording arterial pressure and pressure pulse contours. Anesthesiology 1949;10:125–32

11. Elmquist L. Noninvasive automatic blood pressure machines in the PACU—is there a price? J Clin Monit 1994;10:134–6

12. Frank SM, Norris EJ, Christopherson R, Beattie C. Right- and left-arm blood pressure discrepancies in vascular surgery patients. Anesthesiology 1991;75:457–63.

13. Franklin SS, Weber MA. Measuring hypertensive cardiovascular risk: the vascular overload concept. Am Heart J 1994;128:793–803

14. Gardner RM, Hollingsworth KW. Optimizing the electrocardiogram and pressure monitoring. Crit Care Med 1986;14:651–8

15. Geddes LA. Handbook of Blood Pressure Measurement. Clifton, NJ: Humana Press, 1991

16. Gibbs NM, Larach DR, Derr JA. The accuracy of Finapress™ noninvasive mean arterial pressure measurements in anesthetized patients. Anesthesiology 1991;74:647–52

17. Gravlee GP, Wong AB, Adkins TG, et al. A comparison of radial, brachial, and aortic pressures after cardiopulmonary bypass. J Cardiothorac Anesth 1989;3:20–6

18. Gravlee GP, Brockschmidt JK. Accuracy of four indirect methods of blood pressure measurement, with hemodynamic correlations. J Clin Monit 1990;6:284–98

19. Iyriboz Y, Hearon CM, Edwards K. Agreement between large and small cuffs in sphygmomanometry: a quantitative assessment. J Clin Monit 1994;10:127–33

20. Kinzer JB, Lichtentrhal PR, Wade LD. Loss of radial artery pressure trace during internal mammary artery dissection for coronary artery bypass graft surgery. Anesth Analg 1985;64:1134–6

21. Lumsden T, Marshall WR, Divers GA, Riccitelli SD. The PB3300 intraarterial blood gas monitoring system. J Clin Monit 1994;10:59–66

22. Mangano DT, Hickey RF. Ischemic injury following uncomplicated radial artery catheterization. Anesth Analg 1979;58:55–7

23. Meyer RM, Kimovec MA, Hefner GG. Cable-testing device fails to indicate that hypertension is artifactual. J Clin Monit 1993; 9:54–9

24. Nystrom E, Reid KH, Bennett R, et al. A comparison of two automated indirect arterial blood pressure meters with recordings from a radial arterial catheter in anesthetized surgical patients. Anesthesiology 1985;62:526–30

25. Pauca AL, Hudspeth AS, Wallenhaupt SL, et al. Radial artery-to-aorta pressure difference after discontinuation of cardiopulmonary bypass. Anesthesiology 1989;70:935–41

26. Prys-Roberts C. Arterial manometry under pressure? Anesthesiology 1974;40:1–3

27. Ramsey M. Blood pressure monitoring: automated oscillometric devices. J Clin Monit 1991;7:56–67

28. Ramsey M. Automatic oscillometric NIBP versus manual auscultatory blood pressure in the PACU. J Clin Monit 1994;10:136–9

29. Ream AK. Systolic, diastolic, mean or pulse: which pressure is the best measurement of arterial pressure?, 53–74 In: Gravenstein JS, Newbower RS, Ream AK, et al, eds: Essential Noninvasive Monitoring in Anesthesia. New York: Grune & Stratton, 1980

30. Slogoff S, Keats AS, Arlund C. On the safety of radial artery cannulation. Anesthesiology 1983;59:42–7

31. Stern DH, Gerson JI, Allen FB, Parker FB. Can we trust the direct radial artery pressure immediately following cardiopulmonary bypass? Anesthesiology 1985;62:557–61

32. Urzua J, Sessler DI, Meneses G, et al. Thermoregulatory vasoconstriction increases the difference between femoral and radial arterial pressures. J Clin Monit 1994;10:229–36

33. Van Bergen FH, Weatherhead DS, Treloar AE, et al. Comparison of indirect and direct methods of measuring arterial blood pressure. Circulation 1954;10:481–90

34. Wahr JA, Tremper KK. Continuous intravascular blood gas monitoring. J Cardiothorac Vasc Anesth 1994;8:342–53

35. Wesseling KH, Smith NT. Availability of intraarterial pressure waveforms from catheter-manometer systems during surgery. J Clin Monit 1985;1:11–6

36. Yelderman M, Ream AK. Indirect measurement of mean blood pressure in the anesthetized patient. Anesthesiology 1979;50:253–6

37. Yong PG, Geddes LA. The effect of cuff pressure deflation rate on accuracy in indirect measurement of blood pressure with the auscultatory method. J Clin Monit 1987;3:155–9

38. Young CC, Mark JB, White W, et al. Clinical evaluation of continuous noninvasive blood pressure monitoring: accuracy and tracking capabilities. J Clin Monit 1995;11:245–52

CHAPTER EIGHT *Direct Arterial Blood Pressure Monitoring*

NORMAL WAVEFORMS

WAVEFORM COMPONENTS

The systemic arterial blood pressure (ABP) waveform results from ejection of blood from the left ventricle into the aorta during systole, followed by peripheral arterial runoff of this stroke volume during diastole. Like the venous pressure waveform, the arterial waveform can be divided into systolic and diastolic components (Figs. 8.1 and 8.2). The systolic components follow the ECG R wave, consist of a steep pressure upstroke, peak, and decline, and correspond to the period of left ventricular systolic ejection. The downslope of the ABP waveform is interrupted by the dicrotic notch, which reflects aortic valve closure at end-systole. The remaining decay of ABP occurs during diastole following the ECG T wave, and the ABP reaches its nadir at end-diastole.

Values for systolic and diastolic blood pressure reported by the bedside monitor numeric display are the systolic peak and end-diastolic trough pressures. Mean arterial pressure (MAP) is equal to the area beneath the arterial pressure curve divided by the beat period, and this value is measured and reported by the monitor as well (Fig. 8.2). MAP can be described mathematically as $\int_0^T P(t)\, dt/T$, where P is pressure and T is time. Although MAP is estimated often as diastolic pressure plus one-third times the pulse pressure, this estimation can be misleading. In the example in Figure 8.3, identical values for systolic and diastolic pressure are associated with markedly different values for MAP. At equivalent heart rates, narrow or thin ABP waveforms "spend more time" at lower pressures, resulting in a low MAP, while wide or full ABP waveforms spend more time at higher pressures, resulting in a higher MAP.

Inspection of the ABP waveform on a monitor screen display with a calibrated scale allows rapid estimation of systolic and diastolic pressures, without relying on the numeric display. For example, one can readily determine that the blood pressure is approximately 110/50 mmHg in Figure 8.2, by observing the waveform on the calibrated recording. The clinician can glean this information in an instant, much like glancing at the position of the needle of a car speedometer to determine speed. It is important to maintain consistent scales for the arterial pressure display, so that estimation of arterial pressure can be accomplished at a glance.

Although the systolic and diastolic components of the ABP waveform are readily discerned, their temporal relation to the ECG waveform requires more detailed consideration. Note that the systolic upstroke of the radial artery pressure trace does not appear for 120 to 180 msec after inscription of the ECG R wave (Figs. 8.1 and 8.2). This delay reflects the sum of delays produced by spread of electrical depolarization through the ventricular myocardium, isovolumic left ventricular contraction, aortic valve opening, left ventricular ejection, transmission of the aortic pressure wave to the radial artery, and finally, transmission of the pressure signal from the arterial catheter to the pressure transducer. Consequently, when the radial artery pressure waveform is used to time mechanical cardiac events, these delays must be kept firmly in mind.

EVOLUTION OF THE ARTERIAL WAVEFORM

Pressure waves recorded simultaneously from different arterial sites have different morphologies (Fig. 8.4).[1,6] As the ABP wave travels from the central aorta to the periphery, several characteristic changes occur. The arterial upstroke becomes steeper, the systolic peak becomes higher, the dicrotic notch appears later, the diastolic wave becomes more prominent, and the end-diastolic pressure becomes lower. *Compared with central aortic pressure, peripheral arterial waveforms have higher systolic pressure, lower diastolic pressure, and thus wider pulse pressure.* Furthermore, there is a delay in the arrival of the pressure pulse at peripheral sites, so that the systolic pressure upstroke begins approximately 60 msec later in the radial artery than in the aorta. Again, this temporal delay must be borne in mind when timing cardiac mechanical events from a peripheral arterial waveform. Finally, despite the morphologic and temporal differences between peripheral and central arterial waveforms, the MAP in the aorta is just slightly greater than that in the radial artery.[1,6]

Pressure wave reflection is the predominant factor that influences the shape of the ABP waveform as it travels peripherally.[4-6] As blood flows from the aorta to the radial artery, mean pressure only decreases slightly, as there is little resistance to flow. MAP then falls markedly in the arterioles, owing to the dramatic increase in vascular resistance at this site. This high resistance to flow diminishes the pressure pulsations in small downstream vessels but acts to augment upstream arterial pressure pulses owing to pressure wave reflection.[3,6] Murgo et al[4,5] and O'Rourke and Yaginuma[6] provide detailed explanations of the ABP wave, along with models of the circulation that provide more complete insight into these phenomena. These studies underscore the importance of wave reflection in determining the shape of the arterial pulse recorded from all sites in the body, in health and disease. For example, elderly patients have reduced arterial distensibility, which results in early return of reflected pressure waves, leading to an increased pulse pressure, late systolic pressure peak, and disappearance of the diastolic pressure wave (Fig. 8.5).[3,6] Furthermore, abnormal ABP waveforms seen in conditions such as shock, atrial fibrillation, hypertrophic cardiomyopathy, and aortic valve disease can be explained on the basis of accelerated, delayed, exaggerated, or reduced pressure wave reflection.[6]

From these considerations, it becomes evident that the morphology of the arterial waveform and the precise values for systolic and diastolic blood pressure vary throughout the body under normal conditions in otherwise healthy individuals. *One should expect to record a wider pulse pressure and a higher systolic blood pressure in the radial artery than in the central aorta.*

THE DICROTIC NOTCH

Before leaving this discussion of the normal ABP waveform, the origin and meaning of the dicrotic notch deserves further explanation. From a clinical point of view, identification of the dicrotic notch is important, especially to guide proper timing of aortic counterpulsation using an intraaortic balloon pump. The dicrotic notch recorded directly from the central aorta is termed the *incisura* (from the Latin, *a cutting into*). The incisura is sharply defined and undoubtedly is related to aortic valve closure.[2] In contrast, the peripheral arterial waveform generally displays a later, smoother dicrotic notch, which is more dependent on arterial wall properties than on aortic valve closure (Figs. 8.1, 8.2, and 8.4).[7] Schwid et al[7] provide a more detailed explanation of this phenomenon, using an electrical model of the circulation and computer-generated radial and aortic pressure waveforms.

In summary, the dicrotic notch recorded from a radial artery pressure trace only approximates timing of aortic valve closure. The so-called dicrotic notch seen in peripheral arterial pressure traces results more from reflected pressure waves than from aortic valve closure per se.[7] More accurate determination of the timing of end-systole requires central aortic pressure recording or alternative techniques of measuring aortic blood flow, such as Doppler echocardiography.

Illustrations for Direct Arterial Blood Pressure Monitoring

Figure 8.1 Normal arterial blood pressure (ART) waveform components include (1) systolic upstroke, (2) systolic peak pressure, (3) systolic decline, (4) dicrotic notch, (5) diastolic runoff, and (6) end-diastolic pressure. Arterial blood pressure is 157/63 mmHg in this example. See text for more detail.

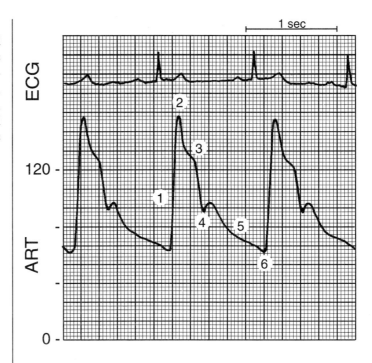

Figure 8.2 Normal arterial blood pressure (ART) waveform, with systolic blood pressure (BP) 111 mmHg and diastolic BP 53 mmHg. Mean arterial pressure is represented by the shaded area beneath the arterial pressure curve divided by the beat period, and it incorporates the systolic (S) and diastolic (D) portions of the cardiac cycle. Note that the systolic pressure upstroke recorded at the radial artery does not begin until 160 msec after inscription of the ECG R wave, owing to a series of normal physiologic events. See text for more detail.

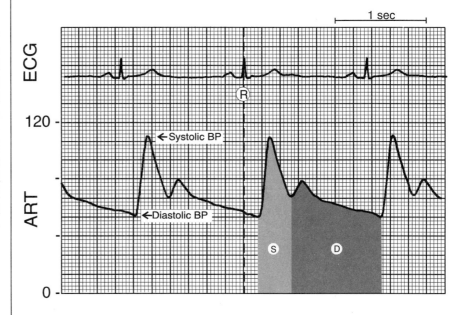

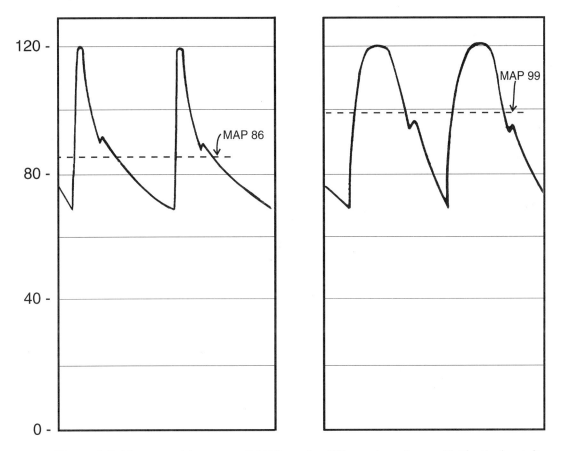

Figure 8.3 Mean arterial pressure (MAP) may be different in patients with identical systolic and diastolic blood pressures. Both panels illustrate the same systolic and diastolic pressure (120/70 mmHg) and the same heart rate, but MAP is lower when the arterial pressure waveform is narrow (*left panel*, MAP 86 mmHg) compared to when the waveform is wide (*right panel*, MAP 99 mmHg). See text for more detail.

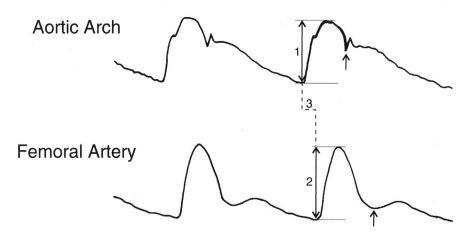

Figure 8.4 Arterial blood pressure waves recorded simultaneously from aortic arch and femoral artery will have different morphologies. The more peripheral femoral artery waveform will have a wider pulse pressure (compare 1 and 2), a delayed upstroke (3), a delayed, slurred dicrotic notch (compare *arrows*), and a more prominent diastolic wave following the dicrotic notch. These changes are exaggerated further in pressure recordings from more distal sites including the radial and dorsalis pedis arteries. See text for more detail. (Modified from O'Rourke and Yaginuma,[6] with permission.)

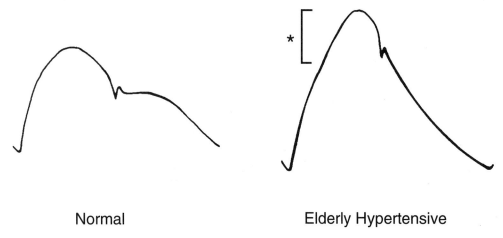

Figure 8.5 Aortic arterial blood pressure waves recorded from a normal subject (*left*) and an elderly hypertensive patient with reduced arterial distensibility (*right*). Early pressure wave reflection results in an increased late systolic pressure peak (*), widened pulse pressure, and disappearance of the diastolic pressure wave. See text for more detail. (Modified from O'Rourke and Yaginuma,[6] with permission.)

References

1. Abrams JH, Cerra F, Holcroft JW. Cardiopulmonary monitoring. In: Wilmore DW, Brennan MF, Harken AH, et al. eds. Care of the Surgical Patient (vol. 1). Critical Care. New York: Scientific American Medicine, 1989: 1–27

2. Braunwald E, Fishman AP, Cournand A. Time relationship of dynamic events in the cardiac chambers, pulmonary artery and aorta in man. Circ Res 1956;4:100–7

3. Franklin SS, Weber MA. Measuring hypertensive cardiovascular risk: the vascular overload concept. Am Heart J 1994;128:793–803

4. Murgo JP, Westerhof N, Giolma JP, Altobelli SA. Aortic input impedance in normal man: relationship to pressure wave forms. Circulation 1980;62:105–16

5. Murgo JP, Westerhof N, Giolma JP, Altobelli SA. Manipulation of ascending aortic pressure and flow wave reflections with the valsalva maneuver: relationship to input impedance. Circulation 1981;63:122–32

6. O'Rourke MF, Yaginuma T. Wave reflections and the arterial pulse. Arch Intern Med 1984;144:366–71

7. Schwid HA, Taylor LA, Smith NT. Computer model analysis of the radial artery pressure waveform. J Clin Monit 1987;3:220–8

CHAPTER NINE *Technical Requirements for Direct Blood Pressure Measurement*

Direct measurement of arterial blood pressure (ABP) requires that the original pressure signal from the cannulated artery be reproduced accurately by the waveform displayed on the bedside monitor. Not surprisingly, the system plumbing, including catheter, tubing, stopcocks, flush devices, and transducer, can distort the pressure signal. This not only changes the shape of the arterial waveform, but also dramatically alters displayed values for systolic and diastolic blood pressure.[2,3,11]

Catheter–transducer systems used in the operating room and intensive care units are described as *underdamped second-order dynamic systems*.[2] Detailed technical descriptions of the underlying physical principals have been provided by other authors.[2,5,6] For our present purposes, it is easiest to think of these catheter–transducer monitoring systems as having three characteristic physical properties: elasticity, mass, and friction. These three properties determine the system operating characteristics, termed the *frequency response*, or *dynamic response*. The dynamic response is characterized by two important system parameters, *natural frequency* (f_n, ω) and *damping coefficient* (ζ, Z, D). The natural frequency and damping coefficient are relatively easy to measure and dramatically influence the appearance of the recorded arterial pressure waveform. Natural frequency describes how rapidly the system oscillates, and the damping coefficient describes how rapidly it comes to rest. Before describing how these parameters can be measured in clinical practice, it is useful to consider briefly why they are important.

FREQUENCY CONTENT OF THE ARTERIAL PRESSURE WAVEFORM

The ABP waveform is a periodic complex wave that can be reproduced by Fourier analysis, a technique that re-creates the original complex pressure wave by summing a series of simpler sine waves of various amplitudes and frequencies.[9,11] The original pressure wave has a characteristic periodicity termed the *fundamental frequency*, which is equal to the pulse rate. Note that the pulse rate is reported normally in beats per minute, while the fundamental frequency is reported in cycles per second or Hertz (Hz). For example, a pulse rate of 60 beats/min equals 1 beat/sec, or 1 cycle/sec, or 1 Hz.

The sine waves that sum to produce the complex wave have frequencies that are multiples, or *harmonics*, of the fundamental frequency. Figure 9.1 provides an example of a crude arterial waveform, with its various components, systolic upstroke, systolic peak, dicrotic notch, etc., reconstructed with reasonable accuracy from two sine waves, the fundamental frequency and the second harmonic. If the original arterial pressure waveform contains high-frequency components such as a steep systolic upstroke or other sharp

details, higher frequency sine waves or harmonics are needed to provide a faithful reconstruction of the original pressure waveform, perhaps 10 harmonics. As a general rule, 6 to 10 harmonics are required to provide good to very good reproduction of most ABP waveforms.[4,9] Hence, accurate reproduction of the ABP waveform in a patient with a pulse rate of 120 beats/min (2 cycles/sec, or 2 Hz) requires a measuring system dynamic response of 12 to 20 Hz. Clearly, the faster the heart rate and the steeper the systolic upstroke or slope of the original pressure waveform, the higher the dynamic response needed in the measuring system to reproduce the arterial waveform faithfully. As a corollary, venous waveforms, which generally do not have steep waves or high-frequency components, do not require monitoring systems with such high-frequency responses.

NATURAL FREQUENCY

It is instructive at this point to consider what will happen if the pressure measuring system does not have an adequate dynamic response. What kind of distortion of the original intravascular pressure signal would we expect if the above described criteria were not met, and the catheter–tubing–transducer measuring system had too low a natural frequency? In simplest terms, the system would now resonate, and the pressure waveform recorded on the bedside monitor would be an exaggerated or amplified version of the true intraarterial waveform. This phenomenon is familiar to all clinicians, when they describe the ABP waveform as displaying *overshoot, ringing,* or *resonance*. This problem is highlighted graphically in Figure 9.2. A blood pressure simulator is attached to a reference transducer, and sine wave pressure signals are faithfully reproduced by this reference transducer as the simulator sends out waves of increasing frequency, from 5 to 50 Hz. Note that regardless of pressure wave frequency, the output signal recorded by this reference transducer has an unchanging amplitude, and the pressure wave is neither amplified nor attenuated. In contrast, the recording in the lower panel in Figure 9.2 is derived when the identical simulated sine pressure wave is recorded through a standard clinical catheter–tubing–transducer system. In this instance, the addition of the catheter and tubing has altered the measuring characteristics of the system. As the frequency of the simulated pressure signal approaches 20 Hz, the recorded output signal is amplified, and peak amplification (distortion) occurs at 20 Hz, the natural frequency of the measuring system. In much the same way, real ABP waveforms are distorted and amplified when the frequency content of the pressure signal approaches the natural resonant frequency of the catheter–tubing–transducer system in use. Again, faster heart rates and steeper arterial upstrokes present the greatest challenge to clinical measurement systems, because the higher frequency contents of these waveforms are more likely to approach the resonant frequency of the measurement system.

DAMPING COEFFICIENT

The bedside monitoring system not only must have a sufficiently high natural frequency, but it must also have an adequate damping coefficient. The consequences of an overdamped or underdamped monitoring system are familiar to clinicians. The *overdamped* arterial pressure waveform has a slurred upstroke, absent dicrotic notch, and loss of overall fine detail. Severely overdamped pressure waves display a falsely narrowed pulse pressure, although the mean arterial pressure value may remain reasonably accurate (Fig. 9.3). In contrast, *underdamped* pressure waveforms display systolic pressure overshoot and contain additional artifactual bumps, which are produced by the measurement system but are not part of the original intravascular pressure waveform (Figs. 9.4 and 9.5). It is a mistake to attach physiologic significance to these waves or bumps, since they are produced by an underdamped monitoring system, which continues to ring or oscillate abnormally in response to the input pressure signal.

ADEQUATE DYNAMIC RESPONSE

Armed with a basic intuitive notion of natural frequency and damping coefficient, we can now consider the way in which these two parameters interact in any given monitoring system to produce the observed waveforms. Most catheter–tubing–transducer systems are underdamped, but they have an acceptable natural frequency that exceeds 12 Hz. If the system natural frequency is less than 7.5 Hz, the pressure waveform may be distorted, and adjustment of the damping coefficient cannot restore the monitored waveform to resemble the original waveform adequately.[2,3] On the other hand, if the system natural frequency can be raised high enough (e.g., 24 Hz), different amounts of damping will have minimal effect on the monitored waveform, and faithful reproduction of the original intravascular pressure wave is achieved more easily (Figs. 9.6 and 9.7). In other words, *the lower the natural frequency of the monitoring system, the more narrow the range of damping coefficients that can be tolerated in order to ensure faithful pressure wave reproduction or adequate dynamic response.* For example, if the monitoring system natural frequency is 10 Hz, the damping coefficient must be between 0.45 and 0.6 for accurate pressure waveform reproduction. In this situation, too low a damping coefficient causes the system to be underdamped, resonate, and provide a factitiously elevated systolic blood pressure. In contrast, too high a damping coefficient produces an overdamped system, where systolic pressure is falsely decreased, and fine detail in the pressure trace is lost (Fig. 9.6).

In summary, a pressure monitoring system will have optimal dynamic response if its natural frequency is as high as possible (Fig. 9.8). In theory, this is best achieved by limiting the length of tubing to that minimally required and only using stiff tubing that is intended for pressure monitoring. Normal intravenous extension tubing should not be used, since it is too compliant and will cause the monitoring system to have too low a natural frequency and be excessively damped. Blood clots and air bubbles contained within the tubing–stopcock–transducer plumbing will adversely affect the dynamic frequency response in a similar fashion (see below, "Regarding Air Bubbles"). Since these foreign bodies are often trapped and concealed in stopcocks and other connection points, it is best to keep the system simple with the fewest necessary components.

MEASURING NATURAL FREQUENCY AND DAMPING COEFFICIENT

Gardner[2] has described use of the *fast flush method* to assess the dynamic response of the monitoring system. Under most conditions, this method yields results that are essentially identical to those generated by the laboratory standard square wave testing method.[7] The fast flush method has a number of practical advantages: it can be performed at the bedside without additional equipment beyond the normal monitors and recorders, and it tests the entire monitoring system, from catheter tip to monitor and recorder. To perform this test, the fast flush valve is opened briefly several times, and the resulting flush artifact is examined. It is best to perform the fast flush test during the diastolic runoff period, so that the flush signal is not distorted by the systolic arterial pressure upstroke or dicrotic notch.

Using this technique, the two relevant parameters that define the dynamic response of the monitoring system can be measured. Recall that natural frequency is a measure of how rapidly the system oscillates. Consequently, the natural frequency is determined by the time or distance between two successive cycles. As seen in Figure 9.9, the distance between two oscillation cycles is 1.7 mm at a recorder speed of 25 mm/sec (standard ECG speed). Going through the calculations, 1 cycle/1.7 mm × 25 mm/sec = 14.7 cycles/sec, or a natural frequency of 14.7 Hz. Note that the distance between successive oscillation cycles (i.e., cycles 1 to 2, 2 to 3, etc.) should be identical, since this is a fundamental characteristic of the measurement system—its natural frequency. *The tighter the oscillation cycles, the higher the natural frequency.* In order to measure natural frequency most accurately, the clinician should choose a faster recording speed (e.g., 50 mm/sec), examine several flush cycles, and then calculate an average value.

The damping coefficient is determined from the flush artifact by measuring the amplitudes of successive oscillation cycles. The amplitude ratio so derived indicates how quickly the measuring system comes to rest, our original definition of damping. *A low-amplitude ratio corresponds to a high damping coefficient, or a system that comes to rest quickly. Conversely, a high-amplitude ratio corresponds to a low damping coefficient, or a system that tends to ring and comes to rest slowly.* The damping coefficient can be calculated mathematically but is usually determined graphically from the measured amplitude ratio.[2,5] In Figure 9.9, the amplitudes of two successive oscillation cycles are 24 mm and 17 mm, giving an amplitude ratio of 17/24, or 0.71, which corresponds to a damping coefficient of 0.11 using the graphic solution shown in Figure 9.10. As in the case for measuring natural frequency, one may use any two adjacent peaks to determine the amplitude ratio, since the ratio of successive peaks should be relatively constant. Again, this is a fundamental characteristic of the measurement system—the damping coefficient.

Note that the example illustrated here (Fig. 9.9) has an adequate natural frequency of approximately 15 Hz, but the system is notably underdamped, with a damping coefficient of 0.11. Consequently, this catheter–tubing–transducer system falls into the underdamped region illustrated in Figure 9.8 (point A), and one would expect to see some systolic pressure overshoot recorded with such a system.

Although the technical requirements for accurate blood pressure measurement are evident from the preceding considerations, it is unclear whether the conditions for adequate dynamic response are met in routine clinical practice. Schwid[10] examined the frequency response of 30 radial artery catheter–transducer systems used in routine intensive care monitoring. Mean values (± standard deviation) for natural frequency (14.7±3.7 Hz) and damping coefficient (0.24±0.07) were worse than values typically reported for measurements made under laboratory conditions, falling instead in the underdamped response region reported by Gardner[2] (Figs. 9.6 and 9.8). Furthermore, the range of frequency responses (10.2 to 25.3 Hz) and damping coefficients (0.15 to 0.44) measured in this setting suggests that distortion of the arterial waveform is common in clinical practice, with exaggerated systolic arterial pressure (overshoot) resulting from a relatively underdamped system being the problem most often seen. Figure 9.11 plots these data from Schwid[10] in the format suggested by Gardner[2] and graphically highlights this situation.

REGARDING AIR BUBBLES

If clinical pressure monitoring systems are typically underdamped, leading to systolic pressure overshoot, why not simply increase the damping in the system by introducing a small *air bubble* into the tubing? In addition to the obvious patient risks resulting from unintentional air embolism,

there are important technical reasons why this is not an acceptable solution to the problem. Air bubbles not only increase system damping, but they simultaneously lower monitoring system natural frequency (Figs. 9.12 and 9.13) and may even have the paradoxic effect of worsening system resonance and further exaggerating systolic pressure overshoot! In this example (Fig. 9.14), a 0.1 ml air bubble markedly dampens the system but lowers natural frequency and causes an artifactual 25 mmHg increase in systolic pressure. As an alternative to placing air bubbles in the monitoring system, devices can be added to augment system damping without lowering natural frequency (Fig. 9.13).[2]

CLINICAL IMPORTANCE OF DYNAMIC RESPONSE

Several practical points for daily clinical monitoring practice clearly emerge from the technical considerations just described. First, one should attempt to keep the catheter–tubing–transducer system as simple as possible, using the minimal length of tubing and number of stopcocks required for patient care purposes, in an attempt to optimize the dynamic response of the monitoring system. Second, one should know how the natural frequency and damping coefficient may be calculated using the fast flush method. This allows the clinician an opportunity to recognize artifactual hypotension caused by a severely damped system. In Figure 9.14 (last panel), note that a large air bubble in the tubing system produces an overdamped system and a spurious reduction in recorded blood pressure. The fast flush test demonstrates a severely overdamped system, with no oscillation in the pressure recording noted after the flush artifact is introduced. In contrast, note the fast flush test in Figure 9.15, which demonstrates a typical underdamped clinical pressure monitoring system, with a natural frequency of 12.5 Hz and a damping coefficient of 0.22. In this example, the hypotension is real, not an artifact of an overdamped monitoring system. In other words, the fast flush test provides the clinician a rapid bedside method to distinguish true arterial hypotension from artifactual hypotension caused by a large air bubble or blood clot in the catheter or tubing.

A third practical point regarding these technical considerations relates to the clinical interpretation of systolic arterial hypertension. Owing to the dynamic response limitations of most clinical pressure monitoring systems, it comes as no surprise that direct measurement of systolic arterial pressure often exceeds indirect noninvasive measurement, simply because of underdamping and resonance. Note in Figure 9.4 that the direct arterial systolic blood pressure measurement (166/56 mmHg) markedly exceeds the indirect noninvasive measurement (126/63 mmHg). (See also Ch. 7, Fig. 7.2). Similar artifactual pressures may be generated with pulmonary artery catheter pressure monitoring, particularly when the catheter is set in motion by the actions of the heart during the cardiac cycle (Fig. 9.5). These spurious pressure waves may be amplified because of the limited dynamic response of the pressure monitoring system. (See also Ch. 5, Figs. 5.2 through 5.6.)

TRANSDUCER SETUP: ZEROING, CALIBRATING, AND LEVELING

Before patient monitoring is initiated, the pressure transducer must be zeroed, calibrated, and leveled to the appropriate horizontal position. The initial step in this process is to expose the transducer to atmospheric pressure by opening the adjacent stopcock to air, pressing the *zero pressure* button on the attached monitor, and thus *establishing the zero pressure reference value* (Fig. 9.16). The transducer now has a reference value, ambient atmospheric pressure, against which all intravascular pressures are measured. This process underscores the fact that the pressure numbers displayed on the bedside monitor are all referenced to atmospheric pressure, outside the body. (See also Ch. 15 for a discussion of transmural pressure.) Although one generally refers to *zeroing the transducer*, it should be recognized that the transducer is exposed to atmospheric pressure via an open stopcock, which is usually affixed to the transducer. To be precise, it is this air–fluid interface at the level of the stopcock that is the zero pressure locus and the point that must be aligned with the patient to determine the correct transducer level.

When a major change in intravascular pressure occurs, prior to initiating therapy, the zero reference value should be rechecked. This can be accomplished very quickly, by exposing the transducer to atmospheric pressure (i.e., opening the stopcock adjacent to the transducer to air) and inspecting the monitor to see that the pressure trace displays a perfectly straight line that overlies the zero pressure line on the calibrated monitor screen (Fig. 9.17). One need not wait for the digital pressure value to return to read the number zero; it is much faster to inspect the pressure trace to see whether the zero value falls on or off the zero line. Clinicians working at the bedside should be in the habit of checking the zero value regularly, especially prior to treating sudden changes in displayed pressures. *Note that* checking *the zero value is different from* establishing *the zero reference, which is done at the beginning of the monitoring procedure.* If the zero value falls on the zero line, the stopcock is then closed to air, and pressure monitoring continues.

Occasionally, the zero value falls above or below the zero line, thus leading to falsely elevated or depressed pressure values. This may occur because of transducer *drift*, caused by problems with membrane dome coupling to the electronic pressure transducing elements, as well as other technical problems with the transducer, the attached electrical cable, or the monitor itself.[2,8] These technical problems appear to be less common now that high-quality disposable transducers are used widely. If transducer zero drift is a problem, and repeated checking of the zero value shows it to be off the zero line, the pressure monitoring components should be checked for loose connections. If the system appears to be intact, the components should be changed sequentially to discover the faulty transducer, cable, or pressure monitoring module.

After the zero reference value has been established, the pressure transducer monitoring system is *calibrated*. Calibration can be considered to be an adjustment of the system gain, or its response to a known reference pressure value. Traditionally, this has been performed using a mercury manometer as the standard.[3] Today, however, disposable pressure transducers meeting industry standards are sufficiently reliable in their factory-set calibration that adjustment of the gain (calibration) of the bedside monitor is not necessary. In general, if a transducer or cable is faulty, the initial zero value cannot be established. Rarely, despite successful zeroing, the recorded pressure values appear erroneous, and a malfunctioning pressure transducer, cable, or monitor must be suspected and replaced.[1,8]

Although transducer calibration with a mercury manometer is no longer performed routinely for clinical monitoring, an alternative rapid, safe, and simple technique can be applied using the saline-filled monitoring tubing itself. If there is a question of accurate transducer gain, a known static input pressure can be applied by holding a known length of the saline-filled tubing above the transducer, with the tip exposed to air, thus establishing a water column of known height (and pressure). When this is done (Fig. 9.18), the pressure reading on the monitor should equal the height of the fluid column. Remember to convert the units, $13.6 \text{ cm H}_2\text{O} = 10 \text{ mmHg}$.

The final step in transducer setup is *leveling* the pressure monitoring zero point to the appropriate position on the patient. In general, zeroing and leveling the transducer are accomplished at the same time, prior to initiating patient monitoring. However, it should be recognized that these are two distinct processes. When zero pressure is established, the transducer is exposed to ambient, atmospheric pressure via an open stopcock. When leveling is performed, this zero reference point is assigned to a specific position on the body. Usually, the midaxillary line in the supine patient is chosen as an estimate of the position of the heart.

A few examples may help to provide some intuitive insight to help distinguish zeroing from leveling. During sitting neurosurgical operations, one might choose to zero and level the arterial pressure transducer at the midaxillary line during induction of anesthesia, while the patient is supine, then readjust the level of the transducer to the sitting patient's head to estimate better cerebral perfusion pressure (Fig. 9.19). The transducer should not need to be rezeroed by pushing the *zero pressure* button on the monitor, since only the reference level has been altered. (In fact, if zero is rechecked, it should be unchanged, regardless of transducer location, since atmospheric pressure changes little over the few inches of height alteration being considered here.) ABP now recorded at the level of the head will be lower than that recorded at the heart, the difference being precisely equal to the hydrostatic pressure difference between the head and the heart (Fig. 9.19).

Often, pressure transducers are attached to a nearby IV pole, and patient position is altered by adjusting the height of the operating room table or intensive care bed. A sudden change in blood pressure is noted and is attributable entirely to the change in transducer level in relation to patient level. Raising the table (patient) above the transducer will produce spuriously high pressures, while lowering the table (patient) below the transducer will produce spuriously low pressures (Fig. 9.20). Again, the error introduced is exactly equal to the hydrostatic pressure difference between patient and transducer. (Do not forget to convert cm H_2O into mmHg.) Although these leveling artifacts are generally of small magnitude (e.g., 10 mmHg) in relation to ABP, they are of critical importance when measuring central venous or pulmonary artery pressures (Figs. 9.20 and 9.21). However, on occasion a pressure transducer will fall from its intended position at the level of the midaxillary line and come to rest near the floor, 100 cm below the patient. In this instance, the blood pressure will be falsely elevated by nearly 80 mmHg! These types of level artifacts can be obviated by attaching pressure transducers directly to the patient and taping the transducer to the side of the chest in the midaxillary line.

A final example that may help to understand the distinction between zeroing and leveling is provided by considering the difference between invasive and noninvasive blood pressure measurement in a patient in the lateral position (Fig. 9.22). While the patient is supine, blood pressure is 120/80 mmHg, measured in both arms by noninvasive cuffs and invasive radial artery catheters. The patient is now placed in the

right lateral decubitus position, the left arm is 20 cm above the heart, and the right arm is 20 cm below the heart. The invasive blood pressure transducers remain leveled to the heart at the midthoracic, cardiac position. What values for blood pressure are now recorded by the two noninvasive cuffs and the two arterial catheters? Blood pressure measured in the left arm by cuff will be lower, 105/65 mmHg, since the left arm is 20 cm above the heart, while blood pressure measured in the right arm by cuff will be higher, 135/95 mmHg. However, blood pressure measured from either the left or right radial catheters will remain unchanged, 120/80 mmHg, since the reference level for zero pressure remains fixed at the heart. Indeed, if the arterial pressure transducers were attached to the arms, the zero reference levels for the transducers would have changed as the patient assumed the lateral position, and pressures recorded from right and left arms would equal those recorded by the noninvasive cuffs.

If the reader remains unconvinced, try a simple experiment. After placing an arterial catheter and establishing invasive pressure monitoring, lift the patient's arm containing the catheter while observing the arterial pressure trace on the monitor. Regardless of the position of the arm, the monitored blood pressure remains unchanged as long as the transducer reference level is fixed at the level of the heart (midaxillary line). Next, lift the pressure transducer above the patient and note that the monitored arterial pressure is factitiously low, because the transducer is above heart level (Fig. 9.23). These experiments demonstrate that the fluid-filled tubes used for direct pressure monitoring behave like *U-tubes* from physics class. Any hydrostatic pressure lost by the ascending limb of the tube is gained by the descending limb, thus producing no net pressure loss or gain.

In summary, accurate direct measurement of blood pressure requires that attention be paid to establishing zero pressure and leveling the transducer to the appropriate point on the patient, usually the midaxillary line. Both the zero value and the transducer level should be checked frequently, especially when patient or transducer positions are altered or when monitored pressures change suddenly. Without question, the most common major mistakes in pressure monitoring involve failure to establish zero, failure to recheck the zero value for transducer drift, and failure to relevel the transducer to the patient's midaxillary line when changes in position occur.[3]

Illustrations for Technical Requirements for Direct Blood Pressure Measurement

Figure 9.1 Arterial blood pressure waveform produced by summation of sine waves. The fundamental wave (*top*) is added to 63% of the second harmonic wave (*middle*), resulting in a pressure wave (*bottom*), which resembles an arterial blood pressure waveform (*box*). (Modified from Geddes,[4] with permission.)

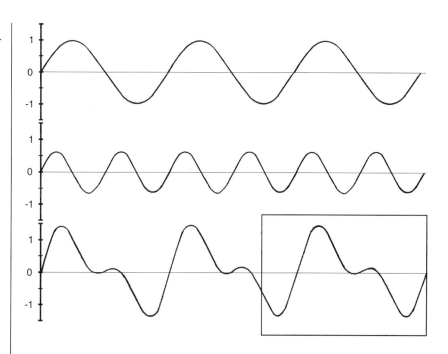

Figure 9.2 Resonance or pressure overshoot demonstrated in a pressure simulator test system. Addition of the catheter and tubing to the transducer in the lower panel results in a distorted output signal recording as the frequency of the sine wave is increased progressively from 5 to 50 Hz. At the natural frequency of this catheter–tubing–transducer system (approximately 20 Hz), the output signal is distorted maximally. Such a monitoring system would likely resonate and produce a small overshoot in systolic pressure. See text for more detail. (Modified from Gardner,[2] with permission.)

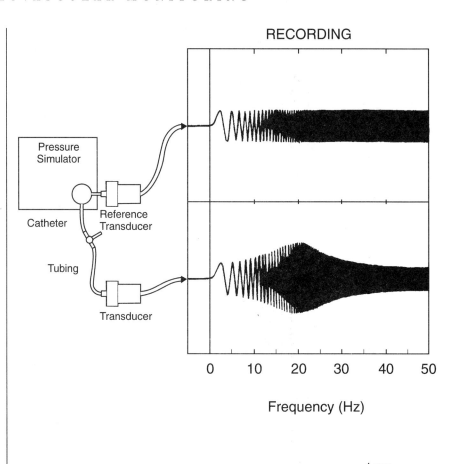

Figure 9.3 Overdamped arterial blood pressure (ART) waveform (A) displays a diminished pulse pressure compared to the normal waveform (B). The slow speed recording (*bottom*) highlights the 3-minute period during which the ART pressure is overdamped (A), but still provides an accurate estimate of the mean arterial pressure. Note that the top and bottom traces were recorded with different pressure scales.

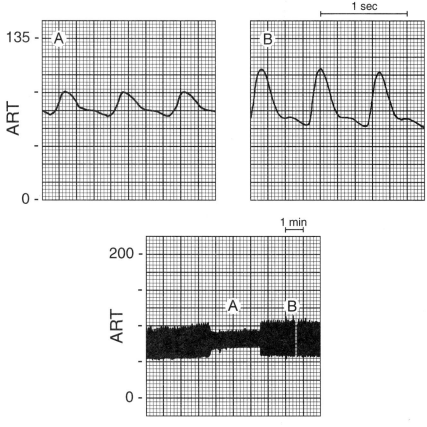

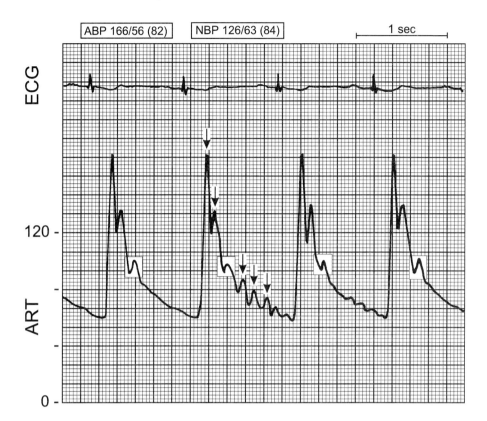

Figure 9.4 Underdamped arterial blood pressure (ART) waveform results in systolic pressure overshoot and displays many additional small nonphysiologic waves (*arrows*). The dicrotic notch (*white boxes*) may be difficult to discern, but it should not be confused with the pressure trough between the first two arrows, which appears because of the underdamped measurement system. The digital values for direct arterial blood pressure (ABP, 166/56 mmHg, mean 82 mmHg) and indirect noninvasive blood pressure (NBP, 126/63 mmHg, mean 84 mmHg) highlight the fact that systolic pressure overshoot occurs in an underdamped monitoring system. This artifact makes it difficult to determine the true value for direct systolic arterial pressure, which is most likely between 176 and 136 mmHg, the first two recorded pressure peaks (*first two arrows*).

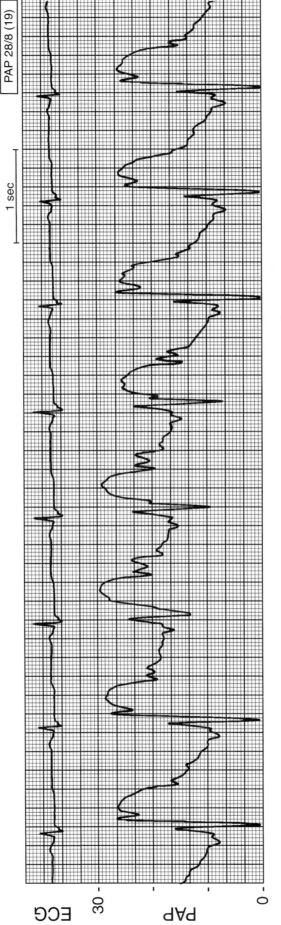

Figure 9.5 Underdamped pulmonary artery pressure (PAP) waveform contains several small, sharp non-physiologic waves, including the prominent end-diastolic/early systolic artifact wave resulting from catheter motion during this phase of the cardiac cycle. Note that the digital values for PAP recorded by the monitor (28/8 mmHg, mean 19 mmHg) provide a reasonable estimate, particularly given the under-damped waveform artifact and the respiratory variation in pressure that are present in this tracing.

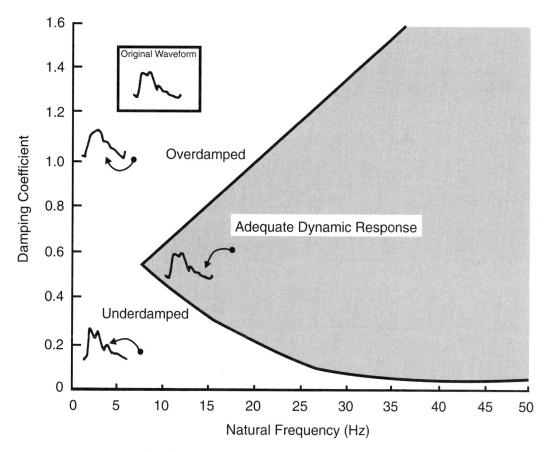

Figure 9.6 Plot of damping coefficients and natural frequencies that do not distort the original arterial pressure waveform shown in the box. The lower the natural frequency of the monitoring system, the more narrow the range of damping coefficients that can be tolerated in order to ensure faithful pressure wave reproduction or adequate dynamic response. In the underdamped region (*lower left*), the pressure waveform will resonate, contain additional nonphysiologic waves, and display systolic overshoot. In the overdamped region (*upper left*), the pressure waveform will appear damped, fine detail in the pressure waveform will be lost, and systolic pressure will be slightly reduced. (Modified from Gardner,[2] with permission.)

Figure **9.7** Interaction between damping coefficient (D) and natural frequency (f$_n$) in pressure waveform recording. (*A*) Underdamped pressure waveform (f$_n$ 10 Hz, D 0.1) displays small, artifactual, nonphysiologic waves and systolic pressure overshoot. (*B*) With the same low f$_n$ (10 Hz), a small increase in D (0.2) diminishes the artifacts seen in the previous waveform. (*C*) Optimal or critical damping (D 0.4) provides an accurate, nearly artifact-free pressure waveform, despite the same low f$_n$ (10 Hz). (*D*) Overdamping results in the loss of fine detail from the pressure waveform and precludes measurement of f$_n$ or D. (See text for more detail on measuring f$_n$ and D.) (*E*) By raising f$_n$ to 20 Hz, the low D (0.1) has little effect and does not distort the pressure waveform. The recorded waveform is nearly artifact free, despite being recorded with the same low D used to record waveform (*A*). (Modified from Gardner,[2] with permission.)

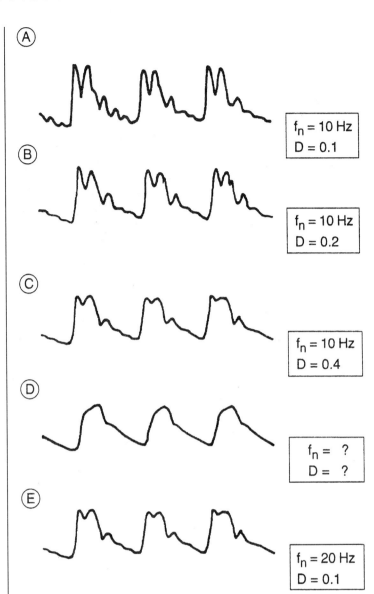

A

f$_n$ = 10 Hz
D = 0.1

B

f$_n$ = 10 Hz
D = 0.2

C

f$_n$ = 10 Hz
D = 0.4

D

f$_n$ = ?
D = ?

E

f$_n$ = 20 Hz
D = 0.1

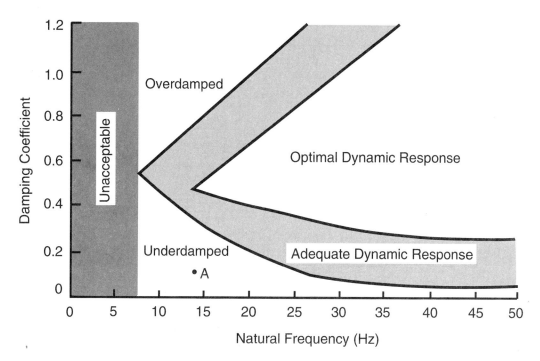

Figure 9.8 Damping coefficient–natural frequency plot showing the five areas into which pressure monitoring systems fall. Catheter–tubing–transducer systems in the *optimal dynamic response* area will record faithfully the most demanding pressure waveforms, such as those from patients with fast heart rates that have steep systolic upstrokes. Systems in the *adequate dynamic response* area will record typical pressure waveforms with minimal distortion. *Overdamped* and *underdamped* areas will introduce the artifacts associated with these technical system limitations. All efforts should be made to avoid using monitoring systems with a natural frequency less than 7 Hz, which falls into the *unacceptable* area. Point A shows the position of the monitoring system evaluated in Fig. 9.9. See text for more detail. (Modified from Gardner,[3] with permission.)

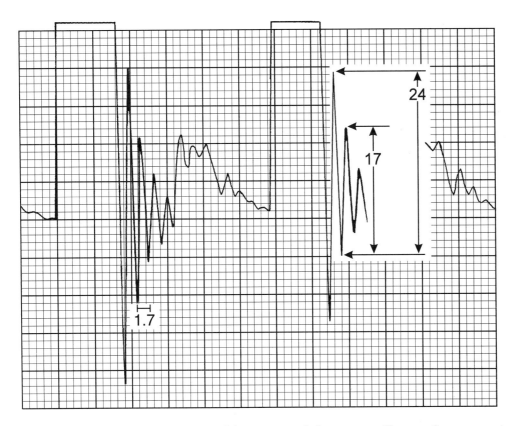

***Figure* 9.9** Calculation of the natural frequency and damping coefficient of a pressure monitoring system using the fast flush method. This tracing is recorded on standard millimeter grid paper at a standard recording speed of 25 mm/sec. It shows the arterial pressure waveform and two *square wave* flush artifacts. Natural frequency is determined by measuring the period of one cycle between adjacent oscillation peaks (1.7 mm) and knowing the recording speed (25 mm/sec). The natural frequency is thus calculated: 25 mm/sec × 1 cycle/1.7 mm = 14.7 Hz. The damping coefficient is determined by measuring the height of adjacent oscillation peaks (17 and 24 mm), calculating the ratio (17/24 = 0.71), and using the graphic solution shown in Fig. 9.10 to arrive at a damping coefficient of 0.11. (Modified from Gardner,[2] with permission.)

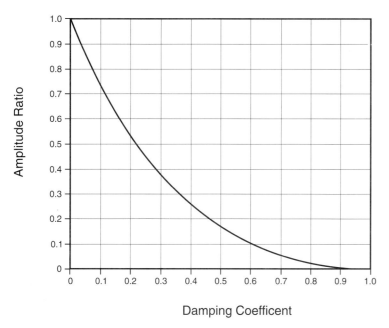

Figure 9.10 Relation between damping coefficient and amplitude ratio of successive peaks of pressure oscillation. This is the graphic solution to the equation for damping coefficient derived by Gardner:[2] $D = -\ln\{(A_2/A_1)\,/\,[\pi^2 + \{\ln(A_2/A_1)\}^2]^{1/2}\}$ where D = damping coefficient, (A_2/A_1) = ratio of successive peaks of pressure oscillation, ln = natural logarithm. For the amplitude ratio shown in Fig. 9.9 (17/24 = 0.71), D = 0.11. See text for more detail. (Modified from Gardner,[2] with permission.)

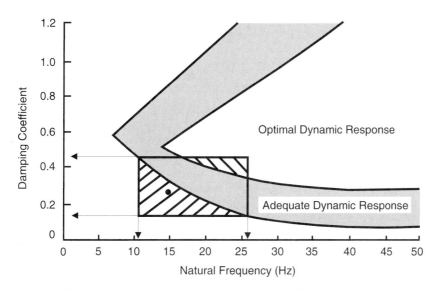

Figure 9.11 Damping coefficient–natural frequency plot with the dynamic response characteristics of transducer systems in routine clinical monitoring practice superimposed in the rectangular hatched box. The data in the rectangular box are taken from Schwid.[10] The point within the hatched box shows that the *mean value* for natural frequency (14.7 Hz) and damping coefficient (0.24) of clinical monitoring systems falls into the underdamped response region, although some systems achieve *adequate dynamic response* and a few achieve *optimal dynamic response*. See text for more detail. (Modified from Gardner,[2] with permission.)

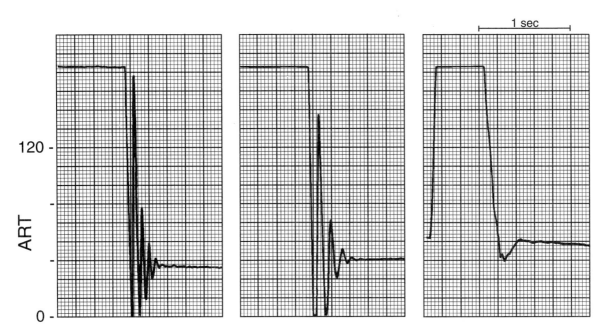

Figure 9.12 Effect of a small air bubble on arterial blood pressure (ART) monitoring system dynamic response evaluated by a fast flush test. In each panel, the square wave flush signal is recorded, followed by the system response. The ART signal is nonpulsatile because it is recorded from a patient during cardiopulmonary bypass. The monitoring system in the left panel has a natural frequency (f_n) of 13 Hz and damping coefficient (D) of 0.15. When a tiny air bubble is introduced into the monitoring system pressure tubing (*middle panel*), D increases as expected (0.22), but f_n simultaneously decreases (8 Hz). Introduction of a larger air bubble (*right panel*) further degrades the dynamic response of the system, and neither D nor f_n can be calculated. See text for more detail.

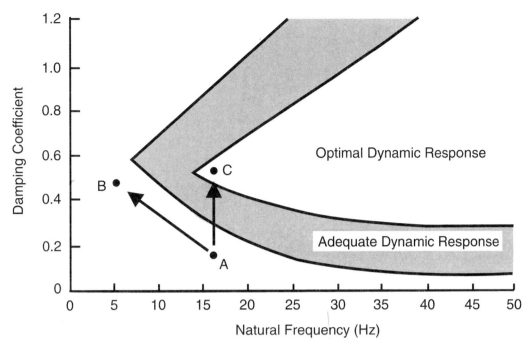

Figure 9.13 Damping coefficient–natural frequency plot showing that air bubbles increase monitoring system damping at the expense of reduced dynamic response. An air bubble would alter dynamic response by changing the monitoring system from point A to point B. Mechanical devices can be added to the monitoring system to increase damping without reducing natural frequency (point A to point C). See Gardner[2] for more detail. (Modified from Gardner,[2] with permission.)

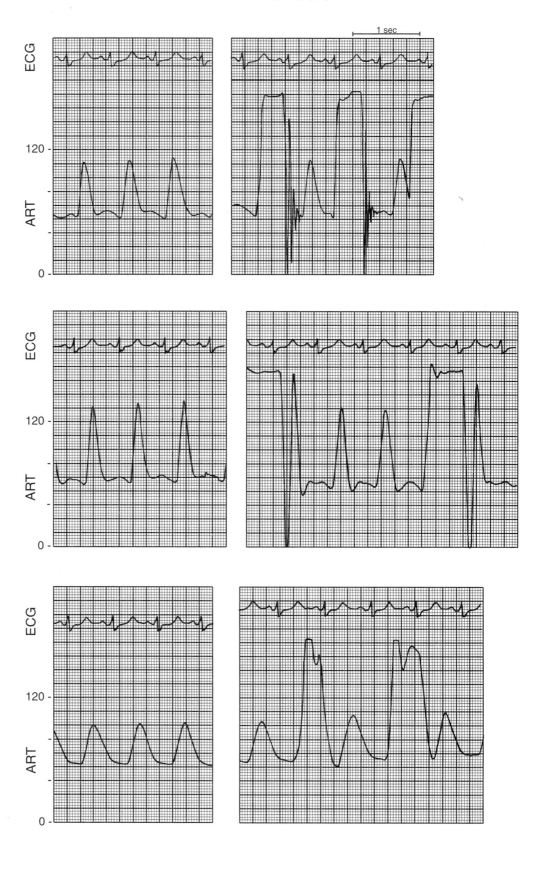

Figure 9.14 Artifactual arterial hypertension produced by a small air bubble in the tubing of a pressure monitoring system. The left panels show arterial blood pressure (ART) waveforms, and the right panels show these waveforms with fast flush square waves superimposed. The original monitoring system (*top two panels*) has a natural frequency (f_n) of 17 Hz and damping coefficient (D) of 0.2 and records ART 111/53 mmHg. When a small air bubble (0.1 ml) is added to the monitoring system (*middle two panels*), ART *paradoxically increases* to 136/61 mmHg. The monitoring system is more damped, but D cannot be calculated from the fast flush test, because there are no adjacent pressure peak oscillations following the flush signal. Natural frequency is decreased to approximately 5 Hz. A larger air bubble (0.5 ml) further degrades dynamic response (*bottom two panels*), and this overdamped system erroneously records arterial hypotension (ART 93/54 mmHg). Neither f_n nor D can be calculated from this fast flush test. See text for more detail.

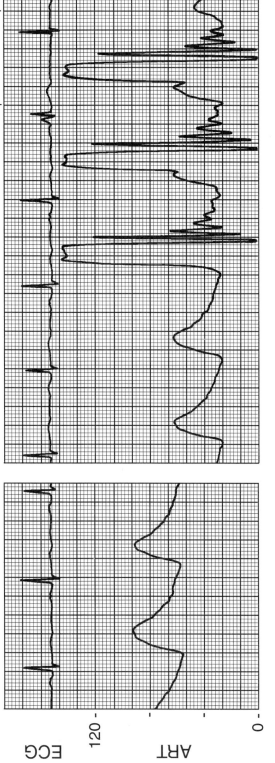

Figure 9.15 Fast flush test demonstrating that arterial hypotension is not the result of an overdamped monitoring system. The initial arterial blood pressure (ART) is 92/55 mmHg (*left panel*) and decreases to 61/27 mmHg (*right panel*). Three fast flush test artifacts are evident (*right panel*), which show the dynamic response of the monitoring system to be in the typical underdamped range, with a natural frequency of 12.5 Hz and damping coefficient of 0.22. Compare with the lower panel of Fig. 9.14.

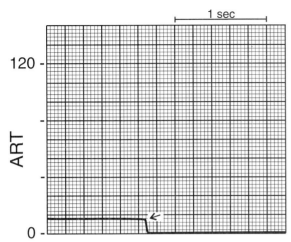

Figure 9.16 The zero pressure reference value for arterial blood pressure (ART) is established by exposing the transducer to atmospheric pressure (*arrow*) and pressing the *zero pressure* button on the bedside monitor.

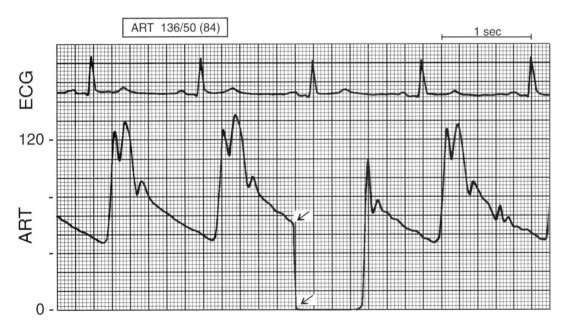

Figure 9.17 Checking the zero pressure reference value for arterial blood pressure (ART) by exposing the transducer to atmospheric pressure through an open stopcock (*top arrow*) and noting that the pressure trace falls to lie on the zero pressure line (*bottom arrow*). Note that ART monitoring is interrupted for less than 1 second to check the zero reference pressure and does not require waiting for the digital pressure display value for ART to return to zero. Instead, the displayed ART is 136/50 mmHg, mean 84 mmHg.

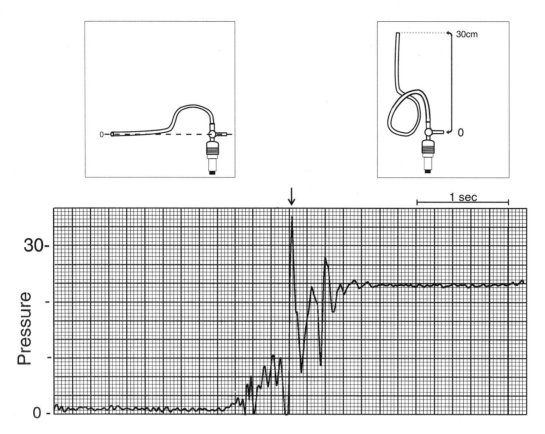

Figure 9.18 Checking transducer gain calibration with saline-filled monitoring tubing. On the left side of the trace, the open tip of the pressure monitoring tubing is held at the zero reference level of the stopcock, and a static pressure of 0 mmHg is recorded. The tubing is moved in the middle of the trace generating a motion artifact (*arrow*). On the right side of the trace, the open tip of the tubing is held 30 cm above the zero reference position, thereby establishing a static fluid column pressure of 30 cm H_2O or approximately 22 mmHg.

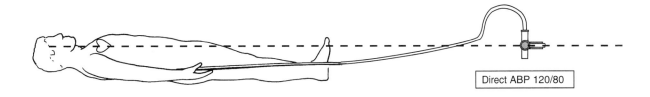

Direct ABP 120/80

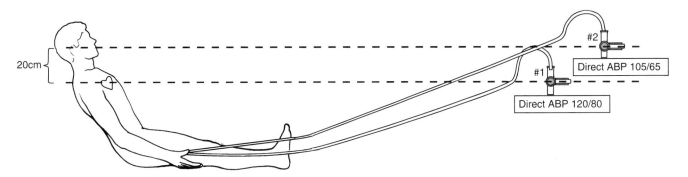

20cm

#2
Direct ABP 105/65

#1
Direct ABP 120/80

Figure 9.19 Adjusting the level of the pressure transducer to estimate cerebral perfusion pressure in a sitting patient. With the patient supine (*top figure*), the level of the brain is considered to be at the same level as the heart, and directly measured arterial blood pressure (direct ABP, 120/80 mmHg) is considered to be the same at both sites. When the patient is placed in the sitting position (*bottom figure*), the brain is now located 20 cm above the heart. If the pressure transducer remains at the level of the heart, the recorded pressure will be unchanged. However, if transducer height is adjusted to the level of the brain, recorded pressure will be lower by an amount exactly equal to the hydrostatic pressure difference between these two transducer positions, which is 20 cm H_2O, or approximately 15 mmHg. Thus, direct ABP will be 105/65 mmHg at the level of the brain. See text for more detail.

Figure 9.20 Change in patient position relative to transducer level affects all invasive pressure measurements. Arterial blood pressure (ART), pulmonary artery pressure (PAP), and central venous pressure (CVP) all change when the patient's bed is lowered suddenly (*arrows*). The small change in pressure of approximately 7 mmHg is identical in each pressure trace but most evident in the CVP trace because of the lower pressure scale.

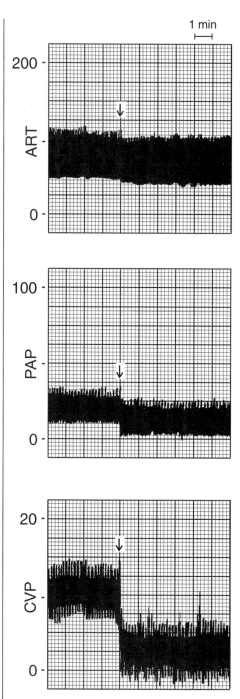

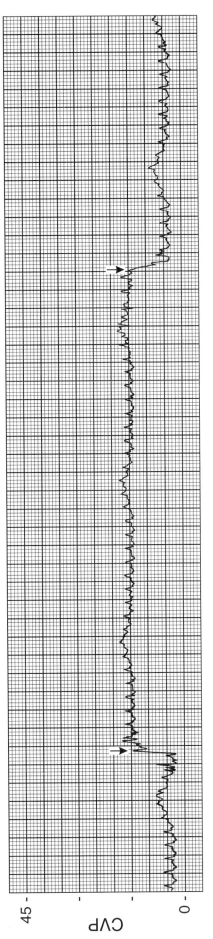

Figure 9.21 Small transducer level changes may produce significant errors in monitoring cardiac filling pressures. A spurious increase in central venous pressure (CVP) from 4 to 15 mmHg occurs when the patient's bed is raised above the level of the pressure transducer (*first arrow*) and persists for 26 seconds until the transducer position is readjusted to the level of the heart (*second arrow*).

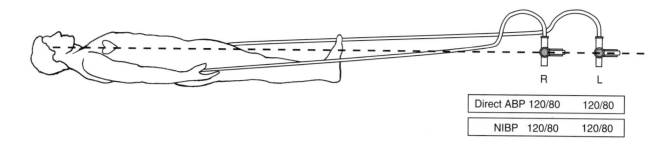

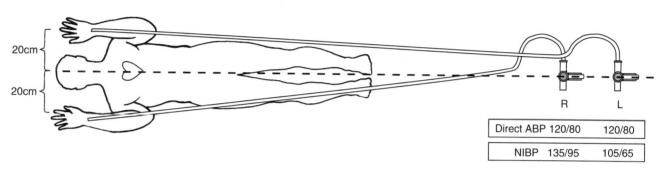

Figure 9.22 Invasive direct arterial blood pressure (direct ABP) compared to noninvasive indirect blood pressure (NIBP) in the supine (*top figure*) and lateral (*bottom figure*) positions. In this example, direct ABP measured from both right (R) and left (L) radial arteries and NIBP measured from both arms all record the same value for blood pressure with the patient in the supine position—120/80 mmHg. When the patient assumes the right lateral decubitus position, both right and left pressure transducers remain at the level of the heart and record the same direct ABP. However, the left arm is now located 20 cm above the heart and the NIBP recorded from this arm will be lower, 105/65 mmHg, while the NIBP recorded from the right arm located 20 cm below the heart will be higher, 135/95 mmHg. See text for more detail.

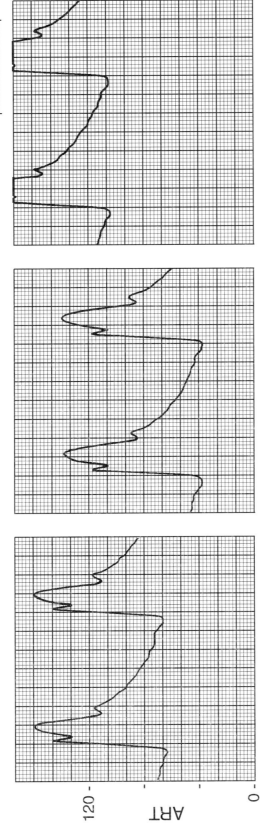

Figure 9.23 Influence of moving the arterial blood pressure (ART) transducer on recorded pressure values. Baseline ART is 160/66 mmHg (*left panel*). Recorded pressure is lower when the transducer is raised above the baseline reference level (*middle panel*) and higher when the transducer is lowered below this reference level (*right panel*). Note that the systolic blood pressure is *clipped* at 173 mmHg, the limit of the recorder output signal.

References

1. Barbieri LT, Kaplan JA. Artifactual hypotension secondary to intraoperative transducer failure. Anesth Analg 1983;62:112–4

2. Gardner RM. Direct blood pressure measurement—dynamic response requirements. Anesthesiology 1981;54:227–36

3. Gardner RM, Hollingsworth KW. Optimizing the electrocardiogram and pressure monitoring. Crit Care Med 1986;14:651–8

4. Geddes LA. Handbook of Blood Pressure Measurement. Clifton, NJ: Humana Press, 1991

5. Geddes LA, Bourland JD. Technical note: estimation of the damping coefficient of fluid-filled, catheter-transducer pressure-measuring systems. J Clin Engin 1988;13:59–62

6. Kleinman B. Understanding natural frequency and damping and how they relate to the measurement of blood pressure. J Clin Monit 1989;5:137–47

7. Kleinman B, Powell S, Gardner RM. Equivalence of fast flush and square wave testing of blood pressure monitoring systems. J Clin Monit 1996;12:149–154

8. Meyer RM, Kimovec MA, Hefner GG. Cable-testing device fails to indicate that hypertension is artifactual. J Clin Monit 1993;9:54–9

9. O'Quin R, Marini JJ. Pulmonary artery occlusion pressure: clinical physiology, measurement, and interpretation. Am Rev Respir Dis 1983;128:319–26

10. Schwid HA. Frequency response evaluation of radial artery catheter-manometer systems: sinusoidal frequency analysis versus flush method. J Clin Monit 1988;4:181–5

11. Shinozaki T, Deane RS, Mazuzan JE. The dynamic responses of liquid-filled catheter systems for direct measurements of blood pressure. Anesthesiology 1980;53:498–504

CHAPTER TEN Basic Electrocardiography

ECG monitoring in the operating room and intensive care unit has several goals: continuous measurement of heart rate, identification of arrhythmias and conduction disturbances, and detection of myocardial ischemia. In the past, monitoring the ECG with the standard bedside device has been considered to be inferior to using a 12-lead ECG machine when a diagnostic question must be answered. For example, one often hears the comment, "there appear to be ST-segment abnormalities on the bedside monitor ECG trace; let's get a *12-lead ECG to see if these are real ischemic changes.*" Although this statement may have had validity in the past,[1] it is becoming less and less true each year. Driven by the needs of clinicians using ECG monitoring equipment, technologic advances in bedside ECG monitors have improved their performance to the point where bedside ECG monitoring now approaches the quality and accuracy of traditional ECG testing.

In order for bedside ECG monitoring to achieve the above-mentioned goals, the clinician must attend to certain details of monitor setup, the most important being lead placement and selection, filter selection, and gain adjustment.

STANDARD LEAD PLACEMENT

The first step in ECG monitoring is to attach the electrode pads securely in the proper positions on the patient. The five color-coded leads have been standardized for the four limbs and a single precordial location (Table 10.1). When trouble-shooting lead placement problems, it is helpful to have committed the lead color code to memory.

Although the limb leads may be attached to the extremities, they are placed more frequently near the shoulders and hips for the sake of convenience. Arm electrodes are placed just inferior to the lateral aspect of the clavicles, and leg electrodes are attached in each anterior axillary line, midway between the costal margin and iliac crest (Fig. 10.1). This torso limb lead placement conforms well to one in widespread use for 12-lead ECG recording during exercise stress testing.[5,17] Whether the limb leads are attached

to the four extremities or the torso will have little influence on the ECG limb lead recordings. However, if one positions a limb lead haphazardly so that it is not outside the cardiac border, the limb lead recordings may be altered dramatically (Fig. 10.2).

In contrast to the limb lead attachments, positioning the single precordial lead requires more attention. A V_5 lead is generally chosen, since this lead has proven to be the most sensitive single lead for detection of myocardial ischemia during exercise stress testing[4,14] and during anesthesia and operation.[11,15,19] The V_5 electrode should be positioned precisely by locating the sternal angle and its immediately inferior interspace (the second), counting down rib interspaces on the anterior chest wall to reach the fifth interspace, and moving laterally to the anterior axillary line[8] (Fig. 10.3). In most patients, the V_5 electrode will be positioned slightly caudad and lateral to the left nipple. Proper placement of this electrode is critical, since misplacement by as little as 1 inch may have profound effects on the sensitivity for detection of ischemic ST-segment shifts.[14]

Often, in the operating room and intensive care unit, the surgical incision or dressing will interfere with the standard five-lead electrode placement described above. When the surgical preparation (but not the incision) involves the intended electrode area, the standard positions may be used, and the electrode pads and leads are covered with plastic tape or a clear plastic drape to maintain good electrode–skin contact. On the other hand, if the incision is to be made where a standard electrode pad resides, an alternative site must be selected. This is rarely a problem for the limb leads, since satisfactory alternative sites exist on the extremities or back of the patient. However, the V_5 electrode is often affected, for example during left thoracotomy. The V_1 electrode position, just right of the sternum in the fourth interspace, may be the only standard lead position outside the surgical field, and this lead is less sensitive for detection of ischemia.[15] As a practical matter, the clinician must recognize that monitoring a nonstandard precordial ECG lead located at a distance from the V_5 position cannot be expected to provide the same sensitivity for detecting ischemic ST-segment changes as a standard lead V_5 recording.

Although precordial lead V_5 is the best single lead to monitor for detection of left ventricular ischemia, evidence of right ventricular ischemia[6] and infarction is best gleaned from right-sided precordial leads, particularly lead V_{4R}, located in the V_4 position but to the right of the sternum[12,13,27] (Fig. 10.4). Lead V_{4R} would not be chosen for routine monitoring, since under most circumstances, left ventricular ischemia is of paramount concern. However, V_{4R} might be selected when right ventricular ischemia or infarction is suspected. This may be appropriate when infe-

Table 10.1 Five-Electrode ECG Color-Code System

LEAD COLOR	LEAD LOCATION
White	Right arm
Black	Left arm
Green	Right leg
Red	Left leg
Brown	Precordium

rior ischemia or infarction is present, since right ventricular infarction accompanies inferior infarction in 50 percent of patients, owing to the common coronary blood supply to these two regions of the myocardium.

ALTERNATIVE LEAD SYSTEMS

When the bedside monitor does not have a five-electrode system, but rather an older three-electrode system, the latter can be adapted to provide a lead configuration that approximates the standard precordial leads. The nomenclature for these modified bipolar limb leads is based upon standard precordial lead terminology. For example, in the CS_5 lead, the CS designates that the central (C) negative right arm electrode is located in the right subclavicular (S) region, the positive left arm electrode is located in the precordial V_5 position (5), and lead I is selected on the monitor to display this modified bipolar lead (Fig. 10.5). Similarly, the CM_5, CB_5, and CC_5 leads all have the positive electrode located in the precordial V_5 position, and consequently, all these leads are reasonable alternatives to the unipolar V_5 lead. In contrast, the MCL_1 lead has its positive electrode located in the V_1 position and is best used for detection of P waves and diagnosis of arrhythmias (Fig. 10.5). In each of these bipolar limb lead systems, the third electrode generally remains in its standard position and serves as a ground.[8] However, since this electrode is not part of the bipolar lead circuit being selected, its precise location is not critical.

While the modified bipolar leads that approximate standard unipolar lead V_5 can be used for detection of myocardial ischemia, differences in R wave amplitude and ST-segment morphology exist and may lead to under- or overestimation of the ST-segment change.[2,5,10,16] Consequently, a standard unipolar precordial V_5 lead is preferred when available. Griffin and Kaplan[8] provide a more detailed description of these modified bipolar limb leads, including their advantages and limitations.

INVASIVE ECG LEADS

In addition to surface electrode recordings, the ECG may be detected from adjacent body cavities or directly from the cardiac chambers. An *esophageal ECG* can be recorded using a modified esophageal stethoscope that incorporates ECG electrodes into its design.[8] Alternatively, a smaller esophageal *pill electrode* has been described for more prolonged ECG recording from the esophagus in awake patients.[3] The esophageal lead has proven useful for diagnosis of arrhythmias because the electrodes are located in close proximity to the cardiac atria. This lead discloses atrial electrical activity that is augmented relative to ventricular electrical activity and often not discernible on the surface

ECG recording (Fig. 10.6).[3,7] Furthermore, this lead may aid detection of posterior left ventricular ischemia or reveal reciprocal changes resulting from right ventricular ischemia,[25] since these diagnoses are difficult to make with standard surface lead recordings. Owing to their invasive nature, esophageal ECG leads have a limited application and are generally reserved for patients undergoing general endotracheal anesthesia or mechanical ventilation. A different invasive ECG lead, an *endotracheal ECG*, has been described for use in infants using a suitably modified endotracheal tube, but experience with this lead site is limited.[8]

A number of methods are available for monitoring an *intracardiac ECG*.[8] Although a saline-filled central venous pressure catheter has been used for ECG recording directly from the heart (Fig. 10.7), this method has been applied primarily to aid positioning of the venous catheter for aspiration of venous air emboli during neurosurgical procedures. More commonly, the electrodes of cardiac pacing catheters are used for direct endocardial ECG recording. A *pacing pulmonary artery catheter* has three atrial electrodes, any of which may be used to make an ECG recording that reveals clear atrial activity and aids diagnosis of arrhythmias. An *atrial paceport pulmonary artery catheter* allows introduction of a special atrial pacing wire, which can be used in a similar fashion. Finally, an atrial lead can be monitored from temporary *epicardial pacing wires* sewn to the right atrial wall during cardiac surgery. In each of these methods, atrial electrodes applied to the endocardial or epicardial surface of the heart for cardiac pacing are used for direct recording of the ECG (Fig. 10.8). Similar to the nomenclature applied to cardiac pacing, a *bipolar atrial electrogram* utilizes two atrial electrodes, and a *unipolar atrial electrogram* is recorded with one atrial electrode and either one skin electrode or the four limb electrodes as a common terminal.

The special leads just described do not replace standard surface ECG monitoring but rather provide supplemental diagnostic information. The clinician must realize that all invasive ECG monitoring carries additional risk, including the potential for mucosal burns of the esophagus or trachea[9] and microshock hazard of inducing cardiac arrhythmias. Methodologic details for recording these special leads can be found elsewhere.[8,20]

LEAD SELECTION AND DISPLAY

Assuming that a five-electrode system is used, and that all six limb leads and one precordial lead are available, which lead or leads should be selected for display on the bedside monitor? In order to diagnose arrhythmias and conduction disturbances, P waves must be discerned clearly, for which inferior leads (II, III, aVF) and anterior precordial leads

(V_1 or MCL_1) are most useful. On the other hand, detection of myocardial ischemia is best accomplished using lead V_5 or one of the comparable modified bipolar limb leads (Fig. 10.5). If the bedside monitor is only capable of displaying a single lead, a decision must be made as to whether arrhythmia or ischemia is more likely and/or more important to detect in a given patient. For instance, a young healthy patient undergoing anesthesia for knee arthroscopy would fall into the former category, while a 76-year-old patient undergoing resection of an abdominal aortic aneurysm would be considered in the latter group.

Fortunately, most newer bedside monitors allow display of two or more leads simultaneously. Selection of leads II and V_5 seems best in this situation, since this improves the likelihood that both arrhythmias and myocardial ischemia can be detected and properly diagnosed.

FILTER SELECTION

Modern bedside monitors offer a selection of filters for ECG signal processing. The two most common choices are called *monitor mode* and *diagnostic mode*. In monitor mode, the ECG typically has a low-frequency filter of 0.5 Hz and a high-frequency filter of 40 Hz, while in diagnostic mode, the corresponding filters are 0.05 and 100 Hz. The low-frequency filter attenuates signals below a certain frequency, only allowing those above the threshold value to pass. Consequently, *low-frequency filters* are known also as *high-pass filters*. By analogy, *high-frequency filters* are also called *low-pass filters*, and filters that eliminate both high and low frequencies are termed *bandpass*. Consequently, the monitor mode ECG display is *more* filtered than the diagnostic mode ECG display, since its filter bandpass is narrower.

Monitor mode filtering gets its name because bedside monitors historically used only these narrower bandpass filters. Increased low-frequency filtering diminishes baseline drift caused by patient movement and respiration.[18,26] This low-frequency filtering helps prevent the ECG trace from disappearing from the display screen as the baseline wanders, thus providing a more continuous signal for arrhythmia monitoring. The high-frequency filter in monitor mode reduces 60-Hz power line noise, thus decreasing signal distortion.[24]

Unfortunately, the additional signal filtering provided by the monitor mode may distort the recorded ST segment by not reproducing accurately the transition from the QRS wave to the ST segment. This problem arises because the ST segment has a flat slope, and thus, this low-frequency component of the ECG trace is altered by the monitor mode low-frequency filter (0.5 Hz). A number of authors[1,21] have shown that the ST-segment shift is exaggerated when a monitor mode filter is employed. As a result, a 0.1 m V ST-segment shift occurs more often when

monitor mode (0.5 Hz) filtering is employed than when diagnostic mode (0.05 Hz) filtering is used. This may lead to the overdiagnosis of myocardial ischemia, simply because the ST-segment shift has been amplified artifactually by the electronic filter used in the monitor.[22,23]

Figure 10.9 shows the effect of filter selection on the ST segment. Artifactual 1 mm ST-segment depression is produced when the ECG signal is recorded with a monitor mode filter, even though the less filtered diagnostic mode recording shows the ST segment to be isoelectric. Varying amounts of ST-segment distortion can appear, depending on the ECG QRS-ST morphology and heart rate. Although the monitor mode filter may cause only J-point depression (Fig. 10.10) or a minor shift in the ST segment, striking ST elevation or depression (Fig. 10.11) may be produced by monitor mode filters. New developments in digital signal processing may combine the benefits of both monitor and diagnostic modes of filtering, providing an ECG trace with both a stable baseline and undistorted ST segments. However, at the present time, accurate interpretation of ST-segment shifts on the bedside monitor requires that diagnostic mode filtering be employed with a low-frequency filter of 0.05 Hz.[18]

Some monitors offer a third ECG filter option, generally termed *filter mode*. This filter uses an even narrower bandpass (eg., 0.5 to 25 Hz) and also incorporates a *notch filter* aimed at eliminating the 60 Hz interference that may arise from the wall power source and the electrical equipment and cords near the patient. In the example in Figure 10.12, note the marked distortion produced by 60 Hz interference when the ECG is recorded in diagnostic mode, some improvement noted in the monitor mode recording, and elimination of the artifact when the ECG is recorded in filter mode. In some instances, this type of filtering must be selected to provide an interpretable ECG trace when the 60 Hz interference cannot be eliminated by other means. However, ST-segment distortion may occur at the same time that the 60 Hz artifact is eliminated.

GAIN ADJUSTMENT

Not only does the bedside monitor allow selection of the ECG leads to be displayed and the filters to be utilized, but the signal gain may also be adjusted. When ECG monitoring is initiated, the displayed signal gain often is selected automatically by the monitor to provide the largest QRS complex that will fit into the allotted space on the screen. This so-called *autogain* feature provides a tall QRS complex, which facilitates heart rate measurement by the monitor and allows the clinician to recognize waveform details. If an autogain feature is not employed by the monitor, the displayed ECG signal may be too small, and the monitor will not accurately detect the R wave or measure the heart rate. In these instances, the ECG signal gain can be increased, or a different lead that displays a taller R wave can be selected. In contrast, when the ECG signal is large, the monitor may double-count the heart rate when a tall T wave or atrial pacing spike is sensed erroneously along with the normal R wave. This problem may be eliminated by reducing the gain of the ECG signal, as well as changing the lead or reducing the pacing spike amplitude by decreasing the current output of a temporary pulse generator box.

Although ECG gain adjustment is useful for these reasons, the clinician must beware that gain changes simultaneously exaggerate or minimize ST-segment shifts. Both the monitor screen display and paper recordings are subject to these gain influences. For example, when we speak of *1, 2 or 3 mm ST-segment depression*, we are really describing the ST-segment depression with reference to the *standard gain* for diagnostic 12-lead ECG recordings, which is *10 mm = 1 mV, or 1 mm = 0.1 mV*. In fact, it would be more informative to describe the ST shift in millivolts (0.1, 0.2, or 0.3 mV) or microvolts (100, 200, or 300 μV) rather than in millimeters, but the use of millimeters seems firmly entrenched in clinical practice. The important point to remember is that, unless the ECG signal gain is specified, the physiologic significance of a given magnitude of ST-segment shift remains undefined—the number of millimeters of ST depression or elevation is meaningless.

Figure 10.13 shows an ECG recording at standard gain (10 mm/mV), half gain (5 mm/mV), and twice normal gain (20 mm/mV). Note that all components of the ECG trace (P, QRS, and T waves) are altered by the gain adjustment. However, the ST segment is isoelectric at standard gain and remains so whether the gain is reduced or increased.

In contrast, when the ST segment is depressed or elevated, alterations in signal gain will change the magnitude in millimeters of the ST-segment shift, making it appear factitiously small or large. Figure 10.14 shows the effect of gain alteration on an ECG trace that displays a 1.5 mm (0.15 mV) ST-segment depression at the standard gain of 10 mm/mV. When the gain is reduced to half standard, 5 mm/mV, the R wave amplitude shrinks from 8 mm to 4 mm, and the ST depression is reduced proportionately and now appears insignificant, measuring less than 1 mm. However, when the ECG signal gain is adjusted to twice standard amplitude, 20 mm/mV, the R wave amplitude becomes 16 mm, and the ST depression measures 3 mm. Clearly, correct diagnosis of myocardial ischemia based upon ST-segment shifts must take account of this gain factor.

The simplest way to avoid this type of misinterpretation is to adjust the bedside monitor ECG signal to a standard gain of 10 mm/mV. Unless there is a specific reason to select a different gain for the ECG trace, use of the standard gain allows the most direct on-line interpretation of ST-segment shifts and obviates the need to correct for the amplified or reduced size of the ECG signal. When a standard gain is employed, a 1 mm ST depression seen on the bedside monitor will have the same meaning that it does when detected on a standard diagnostic 12-lead ECG recording. Most monitors can be set up to provide this standard gain as the default setting, so that standard gain appears automatically each time patient monitoring is initiated.

A note of caution should be interjected regarding comparison of the monitored ECG trace to a *standard* 12-lead ECG recording. Beware that the *standard* 12-lead ECG has not been recorded at *half-standard gain* (5 mm/mV), since this commonly occurs when the patient has left ventricular hypertrophy resulting in high precordial R wave voltage.

Just as the scale of a pressure waveform is displayed on the monitor screen, the ECG scale or signal gain should be evident on both the monitor screen and paper recording so that the clinician is alerted when the gain is not standard. Monitors display this information in either an alphanumeric format (i.e., ECG gain 1.0×, 2.0×, etc.) or by way of a vertical bar on the ECG trace, the height of which represents the standard 1.0 mV calibration signal. Of note, nonstandard ECG signal gain cannot be detected by simple inspection of the ECG R wave amplitude displayed. Figure 10.15 illustrates a subtle example where increasing ECG gain is not evident from inspection of the R wave height. The standard 10 mm/mV recording displays a 16 mm R wave and just under 1 mm ST depression. Note the sharply inscribed R wave peak. At half gain (5 mm/mV), all ECG waveform components are reproduced faithfully at half the original amplitude. However, recordings at two and four times standard gain (20 mm/mV and 40 mm/mV, respectively) show two and four times the magnitude of ST-segment depression, without comparable increases in R wave amplitude. In both of these traces, the maximum limit of the recorder and amplifier has been exceeded, resulting in "clipped" R waves, which measure only 21 mm. The R wave peaks in these traces are flattened, since the actual peak extends past the plateau created by amplifier saturation. In this example, marked increases in ECG gain that exaggerate the magnitude of ST segment depression are not recognized by proportionate increases in R wave amplitude.

In summary, diagnostic quality ECG monitoring is performed easily with bedside monitors as long as attention to the aforementioned technical details is maintained. Proper electrode placement, lead selection, and filter and gain adjustment are required for the full diagnostic potential of ECG monitoring to be realized.

Illustrations for Basic Electrocardiography

Figure 10.1 Standard ECG limb lead placement for patient monitoring. RA, right arm; LA, left arm; RL, right leg; LL, left leg.

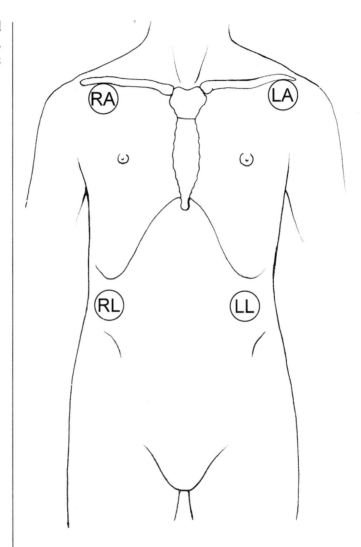

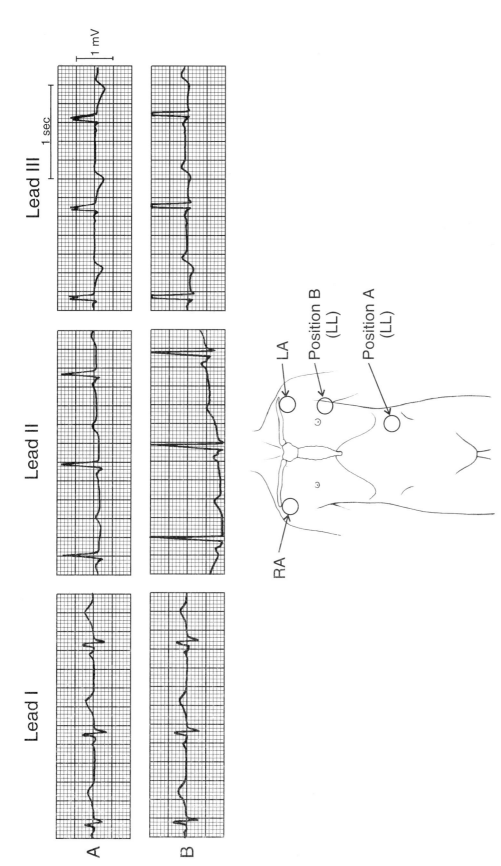

Figure 10.2 Importance of ECG limb lead placement. ECG recording of leads I, II, and III from position A, with the left leg (LL) lead in the standard location below the heart near the left iliac crest compared with position B, with the LL lead placed over the precordium (near the V$_5$ position). Standard ECG limb lead positioning should be outside the cardiac borders, as shown here in position A. If the LL lead electrode is placed inappropriately in position B, the recording of leads II and III will be modified. Note, however, that the recording of lead I is not affected by the misplaced LL lead, since lead I measures the difference between left arm (LA) and right arm (RA) electrodes.

Figure 10.3 Proper anatomic location of the six standard unipolar precordial ECG leads. Precise positioning of the lateral precordial leads is ensured by identifying the fifth intercostal space in the mid-clavicular line (MCL) for lead V_4, moving laterally to the anterior axillary line (AAL) for V_5, and further laterally to the mid-axillary line (MAL) for V_6.

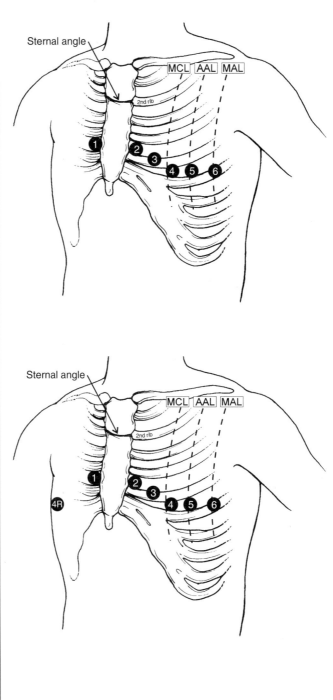

Figure 10.4 Right-sided precordial ECG leads, particularly V_{4R}, may be the most sensitive for evaluating right ventricular ischemia and infarction. Lead V_{4R} is located over the right precordium in the same relative position as lead V_4 on the left. The ECG traces in the box show that ST-segment elevation in lead V_{4R} accompanies similar changes in the inferior limb leads (II, III, and aVF) in a patient with both right ventricular infarction and inferior wall left ventricular infarction. The coexistence of these ECG abnormalities is common, since the right coronary artery provides a common blood supply to both the right ventricle and the inferior wall of the left ventricle in the majority of patients. MCL, mid-clavicular line; AAL, anterior axillary line; MAL, mid-axillary line. (ECG traces modified from Kinch and Ryan,[12] with permission.)

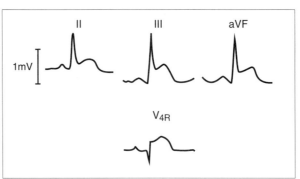

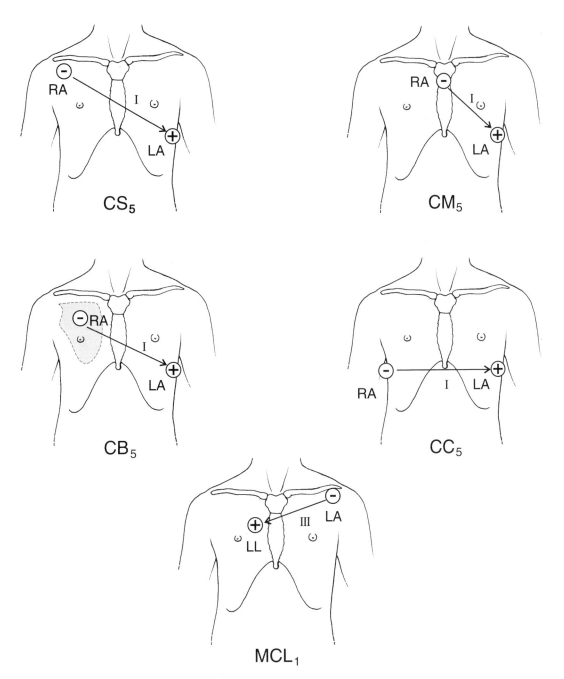

Figure 10.5 When only a three-electrode lead set is available, *modified bipolar limb leads* may be recorded as surrogates for standard precordial unipolar leads. Alternatives to precordial lead V_5 are recorded by selecting lead I on the bedside monitor and placing the positive exploring left arm (LA) electrode in the V_5 position. The nomenclature describing these leads derives from the location of the positive exploring electrode located in the V_5 position and the negative right arm (RA) electrode position being located as follows: (CS) central subclavicular, (CM) central manubrial, (CB) central back (shown overlying the right scapula), and (CC) central chest. In contrast, note that the MCL_1 lead (modified central lead 1) is recorded by selecting lead III on the bedside monitor and placing the positive exploring left leg (LL) electrode in the V_1 position with the negative LA lead in a *modified* position beneath the left clavicle. For more detail, see text and Griffin and Kaplan.[8] (Modified from Griffin and Kaplan,[8] with permission.)

Figure 10.6 Simultaneous recording of ECG lead II and an *esophageal ECG lead* (ESO). Note that atrial electrical activity (*arrow*) inscribes a much larger amplitude signal when recorded from the ESO lead as compared to standard surface lead II. The ESO lead is useful for diagnosis of arrhythmias and detection of ischemia involving the right ventricle or posterior left ventricle. (Modified from Benson,[3] with permission.)

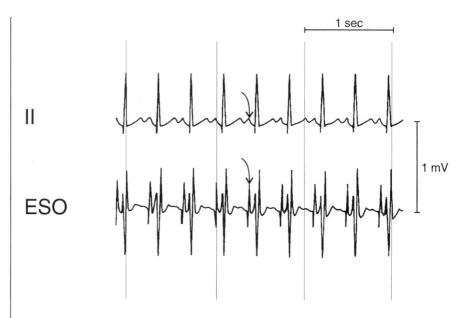

Figure 10.7 Simultaneous recording of ECG lead II and an *intracardiac ECG lead* derived from a saline-filled central venous pressure catheter (CVP lead). Atrial electrical activity is difficult to discern in the surface ECG trace, but clear P waves are revealed in the intracardiac recording (*white boxes*) and help make the diagnosis of sinus tachycardia.

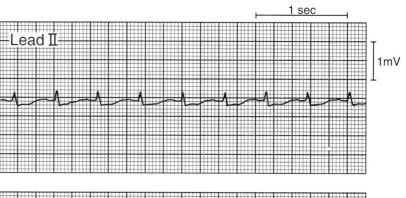

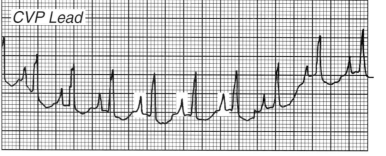

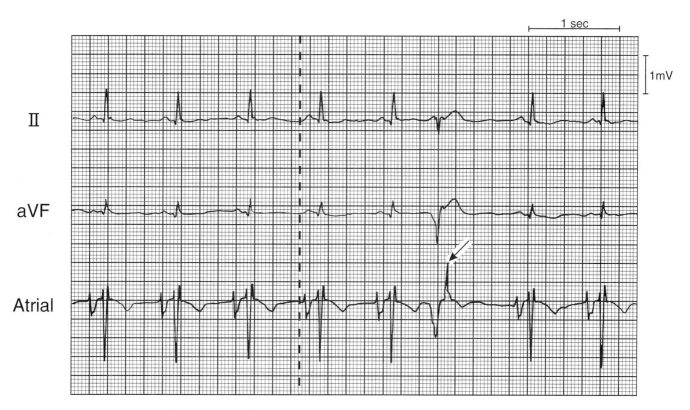

Figure 10.8 Simultaneous recording of surface ECG leads II and aVF and an *atrial epicardial lead* (atrial) recorded from a pacing wire attached to the surface of the right atrium. Onset of atrial electrical activity is denoted by the P wave in the surface leads and marked by the dashed vertical line. Note that the amplitude of the atrial electrical signal is greatest in the atrial lead recording. In addition, the sixth beat is a ventricular premature beat, and the resulting retrograde atrial depolarization is clearly evident in the atrial lead (*arrow*) but not seen as easily in standard surface ECG leads II or aVF.

Figure 10.9 Effect of filter selection on the ST segment. The *monitor mode filter (top panel)* has a narrow bandpass between 0.5 and 40 Hz, while the *diagnostic mode filter (bottom panel)* has a wider bandpass between 0.05 and 100 Hz. Application of the monitor mode filter produces artifactual 1 mm ST-segment depression. Compare the ST segments in the white boxes. See text for more detail.

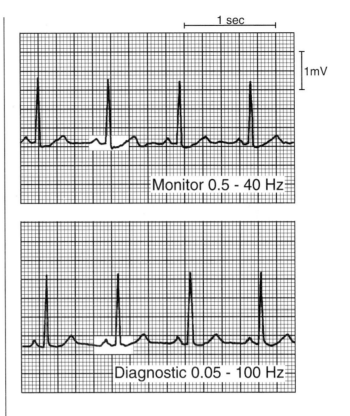

Figure 10.10 Effect of filter selection on the ST segment. Application of the monitor mode filter *(top panel)* produces artifactual J-point depression and up-sloping ST-segment depression *(white box)*. These abnormalities are not seen when the diagnostic mode filter *(bottom panel)* is used to record the ECG.

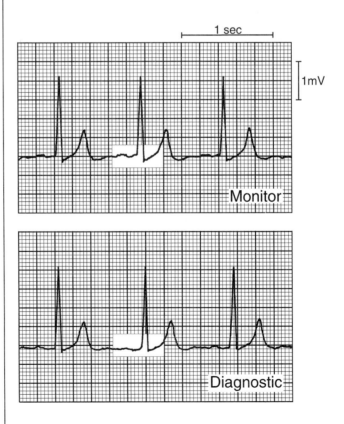

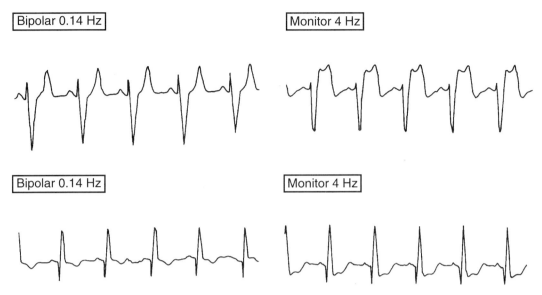

Figure 10.11 Effect of filter selection on the ST segment. Compared to a wider bandpass diagnostic mode filter (bipolar 0.14 Hz) (*upper left panel*), marked artifactual ST-segment elevation results when a monitor mode filter (monitor 4 Hz) (*upper right panel*) is applied to this ECG recording. In contrast, marked ST-segment depression appears in an ECG recording from another patient when the monitor mode filter is applied (*lower panels*). (Modified from Arbeit et al,[1] with permission)

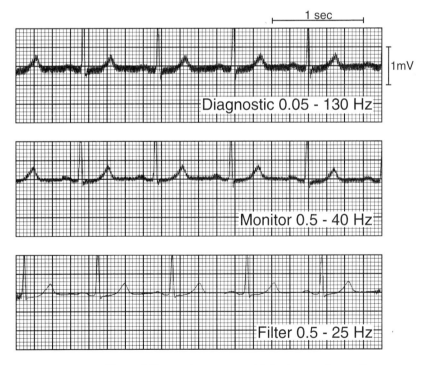

Figure 10.12 Effect of filter selection on ECG electrical interference from the wall power source. Compared to the diagnostic mode filter (bandpass 0.05 to 130 Hz), the narrower bandpass of the monitor mode (0.5 to 40 Hz) reduces this high-frequency artifact, and the filter mode (0.5 to 25 Hz) that incorporates an additional *notch filter* at 60 Hz eliminates this electrical artifact entirely.

Figure 10.13 ECG recording at the standard gain of 10 mm/mV (*top panel*), half standard gain (5 mm/mV, *middle panel*), and twice standard gain (20 mm/mV, *bottom panel*). Each ECG trace is interrupted by a 1 mV electronic calibration signal, which highlights the gain adjustment. Note that all ECG waveform components, including P, R, and T wave amplitudes, vary in direct proportion to overall signal gain. The ST segment remains isoelectric regardless of gain selection.

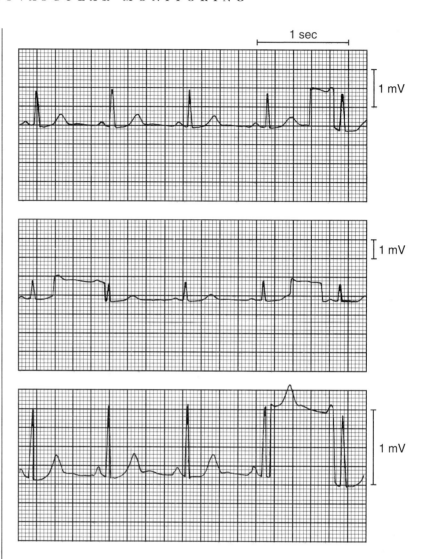

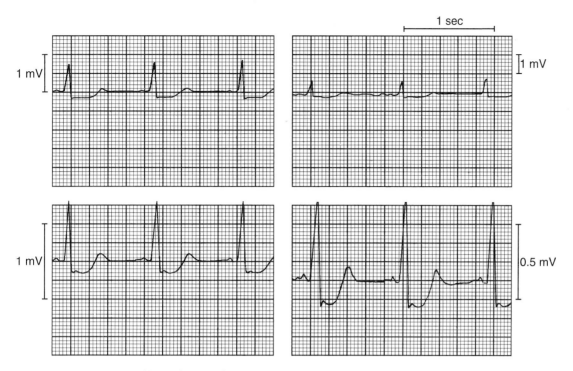

Figure 10.14 Effect of gain adjustment on the magnitude of ST-segment shift. The magnitude of ST-segment depression and R wave amplitude vary in direct proportion to overall signal gain denoted by the vertical calibration signals adjacent to the traces (10 mm/mV, *upper left panel*; 5 mm/mV, *upper right panel*; 20 mm/mV, *lower left panel*; 20 mm/0.5 mV or 40 mm/mV, *lower right panel*). Note that at four times standard gain (*lower right panel*), the ST depression increases to 6 mm but R wave amplitude only increases to 21 mm because the limits of the recorder output have been reached. See text for more detail.

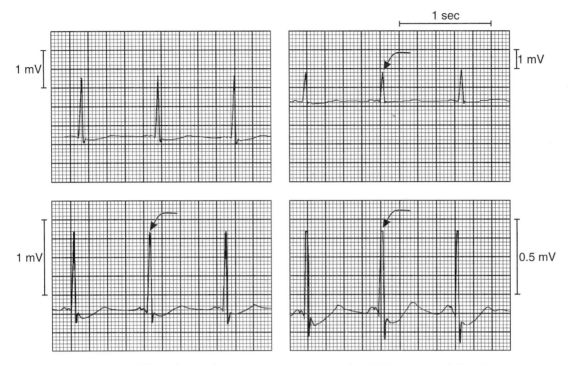

Figure 10.15 Effect of gain adjustment on the magnitude of ST-segment shift. ST-segment depression varies in direct proportion to overall signal gain, denoted by the vertical calibration signals adjacent to the traces (10 mm/mV, *upper left panel*; 5 mm/mV, *upper right panel*; 20 mm/mV, *lower left panel*; 20 mm/0.5 mV or 40 mm/mV, *lower right panel*). Note that R wave amplitudes do not change in proportion to overall signal gain, because the limits of the ECG recorder have been exceeded in the lower two traces, resulting in *clipped* or flattened R waves, 21 mm in height (*arrows*). See text for more detail.

References

1. Arbeit SR, Rubin IL, Gross H. Dangers in interpreting the electrocardiogram from the oscilloscope monitor. JAMA 1970; 211:453–6

2. Bazaral MG, Norfleet EA. Comparison of CB_5 and V_5 leads for intraoperative electrocardiographic monitoring. Anesth Analg 1981;60:849–53

3. Benson DW. Transesophageal electrocardiography and cardiac pacing: state of the art. Circulation 1987;75(Suppl 3):III-86–90

4. Blackburn H, Katigbak R. What electrocardiographic leads to take after exercise? Am Heart J 1964;67:184–5

5. Chaitman BR, Hanson JS. Comparative sensitivity and specificity of exercise electrocardiographic lead systems. Am J Cardiol 1981;47:1335–49

6. De Hert SG, De Jongh RF, Van Den Bossche AO, et al. The detection of intra-operative myocardial ischaemia. Preliminary experience with the right-sided precordial lead. Anaesthesia 1989;44(Part II):881–4

7. Grant AO. Transesophageal electrocardiography and cardiac pacing. Discussion. Circulation 1987;75(Suppl 3):III-91–2

8. Griffin RM, Kaplan JA. ECG Lead Systems. In: Thys DM, Kaplan JA, eds. The ECG in Anesthesia and Critical Care. New York: Churchill Livingstone, 1987:17–30

9. Hayes JK, Peters JL, Smith KW, Craven CM. Monitoring normal and aberrant electrocardiographic activity from an endotracheal tube: comparison of the surface, esophageal, and tracheal electrocardiograms. J Clin Monit 1994;10:81–90

10. Jain U, Rao TLK, Shah K, Kleinman B. Electrocardiographic lead systems. Anesthesiology 1989;70:1026–7

11. Kaplan JA, King SB. The precordial electrocardiographic lead (V_5) in patients who have coronary-artery disease. Anesthesiology 1976;45:570–4

12. Kinch JW, Ryan TJ. Right ventricular infarction. N Engl J Med 1994;330:1211–7

13. Klein HO, Tordjman T, Ninio R, et al. The early recognition of right ventricular infarction: diagnostic accuracy of the electrocardiographic V_4R lead. Circulation 1983;67:558–65

14. Kubota I, Ikeda K, Ohyama T, et al. Body surface distributions of ST segment changes after exercise in effort angina pectoris without myocardial infarction. Am Heart J 1985;110:949–55

15. London MJ, Hollenberg M, Wong MG, et al. Intraoperative myocardial ischemia: localization by continuous 12-lead electrocardiography. Anesthesiology 1988;69:232–41

16. London MJ, Wong MG, Hollenberg M, et al. Electrocardiographic lead systems. Anesthesiology 1989;70:1027–9

17. Mason RE, Likar I. A new system of multiple-lead exercise electrocardiography. Am Heart J 1966;71:196–205

18. Mirvis DM, Berson AS, Goldberger AL, et al. Instrumentation and practice standards for electrocardiographic monitoring in special care units. Circulation 1989;79:464–71

19. Roy WL, Edelist G, Gilbert B. Myocardial ischemia during non-cardiac surgical procedures in patients with coronary-artery disease. Anesthesiology 1979;51:393–7

20. Silvay G, Halperin JL. The ECG following cardiac surgery. In: Thys DM, Kaplan JA, eds. The ECG in Anesthesia and Critical Care. New York: Churchill Livingstone, 1987:203–23

21. Slogoff S, Keats AS, David Y, Igo SR. Incidence of perioperative myocardial ischemia detected by different electrocardiographic systems. Anesthesiology 1990;73:1074–81

22. Slogoff S, Keats AS. How best to monitor for detection of myocardial ischemia? Anesthesiology 1991;74:1172

23. Steinbrook RA, Goldman DB, Mark JB, et al. How best to monitor for detection of myocardial ischemia? Anesthesiology 1991;74:1171–2

24. Tayler DI, Vincent R. Artefactual ST segment abnormalities due to electrocardiograph design. Br Heart J 1985;54:121–8

25. Trager MA, Feinberg BI, Kaplan JA. Right ventricular ischemia diagnosed by an esophageal electrocardiogram and right atrial pressure tracing. J Cardiothorac Anesth 1987;1:123–5

26. Weinfurt PT. Electrocardiographic monitoring: an overview. J Clin Monit 1990;6:132–8

27. Zehender M, Kasper W, Kauder E, et al. Right ventricular infarction as an independent predictor of prognosis after acute inferior myocardial infarction. N Engl J Med 1993;328:981–8

CHAPTER ELEVEN *Myocardial Ischemia*

ECG DETECTION

PATTERNS OF ISCHEMIA: ST-SEGMENT CHANGES

Although the ECG manifestations of myocardial ischemia are myriad, certain ECG features have been used most frequently for perioperative detection of ischemia using the bedside monitor. *Subendocardial ischemia* is characterized by ST-segment depression that is horizontal or downsloping, 1.0 mm (0.1 mV) or greater in magnitude, measured 60 msec after the J-point, and present for at least 1 minute (Fig. 11.1). This pattern of ischemia is the more common one detected during both stress ECG (e.g., treadmill testing) and in the operating room when myocardial oxygen demand increases to exceed the available supply (*demand ischemia*). The subendocardial layer of the left ventricle is most susceptible to demand-related ischemia because of its anatomic location most distant from the epicardial coronary arterial supply.[42]

In contrast, *transmural ischemia*, characterized by ST-segment elevation, occurs when coronary blood flow to a region of the myocardium is totally obstructed (*supply ischemia*) (Fig. 11.2).[43] This pattern is seen typically as a result of coronary thrombosis during acute myocardial infarction,[1] epicardial coronary artery spasm (e.g., Prinzmetal angina[5,29,30]), or coronary artery embolism of air (Fig. 11.3) or particulate debris occurring during cardiac surgery. The precise criteria for using ST-segment elevation as a marker of transmural ischemia are less widely accepted than those applied for ST depression as a sign of subendocardial ischemia. The elevated ST segments typically are horizontal or slope toward the T wave. As a result, the amount of ST-segment elevation is measured at the J-point and should be at least 1.0 mm (0.1 mV) in two or more limb leads or 2.0 mm (0.2 mV) in two or more precordial leads.[43]

Categorizing ST-segment shifts into those caused by subendocardial ischemia or transmural ischemia provides a useful clinical framework but is a significant oversimplification of an extensively studied yet incompletely understood subject. For the reader interested in a more detailed discussion of these issues, Holland and Brooks[12] offer a comprehensive review of the various criteria applied to ST-segment shifts for the diagnosis of myocardial ischemia during stress testing, as well as the physiologic processes that underlie these ECG changes.

When using the ECG to detect ST-segment shifts and diagnose myocardial ischemia, a number of important points should be kept in mind. There must be meticulous attention to the technical details of ECG monitoring, as emphasized in Chapter 10. Proper electrode placement, lead selection, filter selection, and gain adjustment will make it less likely that ischemic events will be missed or overdiagnosed.[36,37,39] For example, inappropriate lead position or reduced signal gain may act to obscure ST-segment changes indicative of ischemia (Fig. 11.4).

Diagnosis of myocardial ischemia based upon ST-segment shifts must take account of the clinical setting and likelihood that the patient has underlying coronary disease or other cardiac conditions in which ischemia commonly occurs. Independent methods to diagnose myocardial ischemia, such as echocardiography, have confirmed that ST-segment depression that develops in a patient undergoing abdominal aortic reconstructive surgery is more likely to represent myocardial ischemia than the same ST-segment change that occurs in a healthy young parturient undergoing cesarean section.[8,24,38] Before diagnosing ischemia and initiating therapy based on this diagnosis, the clinician should consider: Is this a high-risk patient, a high-risk procedure, or both? As succinctly described by Marriott,[23] "the electrocardiogram should always be read in the clearest light of clinical observation. All pertinent data should be in the hands of the interpreter." A more formal Bayesian analysis of ECG detection of ischemia and coronary disease is offered by Rifkin and Hood[28] and Diamond and Forrester[7] and is beyond the scope of this discussion.

It is appealing to consider that the *magnitude* of ST-segment shift reflects the *severity* of ischemia, but this is not necessarily the case. For example, 2 mm ST-segment elevation may suggest more severe ischemia than 3 mm ST-segment depression, insofar as the former involves the full thickness of the myocardium as opposed to just the subendocardial layer. Although clinical outcome studies conducted in patients undergoing coronary artery bypass graft surgery have demonstrated a relation between the magnitude of ST depression and risk of perioperative myocardial infarction,[34,35] other investigations fail to show a strong quantitative correlation between the amount of ST-segment shift and alternative markers of ischemic injury.[12] As a result, when one monitors ST-segment changes in any individual patient (Fig. 11.1), one should not conclude that a larger shift in ST-segment necessarily reflects a greater severity of ischemia, but rather that there is a greater certainty that myocardial ischemia is present.[28]

Just as the magnitude of ST-segment shift does not indicate the severity of ischemia, the number of leads that show these ST abnormalities does not correspond precisely to the anatomic extent of ischemia. This is particularly true for subendocardial ischemia and ST-segment depression. Because the positive poles of most of the standard leads are directed toward the left ventricle, subendocardial ischemia may produce ST-segment depression in the leftward, lateral, and/or inferiorly oriented leads. Consequently, the location of the leads that display the ST depression does not indicate with any great precision the area of left ventricular subendocardium that is ischemic.[42]

In contrast to subendocardial ischemia, the location and extent of transmural ischemia is better predicted by the pattern of ST-segment elevation across ECG leads.[16,43] Continuous 12-lead ECG monitoring of ST-segment elevation has been used to provide a characteristic *fingerprint* of the perfusion territory affected during episodes of transmural myocardial ischemia.[15,16]

Isolated J-point depression and up-sloping ST segments are less specific patterns of ischemia than the standard ST depression and elevation criteria described above.[26,32] Nonetheless, in any individual patient, these ECG changes may indeed represent myocardial ischemia. The clinician must consider the patient's history, symptoms, and other ancillary information before arriving at a diagnosis of ischemia in these instances.

Other conditions confound the electrocardiographic diagnosis of myocardial ischemia. ST-segment depression is a less specific indicator of ischemia in patients with left ventricular hypertrophy, left bundle branch block, previous Q wave infarction, ventricular pacing, Wolff-Parkinson-White syndrome, mitral valve prolapse, electrolyte disorders, and digoxin therapy.[11,33] Unfortunately, it is in just these patients that one often must depend on the ECG to monitor for ischemia. Inasmuch as many of the aforementioned conditions are relatively chronic, it is reasonable to use the patient's baseline ECG as a starting point and consider new ST shifts as suggestive of ischemia, particularly when other evidence corroborating this diagnosis can be found in the ECG trace or through additional hemodynamic monitoring. (See below, ancillary ECG clues, and Ch. 12.) Recent epidemiologic investigations have identified specific ECG features to diagnose myocardial infarction in patients with preexisting left bundle branch block,[31] but these criteria have yet to be applied to the ECG diagnosis of ischemia.

ST-segment abnormalities often are present on baseline ECG traces (Figs. 11.5 and 11.6). In these instances, the diagnosis of myocardial ischemia based upon ST-segment changes is more difficult, and it remains uncertain whether a given *absolute threshold* value for ST-segment depression or a given *change from baseline* should be used as the diagnostic criterion for ischemia.[13,18] For example, if the baseline ECG trace shows 0.5 mm ST depression (Fig. 11.6), should ischemia be diagnosed if the ST depression reaches 1 mm (*absolute threshold*), 1.5 mm (1 mm *change from baseline*), or an even more exclusionary criterion of 2.0 mm? Perhaps the best approach is to consider these ST-segment changes as a continuum with a greater magnitude of ST depression reflecting a greater likelihood that ischemia is present, an approach that has been advocated for ECG stress testing.[28]

PATTERNS OF ISCHEMIA: ANCILLARY ECG CLUES

Although ST-segment depression and elevation are the most common ECG abnormalities associated with myocardial ischemia, other ECG clues may be present. While these ancillary clues to myocardial ischemia are certainly less sensitive and less specific than ST-segment shifts, they may provide useful supplementary diagnostic information in individual cases. In nonoperative settings, *T wave* changes have been associated with myocardial ischemia, particularly T wave inversion caused by subendocardial ischemia.[42] However, during the perioperative period, changes in T wave morphology are extremely common and are not associated with untoward cardiac events or myocardial ischemia.[2] *Pseudonormalization* of chronically inverted T waves may also indicate ischemia in individual patients (Fig. 11.7).[25] It is often difficult to decide whether these changes indicate amelioration of a chronic ischemic pattern, pseudonormalization and worsening of ischemia, or whether they arise on an entirely nonischemic basis. Knowledge that the observed T wave changes accompanied prior episodes of angina pectoris constitutes evidence that these *nonspecific* ECG changes indicate ischemia in an individual patient.

Conduction abnormalities and arrhythmias may provide additional indirect evidence for myocardial ischemia.[27] New onset of *left bundle branch block* has been associated with myocardial ischemia and may portend a poorer outcome after coronary artery bypass surgery.[6] *Ventricular arrhythmias* should be presumed to have an ischemic basis when they develop in the presence of other evidence for ischemia, particularly ST-segment depression (Fig. 11.8). *Bradycardia* and *atrioventricular block* commonly accompany ischemia within the distribution of the right coronary artery (Fig. 11.9), because the blood supply to the sinoatrial and atrioventricular nodes arises from the right coronary artery in most patients.

LIMITATIONS OF INDIVIDUAL LEAD MONITORING

While considerable emphasis has been placed on the use of the V_5 precordial lead for intraoperative ischemia monitoring, one must realize that there are many instances when ST-segment changes are minimal in lead V_5 but striking in other leads (Fig. 11.10), particularly inferior leads II, III, and aVF (Figs. 11.3 and 11.11). This pattern of inferior lead ST elevation is common during cardiac surgery requiring opening of the left heart chambers, like aortic or mitral valve replacement. In these cases, retained intravascular air is likely to embolize into the arterial circulation after emerging from cardiopulmonary bypass. These air bubbles float to the uppermost portion of the aortic root, often enter the right coronary ostium because of its anterior non-dependent location, and cause transient obstruction to right coronary artery blood flow. Arterial air embolism thus results in a pattern of transmural ischemia with ST-segment elevation localized in the inferior ECG leads (Figs. 11.3 and 11.11).

Because coronary atherosclerosis affects portions of the myocardium differentially depending on the pattern of coronary artery obstruction, myocardial ischemia typically develops in a regional pattern in patients with obstructive coronary disease. Furthermore, during coronary artery bypass surgery, specific regions of the myocardium are at risk, depending on the success of territorial revascularization. For example, anterior wall ischemia barely detectable by a laterally positioned V_5 lead may be recognized more readily in an anterior precordial lead. Unfortunately, these anterior leads cannot be used during cardiac surgery, because they interfere with the surgical incision (Fig. 11.12). The clinician must have a high index of suspicion that minor ST changes noted in the one or two monitored leads occasionally may reflect the *tip of the ischemic iceberg* (Fig. 11.13).

CONFOUNDING INFLUENCES DURING THE PERIOPERATIVE PERIOD

As noted earlier, a number of common cardiac conditions may alter the ST segments and make electrocardiographic diagnosis of ischemia more difficult. During the perioperative period, a number of more subtle influences come into play and must be considered when one uses the ECG to detect ischemia.

After the ECG leads are attached to the patient in the operating room, it is advisable to make a short paper recording of the initial intraoperative ECG to provide a baseline for comparison. This helps the clinician to be certain that the electrodes are properly positioned and the lead wires properly attached. If the lead wires are switched unintentionally, the ECG may look markedly different, with Q waves disappearing from some leads and reappearing in new leads (Fig. 11.14). The precordial electrode should be placed carefully in the V_5 position, and the resulting ECG trace should resemble the corresponding recording from the preoperative 12-lead ECG. Although a minor change from the preoperative recording may result if the precordial V_5 electrode is not placed in the *exact* location where the corresponding electrode had been positioned for the 12-lead ECG recording (Fig. 11.15), larger changes in the ST segment may

reflect new or worsened myocardial ischemia (Fig. 11.16). The only method to ensure reproducible precordial electrode placement is to mark the lead positions on the patient's skin or leave the same electrodes affixed to the skin throughout the perioperative period.

Hypothermia causes striking changes in the ECG ST segment that mimic the changes of myocardial ischemia. The Osborne wave[10] appears as ST-segment elevation that begins with the J-point and distorts the terminal portion of the QRS (Fig. 11.17). These waves develop when the myocardial temperature is less than 30°C, and they are seen typically in multiple leads, particularly the inferior and mid-precordial leads. Osborne waves are observed commonly during onset of hypothermic cardiopulmonary bypass (Fig. 11.18). On occasion, the heart may be cooled unintentionally, and a similar striking change in the ST segment is recorded (Fig. 11.19).

Although the standard 12-lead ECG is recorded with the patient in the supine position, intraoperative ECG monitoring frequently must be conducted with the patient in the prone, sitting, or lateral decubitus position. When the patient assumes these positions, the heart moves within the thorax, and the ECG thus recorded may be altered unpredictably.[17,40] In some individuals, changes in body position will have little influence on the ECG (Fig. 11.20), while in others, identical changes in position are accompanied by dramatic alterations in R wave amplitude and ST-segment shift (Fig. 11.21). In both of the examples shown in Figures 11.20 and 11.21, the left lateral position produces an increased R wave amplitude in the precordial lead as the heart shifts toward the recording electrode. In a patient with no preexisting ST deviation seen in the supine ECG recording, the ST segments remain isoelectric even when the patient rolls onto the left side (Fig. 11.20). In contrast, the ECG that shows 1.0 mm ST depression when recorded with a patient in the supine position changes to reveal 2.0 mm ST depression when the ECG is recorded with the patient on the left side (Fig. 11.21). Note that the amount of ST-segment shift is *proportional* to the ECG R wave amplitude. Thus, changes in body position influence the ST segment by altering overall ECG signal amplitude, including the height of the R wave, much the same as the gain control knob on the bedside monitor changes the R wave amplitude and the corresponding ST-segment shift (see Ch. 10, Figs. 10.13 to 10.15).

Surgical packs and retractors also may influence the ECG recording, at least in part by altering the spatial relationship between the heart and the recording electrodes. Sternal retractors used during cardiac surgery displace the precordial ECG electrode fixed to the chest wall, so that a V_5 lead position may change to resemble V_4 or V_6 more closely. Sudden changes in the precordial QRS waves and ST segments accompanying sternal retraction simply may reflect this mechanical repositioning of the precordial electrode. Furthermore, these retractors can have a marked influence on R wave amplitude and cause a proportional change in the magnitude of ST-segment deviation (Fig. 11.22).[21] Finally, the respiratory cycle may alter the recorded ECG, in part by changing cardiac axis and R wave amplitude (Figs. 11.23 and 11.24). Each of these examples serves to highlight that accurate interpretation of ST-segment shifts must take account of these mechanical influences upon the ECG. While mechanical acts (body position changes, retractor placement, respiratory cycle) may alter the ECG by reducing or amplifying the ECG R wave amplitude, causing proportional changes in the magnitude of ST deviation, these actions may influence the ECG through other mechanisms.[44] Changes in autonomic nervous system activity, ventricular volume,[3,9] myocardial perfusion, and thoracic electrical resistance may all play a role in changing the ECG recorded at the skin surface.[20,40,41]

COMPUTER-AIDED ST-SEGMENT MONITORING

Many current bedside monitors continuously measure and display the amount of ST-segment displacement in one or more leads. At the onset of the monitoring period, a baseline representative ECG complex is stored, and the amount of ST-segment elevation or depression is measured to the nearest 0.1 mm (0.01 mV or 10 μV). Very small amounts of ST-segment deviation can be measured accurately and serve as a reminder to the clinician of these ST changes before they reach clinical significance. In the example in Figure 11.25,[22] minor deviations of the ST segments in leads I, II, and V$_5$ are displayed by the monitor and confirmed by visual inspection of the ECG complexes. Note that ST elevation is displayed as a positive number (0.1 mm in lead I), and ST depression is displayed as a negative number (–0.6 mm in lead II, –0.8 mm in lead V$_5$). Although none of these ST-segment deviations have reached standard clinical threshold values for ischemia (1.0 mm), the ST segment in V$_5$ clearly is abnormal compared to the trace recorded at the beginning of the monitoring session (Fig. 11.25, top panel).

An additional feature of the ST-segment monitoring display shown here is the trend line presented to the right of the individual ECG complexes (Fig. 11.25, middle and bottom panels). The trend line illustrates that the *sum* of the ST deviations in the three monitored leads has increased progressively over the previous 10 minutes. This type of trend display presents the *sum of the absolute values* of the ST deviations, so that ST elevation (a positive value) does not cancel ST depression (a negative value). The trend line does not indicate which of the three monitored leads manifest the ST segment changes. Identical trend lines would be produced by small, 0.5 mm ST-segment displacements in all three monitored leads or a larger, 1.5 mm displace-

ment in a single monitored lead. This distinction is made by inspecting the individual ECG complexes.

Different bedside monitors employ unique technical methods for acquiring and displaying this computer-aided ST-segment information. However, all of the clinically useful monitors provide a simple ECG waveform display, which indicates the point for measurement of the ST segment and the point for measurement of the isoelectric baseline used for comparison (Fig. 11.26). This allows the clinician to confirm these ST-segment measurements visually and quickly recognize artifactual values.

In general, the ST-segment monitoring software identifies the QRS complex or the R wave in the ECG, then measures the isoelectric baseline and ST segment at predefined points relative to this identified marker. For example, a typical default measurement that uses the QRS complex would place the isoelectric point 40 msec prior to QRS onset and the ST-segment measuring point 60 msec after QRS offset (or J-point). Alternatively, an algorithm based on the R wave would place the isoelectric point 80 msec before the R wave peak and the ST-segment measuring point 108 msec after the R wave peak. In most circumstances, use of these empiric predefined measurement points will allow accurate detection of ST-segment shifts.

Occasionally, the displayed ST-segment data will be erroneous, either because the isoelectric point or the ST-segment measurement point has been identified inaccurately. For instance, the onset of isorhythmic atrioventricular dissociation or an unusually short PR interval may cause the ST-segment monitor to place the isoelectric point at the peak of the P wave, which will produce artifactual ST-segment depression relative to this spurious baseline (Fig. 11.27). Alternatively, the ST segment may not be identified properly (Fig. 11.28). When artifacts of this sort are recognized, the clinician can adjust the isoelectric or ST-segment measurement points (Fig. 11.28) so that the displayed ST-segment data regain their validity. *As emphasized throughout the text, the analog waveform serves as the primary source of information. This is just as important for ST-segment monitoring as it is for monitoring heart rate, blood pressure, or any other hemodynamic variable. Any ST-segment abnormality detected by computer-aided ST-segment monitoring must be corroborated by inspection of the analog ECG waveform.*[4,19]

Other visual aids that may assist clinical interpretation of computer-aided ST-segment monitoring include a display format that superimposes or juxtaposes current ECG complexes on top of or adjacent to a baseline ECG template. This helps the viewer identify morphologic changes by direct visual comparison of current and historic ECG complexes (Fig. 11.29).[15] In circumstances where there are ST-segment abnormalities on the baseline ECG, this superimposition display format allows rapid recognition of a change in the ST segment (Fig. 11.29) or confirms the absence of such a change (Fig. 11.30). Furthermore, changes in R wave amplitude that confound interpretation of ST-segment changes may be recognized in these direct comparison display formats (Figs. 11.31 and 11.32).

Trend displays allow a rapid review of the direction, magnitude, and duration of ST-segment changes during previous minutes or hours (Fig. 11.33). Short-lived ischemic episodes (Fig. 11.33) can be distinguished from protracted periods of ischemia (Fig. 11.34). Marked cyclic variation in ST-segment shifts are identified occasionally in the perioperative period (Fig. 11.35) and presumably reflect waxing and waning ischemia, much like the pattern described in patients experiencing coronary reocclusion after thrombolysis or angioplasty.[15,16]

ST-segment trend displays assume even greater value when these displays are accompanied by trends of other relevant hemodynamic values. Such displays integrate the data and assist the clinician in deciding whether the ischemic ST-segment shifts are associated with hemodynamic changes (Fig. 11.36) or are essentially unrelated to altered heart rate or blood pressure (Fig. 11.37), as is most often the case.[14,34,35,39]

Finally, one must recognize that pseudonormalization of a chronically depressed or elevated ST segment will be indistinguishable from true improvement toward the isoelectric baseline. As the ST segment changes from depression to elevation (Fig. 11.38), it crosses through zero (the isoelectric line), and the ST trend line appears to show *improvement* during this period, as new ST-segment abnormalities develop.

Illustrations for Myocardial Ischemia

Figure 11.1 Subendocardial ischemia produces ST-segment depression. As heart rate increases progressively from 63 beats/min (*top panel*) to 75 beats/min (*middle panel*) and finally to 86 beats/min (*bottom panel*) in this patient with left main coronary artery disease, the ST segment becomes more depressed and more downsloping, owing to an increase in myocardial oxygen demand. See text for more detail.

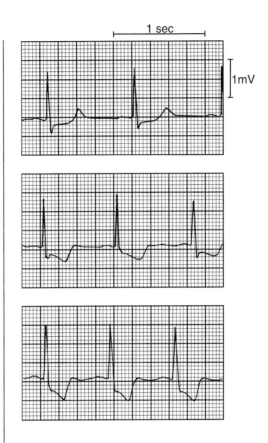

Figure 11.2 Transmural ischemia produces ST-segment elevation. Occlusion of a patent saphenous vein graft during repeat coronary artery bypass surgery causes an abrupt reduction of coronary blood supply and results in progressive ST-segment elevation (*middle and bottom panels*). See text for more detail.

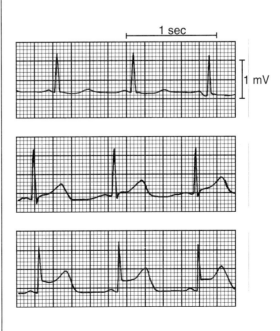

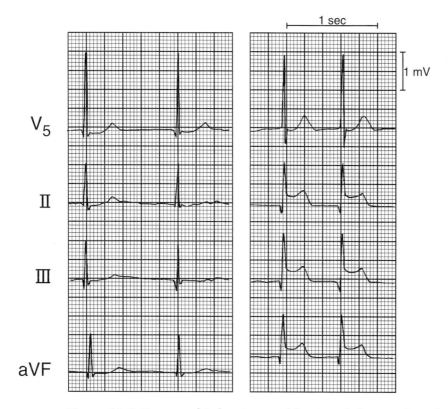

Figure 11.3 Transmural ischemia caused by air embolism to the right coronary artery. Compared to baseline ECG traces (*left panel*), sudden ST elevation isolated to ECG leads II, III, and a VF (*right panel*) suggests acute transmural ischemia of the inferior wall of the left ventricle. These traces were recorded from a 68-year-old woman who had just undergone mitral valve replacement. Air bubbles retained in the left heart chambers after this procedure commonly enter the aorta and the orifice of the right coronary artery, owing to the anterior, nondependent location of the latter. These air bubbles may occlude right coronary blood flow transiently and produce transmural ischemia of the inferior wall of the left ventricle. See text for more detail.

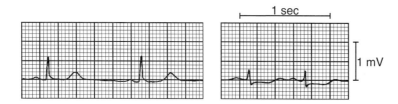

Figure 11.4 Preoperative (*left panel*) and intraoperative (*right panel*) recordings of ECG lead V_5 show different QRS morphologies. The intraoperative recording displays reduced R wave amplitude and an S wave. Whether these differences are caused by lead electrode placement or monitor gain adjustment, they confound interpretation of the 1 mm ST-segment shift seen in the intraoperative trace. However, since this ST depression is observed in association with an increase in heart rate from 59 beats/min to 97 beats/min, it likely represents subendocardial ischemia in this patient with known coronary artery disease.

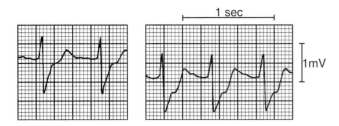

Figure 11.5 Baseline ST-segment abnormalities confound the ECG diagnosis of ischemia. The preoperative ECG trace (*left panel*) recorded from an asymptomatic patient with known coronary artery disease shows right bundle branch block and 1 mm ST-segment depression. Intraoperative recording of the same lead (*right panel*) shows 4 mm ST-segment depression associated with an increase in heart rate from 94 to 111 beats/min. Although these ST changes probably result from myocardial ischemia, the ECG diagnostic criteria are less certain in the presence of these baseline abnormalities.

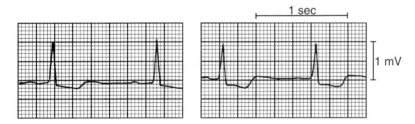

11.6 Baseline ST-segment abnormalities confound the ECG diagnosis of ischemia. At baseline (*left panel*), there is 0.5 mm ST depression, compared with 1.5 mm ST depression recorded intraoperatively (*right panel*). Is this magnitude of change diagnostic of myocardial ischemia? See text for more detail.

Figure 11.7 Myocardial ischemia manifested as pseudonormalization of chronic T wave inversion. At baseline (*top panel*), T wave inversion is present in the ECG. Intraoperative recordings show T wave flattening (*middle panel*) and then upright T waves (*bottom panel*). This pattern mimicked preoperative ECG changes that occurred each time this patient developed anginal chest pain.

Figure 11.8 Ventricular ectopic beats associated with myocardial ischemia. Intraoperative hypertension and tachycardia result in 2 mm horizontal ST depression, suggesting onset of myocardial ischemia (*top panels*). Ventricular bigeminy develops, and the ST segments become downsloping, providing further evidence of ischemia (*middle panel*). Treatment of myocardial ischemia eliminates the ventricular ectopy and improves the ST segments toward baseline values (*bottom panels*).

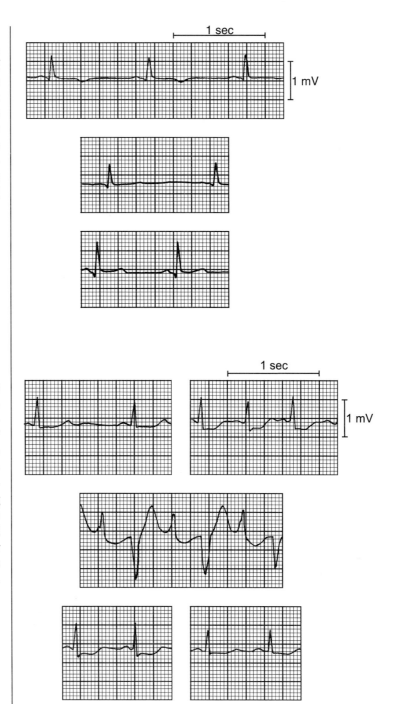

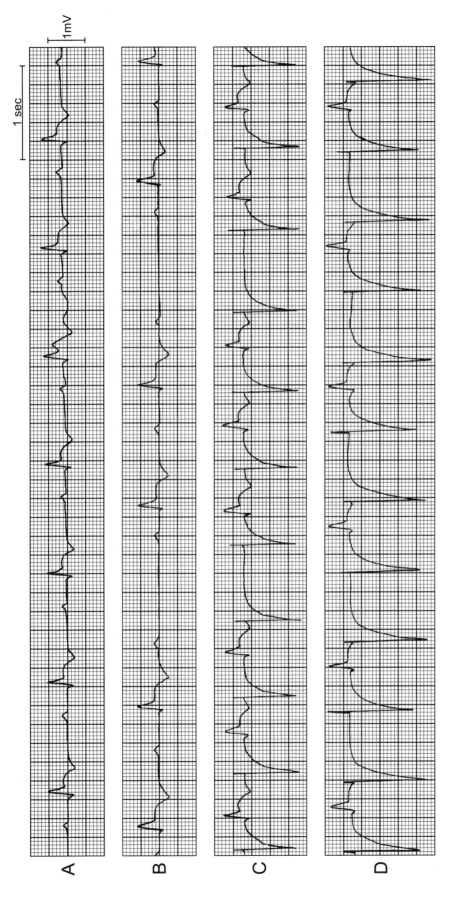

Figure 11.9 Bradycardia and atrioventricular (AV) conduction abnormalities often accompany ischemia or infarction in the distribution of the right coronary artery. Note the Q waves, ST-segment elevation, and inverted T waves in these lead II tracings, consistent with evolving inferior wall transmural infarction. (A) Bradycardia, heart rate 51 beats/min, and first-degree AV block, PR interval 340 msec. (B) Bradycardia, heart rate 40 beats/min, and second-degree AV block, Mobitz type I (Wenckebach) with 3:2 AV conduction. (C) Atrial pacing at 75 beats/min and second-degree AV block, Mobitz type I (Wenckebach) with 4:3 AV conduction. (D) Atrial pacing at 82 beats/min and second-degree AV block with 2:1 AV conduction, resulting in bradycardia, heart rate 41 beats/min. With 2:1 block, it is impossible to distinguish between Mobitz type I and II blocks.

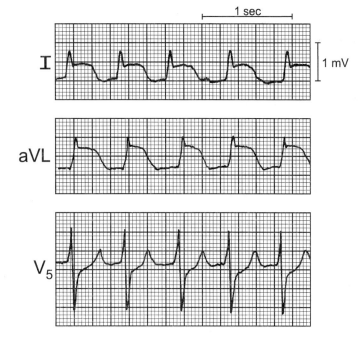

Figure 11.10 Limitations of single-lead ECG monitoring for ischemia. Lead V₅ displays rather nonspecific abnormalities consisting of 1.5 mm upsloping ST-segment depression. In contrast, there is 4 to 5 mm ST-segment elevation in leads I and aVL, consistent with acute transmural ischemia of the lateral wall of the left ventricle. Isolated ST-segment changes confined to lateral leads I and aVL are uncommon in the intraoperative setting.

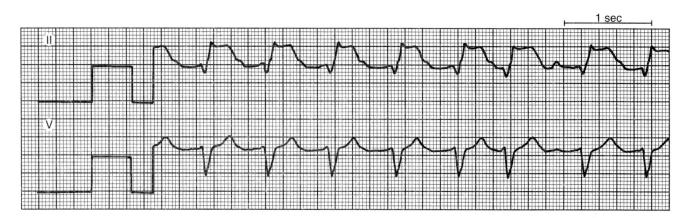

Figure 11.11 Limitations of single-lead ECG monitoring for ischemia. Inferior wall transmural ischemia manifested as 5 mm ST-segment elevation in lead II occurs coincident with nearly isoelectric ST segments in lead V₅. These ECG changes occurred after cardiopulmonary bypass in a patient who underwent repair of an atrial septal defect complicated by repeated episodes of ventricular fibrillation. Both the ventricular fibrillation and the ST-segment changes in lead II resulted from air embolism to the right coronary artery, owing to incomplete evacuation of residual air bubbles from the left side of the heart prior to the end of bypass. Also see Fig. 11.3. See text for more detail.

Figure 11.12 Limitations of single precordial lead ECG monitoring for ischemia. Following coronary artery bypass surgery, a postoperative 12-lead ECG recording demonstrates ST-segment elevation in leads V_2 (3 mm) and V_3 (5 mm), suggesting anterior wall transmural ischemia. The only precordial ECG lead available intraoperatively was lead V_5, which showed less than 1 mm ST-segment elevation and was not considered diagnostic for ischemia.

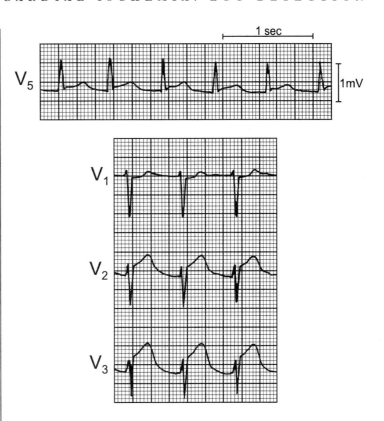

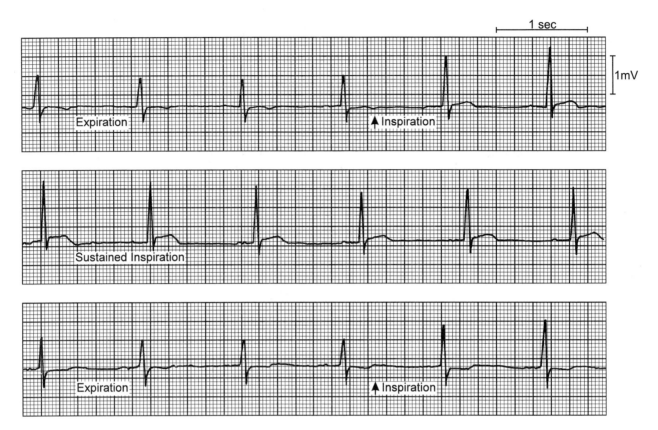

Figure 11.13 Limitations of single precordial lead ECG monitoring for ischemia. Lead V₅ is monitored in this unusual intraoperative example of myocardial ischemia detected during positive pressure mechanical ventilation. ST-segment elevation is not evident until onset of inspiration, when the lead V₅ recording shows an increase in R wave amplitude and 1 mm ST elevation (*top panel*). When inspiration is sustained for 6 seconds, the taller R waves and the ST-segment abnormality are clear (*middle panel*). After treatment for myocardial ischemia, a different ECG pattern is evident (*bottom panel*). Inspiration still increases lead V₅ R wave amplitude, but the associated ST-segment elevation is no longer present. See text for more detail.

Figure 11.14 Importance of proper lead electrode attachment. Preoperative ECG limb lead recording (*top ECG panels*) shows inferior Q waves and an axis of + 102 degrees. The initial intraoperative recording (*bottom ECG panels*) shows new left axis deviation (–36 degrees), and evidence for inferior wall infarction has disappeared! Unintentional switching of left arm and left leg lead electrodes caused this problem. Note that *preoperative* recordings of leads I and II are identical to *intraoperative* recordings of leads II and I, respectively. Furthermore, the preoperative recording of lead III is inverted compared to the intraoperative recording of this same lead. The diagram of Einthoven's triangle shown below the ECG traces helps explain how this lead switch produced the ECG changes recorded.

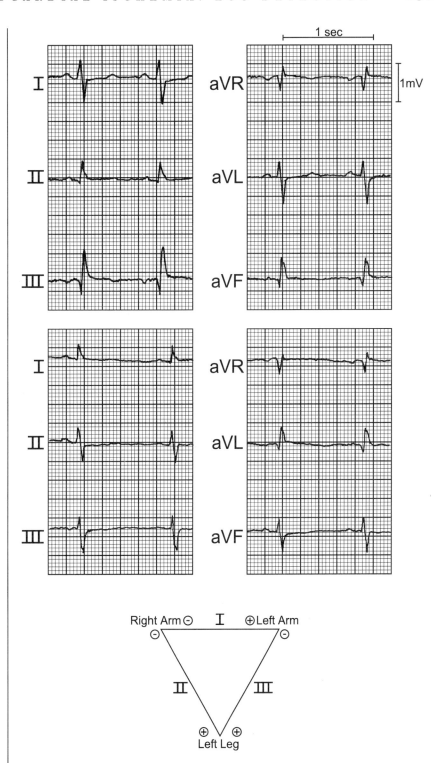

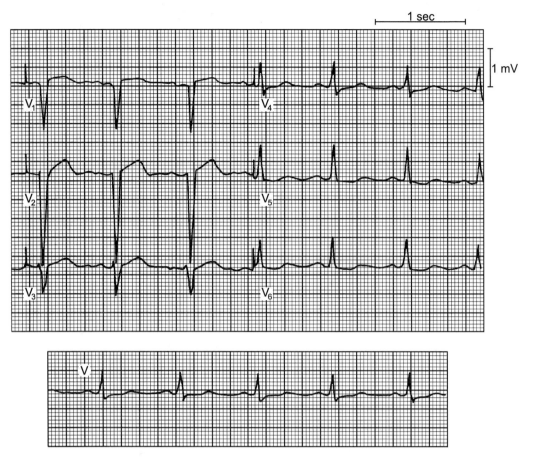

Figure 11.15 Intraoperative precordial lead electrode placement should provide a lead V₅ trace similar to that seen on the preoperative 12-lead recording (*top panel*). The intra-operative V lead trace (*bottom panel*) is intended as a V₅ lead but more closely resembles lead V₄ in terms of R wave amplitude and QRS morphology.

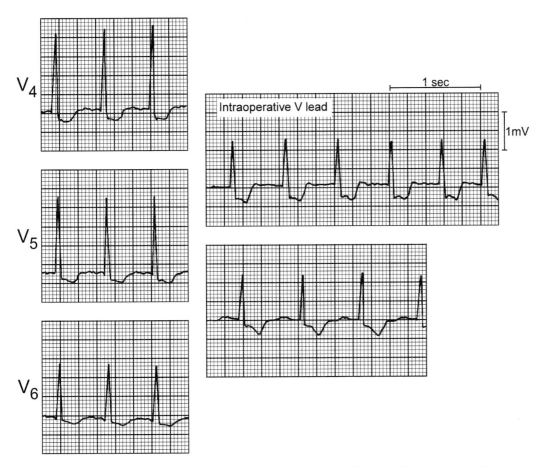

Figure 11.16 Importance of intraoperative precordial lead electrode placement. The initial intraoperative V lead recording displays a 12 mm R wave and a 3.5 mm ST-segment depression (*upper right panel*). This initial V lead trace does not resemble any of the precordial leads on the preoperative 12-lead ECG recording, including antero-lateral leads V₄, V₅, or V₆ (*left panels*). In terms of R wave amplitude, the intraoperative V lead trace most resembles preoperative lead V₆, although the ST depression is much greater in the initial intraoperative trace. The patient whose ECG traces are illustrated here arrived in the operating room for coronary artery surgery anxious, hypertensive, and tachycardic, with a heart rate of 107 beats/min. Reduction in heart rate and blood pressure associated with induction of general anesthesia produced marked improvement in the ST-segment depression (*lower right panel*). This example emphasizes the importance of comparing the initial monitored ECG traces with baseline preoperative 12-lead recordings.

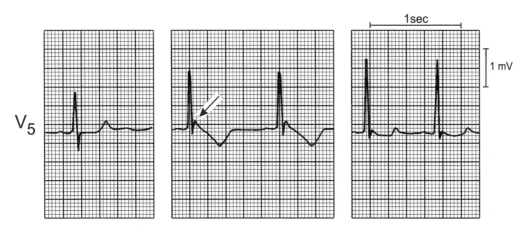

Figure 11.17 Hypothermia produces ECG changes that may be confused with myocardial ischemia. The Osborne wave appears as J-point elevation (*arrow*). See text for more detail.

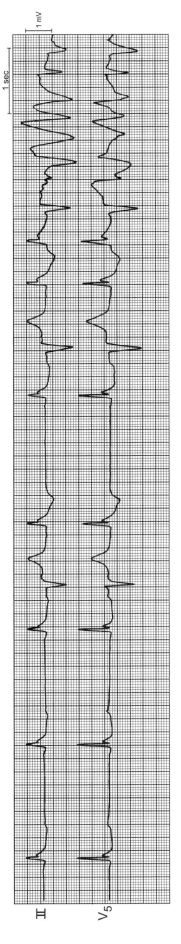

Figure 11.18 ECG changes during hypothermia. Bradycardia with Osborne waves, or J-waves, ventricular ectopic beats, and ventricular fibrillation appear in rapid succession during onset of cooling associated with the initiation of cardiopulmonary bypass. At the time these traces were recorded, bladder temperature was 35.8°C and nasopharyngeal temperature was 31.4°C. Presumably, aortic blood and myocardial temperatures were even cooler than the nasopharyngeal temperature, as a result of rapid core cooling produced by the bypass pump through the arterial inflow cannula placed in the ascending aorta.

Figure 11.19 Unintentional cardiac hypothermia during extrapleural pneumonectomy. A 1-hour trend recording of ST-segment deviations, displayed as millimeters of ST displacement in lead II, illustrates the ECG changes during this event (*top panel*). Irrigation of the surgical field with room temperature saline (*thin arrow*) causes sudden cooling of the heart and results in transient but striking 4 mm ST-segment elevation in lead II (*thick arrow*), which improves over 10 minutes. These ST-segment abnormalities are seen in multiple leads (*bottom panel*). Note also the two brief periods in the ST-segment trend recording (*top panel*) where artifacts interrupt the recording and appear as sudden 6 mm ST depression.

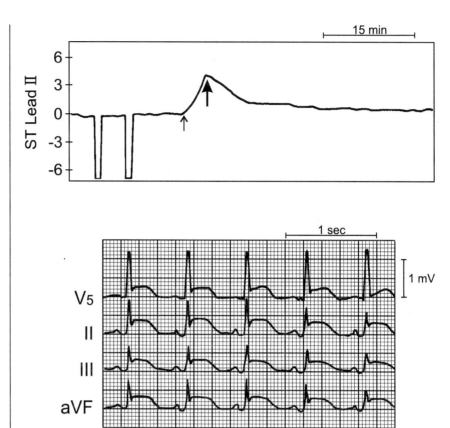

Figure 11.20 Effect of changing body position on the ECG in a patient without preexisting ST-segment abnormalities. Lead CC$_5$, a bipolar lead surrogate for unipolar lead V$_5$, is recorded with the patient in four different positions: supine, standing, right (R) side down, and left (L) side down. Despite changes in R and T wave amplitudes, the ST segments remain isoelectric. Compare with Fig. 11.21. See text for more detail.

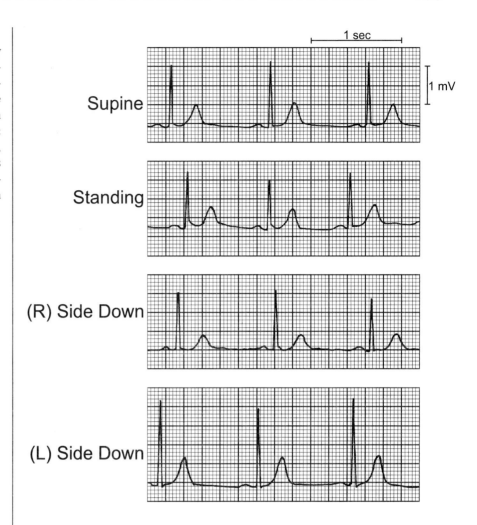

Figure 11.21 Effect of changing body position on the ECG in a patient with preexisting ST-segment depression. Lead CC$_5$, a bipolar lead surrogate for unipolar lead V$_5$, is recorded with the patient in four different positions: supine, standing, right (R) side down, and left (L) side down. The magnitude of ST-segment depression changes in direct proportion to the R wave amplitude. Compare with Fig. 11.20. See text for more detail.

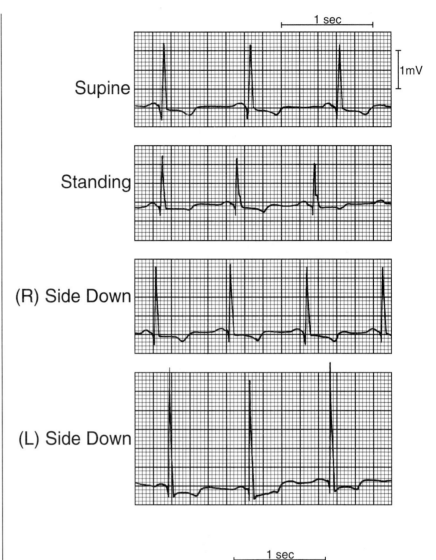

Figure 11.22 Effect of surgical retraction on the ECG. Baseline lead V$_5$ recording shows 2 mm ST-segment depression and 27 mm R wave amplitude (*top panel*). Placement of a sternal retractor during cardiac surgery displaces the precordial lead electrode relative to the heart, resulting in a marked reduction in R wave amplitude to 10 mm and a proportional reduction in the magnitude of ST-segment displacement (*bottom panel*). (Modified from Mark et al,[21] with permission.)

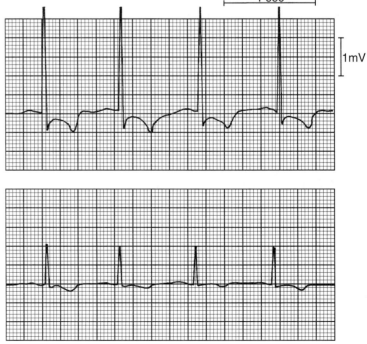

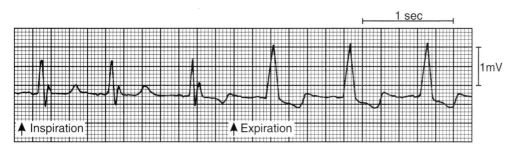

Figure 11.23 Effect of the respiratory cycle on the ECG. Recorded from a 79-year-old patient with aortic stenosis, this lead V_5 ECG trace shows left bundle branch block and a marked change in morphology over the respiratory cycle while the patient's lungs are mechanically ventilated. These changes confound interpretation of the ECG. See text for more detail.

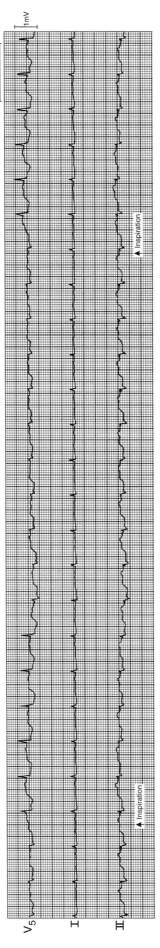

Figure 11.24 Effect of the respiratory cycle on the ECG. This tracing is recorded from a 51-year-old woman undergoing repeat coronary artery bypass surgery. During the inspiratory phase of positive pressure mechanical ventilation, lead V_5 morphology changes significantly, although the respiratory cycle has little effect on limb leads I and II. See text for more detail.

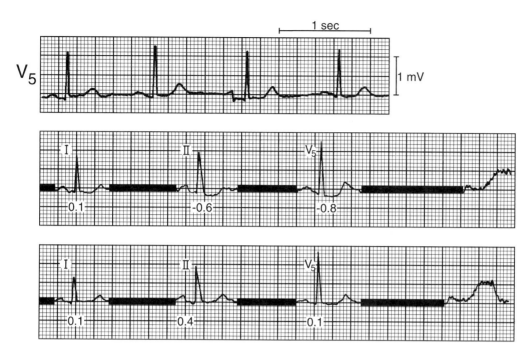

Figure 11.25 Computer-aided continuous ST-segment monitoring. A baseline recording of lead V₅ shows isoelectric ST segments (*top panel*). Shortly after induction of anesthesia, the ST-segment monitoring display shows the three monitored leads I, II, and V₅ and the absolute amount of ST-segment elevation (0.1 mm in lead I) or depression (–0.6 mm in lead II, –0.8 mm in lead V₅) in each lead (*middle panel*). A trend line is displayed on the right side of the panel and demonstrates that the sum of ST-segment deviations in these three monitored leads has increased and reached a plateau over the previous few minutes. Another ST-segment display recorded 5 minutes later shows resolution of these subtle ST changes (*bottom panel*). Note that the appearance of lead V₅ in this last display closely resembles the baseline recording and that the trend line has returned to an isoelectric baseline. See text for more detail. (Modified from Mark,[22] with permission.)

Figure 11.26 Enlarged display of ECG lead V, showing the isoelectric (ISO) and ST-segment (ST) measurement points during continuous computer-aided ST-segment monitoring. The ECG R and T waves are also identified. This V lead ECG complex is shown at standard gain (10 mm/mV) in the upper right corner of the panel. The computer measures and displays 0.1 mm of ST-segment elevation in this lead.

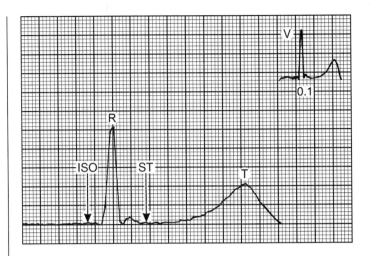

Figure 11.27 Erroneous identification of the isoelectric (ISO) measurement point during computer-aided continuous ST-segment monitoring. A 1 hour trend recording of ST-segment deviations in lead II, displayed as millimeters of ST displacement, shows approximately 15 minutes of ST-segment depression, which reaches 3 mm in magnitude during this episode (*top panel*). The enlarged display of ECG lead II showing the isoelectric (ISO) and ST-segment (ST) measurement points during the episode of ST-segment depression reveals that the ISO point is placed inappropriately at the peak of the P wave, thereby producing artifactual ST-segment depression (*bottom panel*). This episode of artifactual ST-segment depression is caused by isorhythmic atrioventricular dissociation, as evidenced by the short PR interval that develops when the P wave merges with the QRS complex.

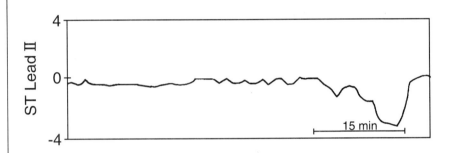

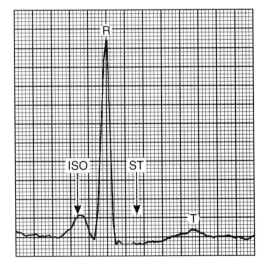

Figure 11.28 Erroneous identification of the ST-segment (ST) measurement point during computer-aided continuous ST-segment monitoring. Atrial pacing provides a challenge to the monitoring computer, since the pacing signal (A spike) is large and easily confused with the QRS complex. Initially, the monitor places the isoelectric (ISO) and ST measurement points before and after the A spike rather than the QRS complex (*top panel*). As a result, the computer measures and reports artifactual 1.6 mm ST-segment elevation in lead V (*top panel*). By adjusting the ST measurement point to fall 60 msec after the QRS complex, a better estimate of ST-segment deviation is monitored (*bottom panel*), and the monitor now displays minor ST-segment depression (–0.2 mm). Note that the ISO point is not placed in its normal position in the PQ segment in this example but instead is located in the TP segment, prior to inscription of the A spike. In this case, placement of the ISO point between the A spike and the QRS would be an inappropriate isoelectric baseline owing to the repolarization abnormality following the tall A spike. Instead, use of the TP segment as the isoelectric baseline is preferred, since the TP and PQ segments should be horizontal and collinear.[12]

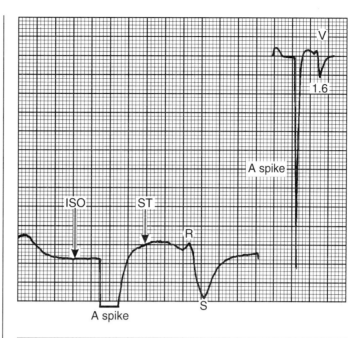

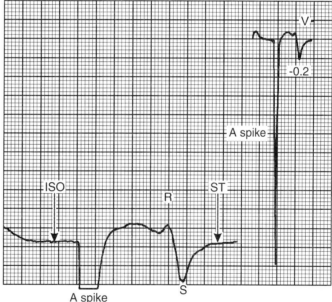

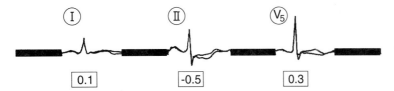

Figure 11.29 Superimposition display format for computer-aided continuous ST-segment monitoring. By overlaying current ECG complexes from leads I, II, and V₅ on top of those recorded at initiation of monitoring, subtle morphologic changes in the ST segments and T waves may be appreciated. In this example, lead I is unchanged (0.1 mm ST elevation), while there is improvement in lead II and lead V₅ (currently, –0.5 mm ST depression and 0.3 mm ST elevation, respectively). This type of superimposition display format is seen much more easily on the monitor screen than shown here in a black and white illustration, since the monitor screen can present the current ECG complexes in a different color or line intensity to distinguish them from the underlying baseline ECG complexes.

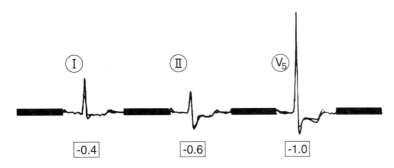

Figure 11.30 Superimposition display format for computer-aided continuous ST-segment monitoring. Current ECG complexes show no significant change in the magnitude of ST-segment depression compared to the ECG recorded at baseline, hours earlier (–0.4 mm in lead I, –0.6 mm in lead II, and –1.0 mm in lead V₅).

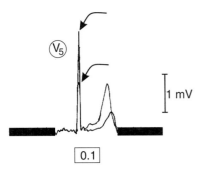

Figure 11.31 Superimposition display format for computer-aided continuous ST-segment monitoring allows rapid recognition of confounding R wave amplitude changes. The current lead V₅ complex is nearly isoelectric (0.1 mm ST elevation) in contrast to the baseline complex, which demonstrated 1.5 mm ST-segment elevation. However, the current ECG R wave is only half of its baseline amplitude (13 vs. 26 mm) (*arrows*). This change confounds interpretation of the apparent ST-segment improvement. Compare with Fig. 11.32. See text for more detail.

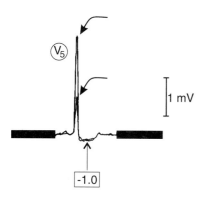

Figure 11.32 Superimposition display format for computer-aided continuous ST-segment monitoring allows rapid recognition of confounding R wave amplitude changes. The current lead V₅ complex shows the same amount of ST-segment depression (−1.0 mm, *vertical arrow*) as seen at baseline, despite the fact that the R wave amplitude has decreased from 26 to 10 mm (*curved arrows*). In the face of a much smaller R wave, might this unchanged 1 mm ST depression indicate a greater degree of myocardial ischemia? Compare with Fig. 11.31. See text for more detail.

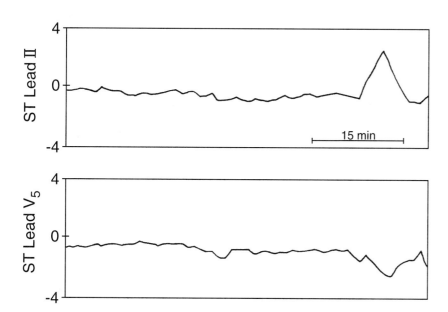

Figure 11.33 One-hour trend displays for computer-aided continuous ST-segment monitoring in leads II and V₅. The magnitude of ST-segment depression (0 to −4 mm) or elevation (0 to 4 mm) is plotted against time. A brief ischemic episode consisting of ST elevation in lead II and ST depression in lead V₅ occurs near the end of the monitoring period. Compare with Fig. 11.34.

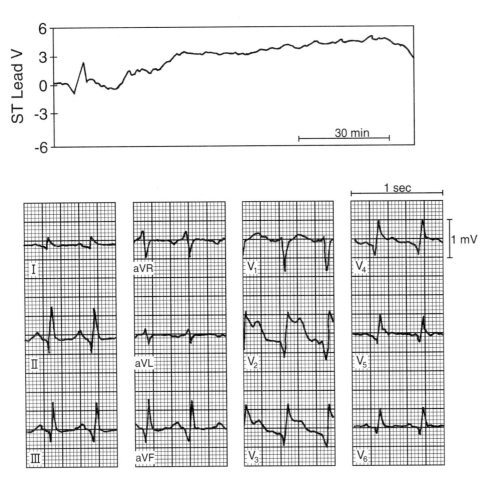

Figure 11.34 Two-hour trend display for computer-aided continuous ST-segment monitoring in lead V showing persistent 4 mm ST-segment elevation (*top panel*). A 12-lead ECG recorded at the end of the monitoring period confirms the presence of anterior wall transmural ischemia. These traces were recorded from a 65-year-old woman undergoing coronary artery bypass surgery, in whom attempts at aortic cannulation produced arterial dissection leading to occlusion of the left main coronary artery. Compare with Fig. 11.33.

Figure 11.35 One-hour trend display for computer-aided continuous ST-segment monitoring in lead V showing cyclic variation in the ST segments (*top panel*). These ST-segment changes are large in magnitude and occur rapidly. Electrocardiographic complexes recorded at time points A and B confirm the nonartifactual nature of this unusual pattern. At point A, lead V displays marked ST-segment elevation (2.9 mm), and at point B, this same lead displays ST-segment depression (−0.8 mm). See text for more detail.

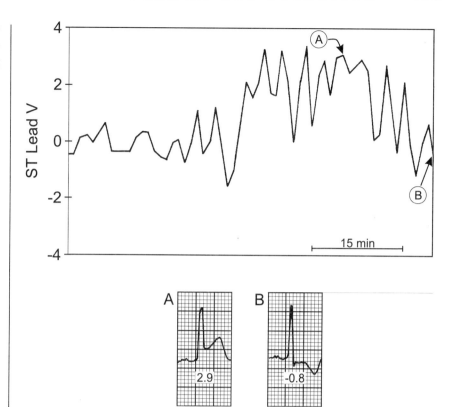

Figure 11.36 One-hour trend displays for computer-aided continuous ST-segment monitoring in lead V₅ and heart rate (HR, beats/min). A 15-minute episode of worsened ST-segment depression occurs at the same time that HR increases from 65 to 105 beats/min (*arrows*). Compare with Fig. 11.37.

Figure 11.37 One-hour trend displays for computer-aided continuous ST-segment monitoring in lead V₅, heart rate (HR, beats/min), and mean arterial pressure (MAP, mmHg). A 15-minute episode of ST-segment depression (*arrows*) occurs without significant accompanying changes in HR or MAP. These trends were recorded from a 40-year-old man during coronary artery bypass surgery and highlight the fact that most episodes of perioperative myocardial ischemia occur without any clear change in hemodynamic variables. Compare with Fig. 11.36.

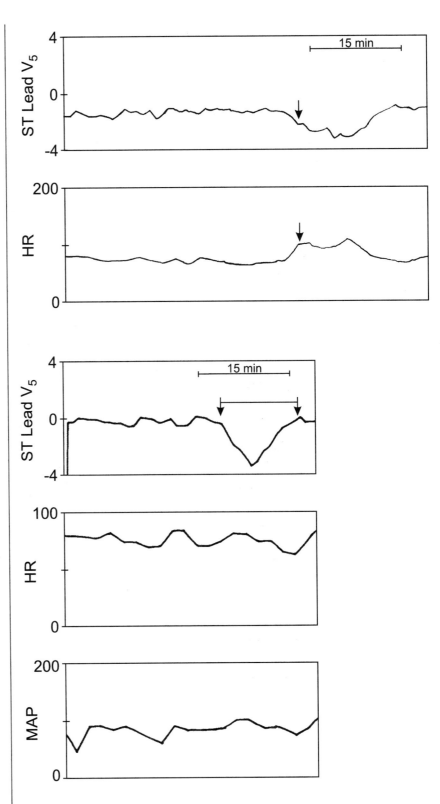

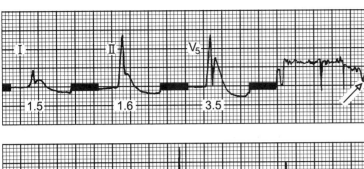

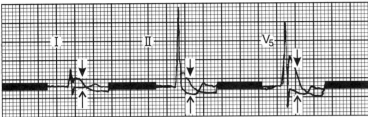

Figure 11.38 Pseudonormalization of ST-segment depression during computer-aided continuous ST-segment monitoring. All three ECG leads display ST-segment elevation at the present time (1.5 mm in lead I, 1.6 mm in lead II, and 3.5 mm in lead V₅) (*top panel*). The ST-segment trend line shows apparent transient improvement in the ST deviations (*open arrow, top panel*) followed by deterioration away from the isoelectric baseline. A superimposition display (*bottom panel*) compares the current ECG complexes with those recorded at baseline. Note that the initial ECG complexes displayed ST-segment depression, particularly in leads II and V₅ (*up arrows, bottom panel*), whereas the current ECG complexes display ST-segment elevation (*down arrows, bottom panel*). As the ST-segments shift from depression to elevation, they cross the isoelectric baseline, thereby giving the false impression of improvement seen in the ST-segment trend (*open arrow, top panel*).

References

1. Anderson HV, Willerson JT. Thrombolysis in acute myocardial infarction. N Engl J Med 1993;329:703–9

2. Breslow MJ, Miller CF, Parker SD, et al. Changes in T-wave morphology following anesthesia and surgery: a common recovery-room phenomenon. Anesthesiology 1986;64:398–402

3. Brody DA. A theoretical analysis of intracavitary blood mass influence on the heart-lead relationship. Circ Res 1956;4:731–8

4. Brooker S, Lowenstein E. Spurious ST segment depression by automated ST segment analysis. J Clin Monit 1995;11:186–8

5. Buxton AE, Goldberg S, Harken A, et al. Coronary-artery spasm immediately after myocardial revascularization. Recognition and management. N Engl J Med 1981;304:1249–53

6. Caspi Y, Safadi T, Ammar R, et al. The significance of bundle branch block in the immediate postoperative electrocardiograms of patients undergoing coronary artery bypass. J Thorac Cardiovasc Surg 1987;93:442–6

7. Diamond GA, Forrester JS. Analysis of probability as an aid in the clinical diagnosis of coronary-artery disease. N Engl J Med 1979;300:1350–8

8. Eisenach JC, Tuttle R, Stein A. Is ST segment depression of the electrocardiogram during cesarean section merely due to cardiac sympathetic block? Anesth Analg 1994;78:287–92

9. Ellestad MH. The mechanism of exercise-induced R-wave amplitude changes in coronary heart disease. Still controversial. Arch Intern Med 1982;142:963–5

10. Fisch C. Electrocardiography and vectorcardiography. In: Braunwald E, ed. Heart Disease. A Textbook of Cardiovascular Medicine (4th ed). Philadelphia: WB Saunders, 1992:116–60

11. Hammill SC, Khandheria BK. Silent myocardial ischemia. Mayo Clin Proc 1990;65:374–83

12. Holland RP, Brooks H. TQ-ST segment mapping: critical review and analysis of current concepts. Am J Cardiol 1977;40:110–29

13. Kligfield P, Okin PM. Evolution of the exercise electrocardiogram. Am J Cardiol 1994;78:1209–10

14. Knight AA, Hollenberg M, London MJ, et al. Perioperative myocardial ischemia: importance of the preoperative ischemic pattern. Anesthesiology 1988;68:681–88

15. Krucoff MW: Electrocardiographic monitoring and coronary occlusion. Fingerprint pattern analysis in dimensions of space, time, and mind. J Electrocardiol 1989;22(Suppl):232–7

16. Krucoff MW, Croll MA, Pope JE, et al. Continuously updated 12-lead ST-segment recovery analysis for myocardial infarct artery patency assessment and its correlation with multiple simultaneous early angiographic observations. Am J Cardiol 1993;71:145–51

17. Lachman AB, Semler HJ, Gustafson RH. Postural ST-T wave changes in the radioelectrocardiogram simulating myocardial ischemia. Circulation 1965;31:557–63

18. London MJ, Hollenberg M, Wong MC et al: Intraoperative myocardial ischemia: localization by continuous 12-lead electrocardiography. Anesthesiology 1988;69:232-41

19. London MJ, Ahlstrom LD. Validation testing of the SpaceLabs PC2 ST-segment analyzer. J Cardiothorac Vasc Anesth 1995;9:684–93

20. Manger D, Lightly GW, Camporesi EM. Electrocardiographic changes associated with the prone position. J Clin Monit 1992;8:92–3

21. Mark JB, Chien GL, Steinbrook RA, Fenton T. Electrocardiographic R-wave changes during cardiac surgery. Anesth Analg 1992;74:26–31

22. Mark JB. Anesthesia for cardiac surgery. In: Lee RT, Lee TH, Peigh PS, eds. Overview of Cardiac Surgery for the Cardiologist. New York: Springer-Verlag, 1994;1–17

23. Marriott HJL. Practical Electrocariography (4th ed). Baltimore: Williams and Wilkins, xiii, 1968

24. McLintic AJ, Pringle SD, Lilley S, et al. Electrocardiographic changes during cesarean section under regional anesthesia. Anesth Analg 1992;74:51–6

25. Noble RJ, Rothbaum DA, Knoebel SB, et al. Normalization of abnormal T waves in ischemia. Arch Intern Med 1976;136:391–5

26. Okin PM, Bergman G, Kligfield P. Effect of ST segment measurement point on performance of standard and heart rate-adjusted ST segment criteria for the identification of coronary artery disease. Circulation 1991;84:57–66

27. Pires LA, Wagshal AB, Lancey R, Huang SKS. Arrhythmias and conduction disturbances after coronary artery bypass graft surgery: epidemiology, management, and prognosis. Am Heart J 1995;129:799–808

28. Rifkin RD, Hood WB. Bayesian analysis of electrocardiographic exercise stress testing. N Engl J Med 1977;297:681–6

29. Selzer A, Langston M, Ruggeroli C, Cohn K. Clinical syndrome of variant angina with normal coronary arteriogram. N Engl J Med 1976;295:1343–7

30. Selzer A. Cardiac ischemic pain in patients with normal coronary arteriograms. Am J Med 1977;63:661–5

31. Sgarbossa EB, Pinski SL, Barbagelata A, et al. Electrocardiographic diagnosis of evolving acute myocardial infarction in the presence of left bundle-branch block. N Engl J Med 1996;334:481–7

32. Sheffield LT. Upsloping ST segments. Easy to measure, hard to agree upon. Circulation 1991;84:426–8

33. Shub C. Stable angina pectoris: 2. Cardiac evaluation and diagnostic testing. Mayo Clin Proc 1990;65:243–55

34. Slogoff S, Keats AS: Does perioperative myocardial ischemia lead to postoperative myocardial infarction? Anesthesiology 1985;62:107-14

35. Slogoff S, Keats AS: Further observations on perioperative myocardial ischemia. Anesthesiology 1986;65:539-42

36. Slogoff S, Keats AS, David Y, Igo SR. Incidence of perioperative myocardial ischemia detected by different electrocardiographic systems. Anesthesiology 1990;73:1074-81

37. Slogoff S, Keats AS. How best to monitor for detection of myocardial ischemia? Anesthesiology 1991;74:1172

38. Smith JS, Cahalan MK, Benefiel DJ, et al. Intraoperative detection of myocardial ischemia in high-risk patients. Circulation 1985;72:1015-21

39. Smith H, Nathan H, Harrison M. Failure to predict intraoperative myocardial ischaemia in patients with coronary artery disease. Can J Anaesth 1989;36:539–44

40. Steinbrook RA, Goldman DB, Mark JB, et al. How best to monitor for detection of myocardial ischemia? Anesthesiology 1991;74:1171-2

41. Sutherland DJ, McPherson DD, Spencer CA, et al. Effects of posture and respiration on body surface electrocardiogram. Am J Cardiol 1983;52:595–600

42. Toyama J, Okada A, Nagata Y, et al. Electrocardiographic changes in pulmonary emphysema: effects of experimentally induced over-inflation of the lungs on QRS complexes. Am Heart J 1974;87:606–13

43. Wagner GS. Ischemia due to increased myocardial demand. In: Wagner GS, ed. Marriott's Practical Electrocardiography (9th ed.) Baltimore: Williams & Wilkins, 1994:121–35

44. Wagner GS. Ischemia due to insufficient blood supply. In: Wagner GS, ed. Marriott's Practical Electrocardiography (9th ed). Baltimore: Williams & Wilkins, 1994:137–51

45. Wang LTS, Milne B, Knight J. Electrocardiographic ST segment changes associated with the inspiratory phase of positive-pressure ventilation after myocardial revascularization. J Cardiothorac Vasc Anesth 1992;6:62–4

CHAPTER TWELVE Myocardial Ischemia

HEMODYNAMIC DETECTION

PULMONARY ARTERY CATHETER DETECTION OF ISCHEMIA: BACKGROUND

During the 1980s, perioperative myocardial ischemia was identified as an important predictor of adverse cardiac events.[23,27–29,35,42,43] Most investigators and clinicians based the diagnosis of ischemia on electrocardiographic signs, particularly ST-segment depression, because this had been the standard method used in coronary care units and during exercise stress testing. Notably in these studies, perioperative myocardial ischemia was clearly associated with significant morbidity or mortality, in contrast to ischemia observed in the controlled setting of exercise stress testing.[6] Consequently, attempts to reduce perioperative cardiac morbidity focused on finding alternative, more sensitive methods for detecting perioperative myocardial ischemia, including the use of the pulmonary artery catheter in selected high-risk patients.[1,19,20,37,38,40] How might the pulmonary artery catheter provide an early clue to the development of myocardial ischemia?

DIASTOLIC DYSFUNCTION: ELEVATED WEDGE PRESSURE, PROMINENT a WAVE

Myocardial ischemia is accompanied by a number of physiologic abnormalities, some of which are detectable with the pulmonary artery catheter. Ischemia impairs or delays left ventricular relaxation.[49] This *diastolic dysfunction is particularly characteristic of demand ischemia* associated with tachycardia or induced by rapid atrial pacing.[4,8,9,15,33,49]

Impaired ventricular relaxation results in a stiffer, less compliant left ventricle in diastole, causing left ventricular end-diastolic pressure (LVEDP) to rise. Not only does this increased LVEDP lead to an elevation in left atrial pressure and pulmonary artery wedge pressure (PAWP), but the *morphology of the PAWP trace becomes abnormal.* Although abnormalities of the wedge pressure waveform in myocardial ischemia have been emphasized by a number of investigators,[16,19,20,36] this important point seems to have gone largely unnoticed by many clinicians. Myocardial ischemia causes an increase in mean PAWP,[1,47] and the phasic a and v wave components become more prominent as diastolic filling pressure rises.[19,20] In the example in Figure 12.1, onset of myocardial ischemia causes doubling of the mean wedge pressure (10 to 23 mmHg), accompanied by a change in waveform morphology, with prominent a and v waves now present. Despite these changes in wedge pressure, note that the ECG is unchanged (although the ST segments are difficult to interpret, owing to baseline ST-T wave abnormalities). In the example in Figure 12.2, ischemia causes a smaller relative change in mean wedge pressure (17 to 26 mmHg), but again, prominent a and v

waves are clearly seen. Although myocardial ischemia will often be detectable as a rise in pulmonary artery pressure (diastolic, mean, or even systolic pressure), these changes are generally less striking than the accompanying change in wedge pressure and the appearance of tall a and v waves in the wedge pressure trace (Fig. 12.3).

A striking feature of the PAWP trace in patients with myocardial ischemia is the *prominent a wave* (Fig. 12.4). Recall that the a wave arises from atrial contraction at end-diastole. This atrial kick or booster pump mechanism is particularly important in patients with left ventricular diastolic dysfunction caused by myocardial ischemia. In these patients, left atrial contraction at end-diastole provides a larger than normal contribution to left ventricular filling.[12,36,45] Since the atrial contraction is confined to the end of diastole, it ensures adequate left ventricular end-diastolic pressure and volume, yet mean left ventricular diastolic filling pressure can remain at a lower level. Adequate left ventricular preload is established, while at the same time, mean left atrial pressure does not need to rise to the level where cardiogenic pulmonary edema would develop. Consequently, patients with ischemia-induced left ventricular diastolic dysfunction have a prominent PAWP a wave, reflecting this end-diastolic atrial contraction into a stiff, incompletely relaxed left ventricle (Fig. 12.3 to 12.5).

A corollary to this observation is that LVEDP is *underestimated* by the mean wedge pressure or pulmonary artery diastolic pressure in patients with ischemia-related left ventricular diastolic dysfunction.[12,36] However, the wedge pressure a wave peak pressure provides a good estimate for LVEDP, since this measurement accounts for the added filling provided by atrial contraction.[12,36] (See Ch. 6, Figs. 6.2 to 6.6, for further discussion of the relation between PAWP and LVEDP in patients with diastolic dysfunction.)

Recognizing that prominent PAWP a waves are present in patients with ischemic left ventricular dysfunction provides a useful insight to a common but confusing observation made during cardiac catheterization. Figure 12.6 displays the preliminary catheterization report from the patient whose hemodynamic traces are shown in Figure 12.5. This patient has severe coronary artery disease, including occlusion of previously placed coronary artery bypass grafts. Despite anterior wall hypokinesia, his *overall systolic function is preserved* (ejection fraction of 72 percent), and the measured and calculated hemodynamic values are mostly normal. Note, however, that the *wedge pressure (mean 7 mmHg) is lower than the LVEDP (15 mmHg).* How can this be? The answer lies with the atrial kick and the prominent wedge pressure a wave. In a patient such as this one, who manifests left ventricular diastolic dysfunction, the PAWP a wave peak pressure (15 mmHg) is the best predictor of

LVEDP (15 mmHg). (See Ch. 6, Figs. 6.1 and 6.5 for a more complete discussion of the relation between wedge pressure and LVEDP.)

A PAWP trace displaying prominent a and v waves may be suspected by observing the unwedged pulmonary artery pressure (PAP) trace (Fig. 12.7) (see also Ch. 4, Figs. 4.9 to 4.11). The tall a wave will distort the systolic upstroke, and the tall v wave will obscure the dicrotic notch of the PAP trace. Thus, the first clue to the presence of myocardial ischemia might be seen in the unwedged, but continuously monitored PAP trace. PAP will be elevated, and its normal morphology will be distorted by the prominent a and v waves reflected back from the left atrium (Figs. 12.3 to 12.5 and 12.7).

Although the hallmark of left ventricular diastolic dysfunction is an elevated LVEDP, this *pressure elevation* generally accompanies *reduced left ventricular end-diastolic volume*.[8,9] Ventricular compliance is decreased in this situation, and the clinician must realize that the elevated pulmonary artery diastolic or wedge pressure does not indicate increased left ventricular preload. Therapy must be directed at the underlying myocardial ischemia, rather than toward reducing left ventricular volume by using a diuretic, which may further decrease left ventricular diastolic filling.

SYSTOLIC DYSFUNCTION: PROMINENT v WAVE

Myocardial ischemia produces a characteristic pattern of left ventricular systolic dysfunction in addition to the diastolic abnormalities noted above. *Systolic dysfunction is the hallmark of supply ischemia*, caused by a sudden reduction or cessation of coronary blood flow to a region of the myocardium.[15,52] For example, balloon inflation during coronary angioplasty induces transient, focal, transmural ischemia, and the affected region of the myocardium rapidly develops abnormal systolic wall motion.[17,52] During episodes of perioperative myocardial ischemia, this systolic dysfunction is detected readily by transesophageal echocardiography[22,44,47] and is manifested by loss of normal systolic thickening of the myocardium and hypokinetic, akinetic, or dyskinetic wall motion.

If this systolic dysfunction is severe enough, changes in global left ventricular pump performance may be detected with hemodynamic monitoring. As ejection fraction falls, left ventricular end-diastolic volume and pressure will rise. This situation is characterized by the combination of systemic arterial hypotension and elevated pulmonary artery diastolic and wedge pressures (Fig. 12.8). This hemodynamic pattern is uncommon during anesthesia and surgery[24,42,43] and suggests severe systolic myocardial dysfunction.

A different situation arises when left ventricular geometry is distorted[39] or when the region of ischemic myocardium overlies a papillary muscle. Acute mitral valve regurgitation may result, not because of any inherent abnormality of the mitral valve leaflets, but rather because of critical alterations in the supporting structures of the mitral valve. These include the mitral annulus, chordae tendinae, papillary muscles, and underlying left ventricular myocardium (Fig. 12.9). Left ventricular systolic dysfunction, which leads to an increase in ventricular volume, may distort the mitral valve annulus, resulting in failure of leaflet coaptation during systole and valvular regurgitation (Fig. 12.9B). In addition, failure of normal systolic inward motion of regions of the left ventricle underlying either papillary muscle may tether the papillary muscle and its chordal attachments to one or both mitral leaflets, thereby *restricting leaflet motion during systole*, preventing leaflet coaptation and valve closure, and resulting in mitral regurgitation (Fig. 12.9C).[25,39] In either case, acute mitral regurgitation is a condition detectable with the pulmonary artery catheter.

Mitral valve regurgitation produces abnormal retrograde filling of the left atrium during systole through the incompetent mitral valve. As a result, a tall systolic c-v wave is inscribed in the left atrial pressure and PAWP traces (Fig. 12.10). Note that the x descent is obliterated and the c and v waves merge, owing to the holosystolic regurgitation of blood. It is not always possible to distinguish a prominent *antegrade* v wave of systolic left atrial filling from a prominent *retrograde* v wave of mitral regurgitation, but the taller the v wave relative to the mean atrial pressure, the more likely that it signifies mitral regurgitation. (See Ch. 17 for more detail on detection of mitral regurgitation and other valvular heart diseases.)

In the clinical setting, onset of mitral regurgitation and its accompanying pathologic c-v wave may be detected from careful examination of the PAP trace itself. Any prominent wedge pressure wave, including a regurgitant c-v wave, is often suspected first by noting the abnormal morphology of the unwedged PAP trace, since this is the waveform that is displayed continuously on the bedside monitor. Consequently, the clinician may first suspect mitral regurgitation by noting a distorted PAP waveform, then wedging the catheter to reveal the tall c-v wave in the wedge pressure trace (Figs. 12.11 and 12.12). (See also Ch. 4, Figs. 4.9 and 4.11.)

UTILITY OF THE WEDGE PRESSURE FOR DETECTING ISCHEMIA: CAUSE OR EFFECT?

Whether the pulmonary artery catheter should be used in all high-risk patients as a supplemental monitor for detection of myocardial ischemia remains debatable,[2,21,38,50] but similar controversy surrounds the role of other technologic tools like transesophageal echocardiography used for similar monitoring purposes in the perioperative period.[5,10,32] Independent of this debate, however, is the question of *how* to use the pulmonary artery catheter to detect ischemia, which is the subject considered in the preceding paragraphs. In particular, emphasis here is placed on describing how changes in PAP, and particularly the development of prominent a and v waves in the PAWP trace, may alert the clinician to the presence of either diastolic or systolic left ventricular dysfunction accompanying myocardial ischemia. The physiologic basis for these hemodynamic changes has been reviewed, and the morphologic characteristics of the pathologic waveforms have been described.

It is clear that changes in PAP or PAWP have many causes other than myocardial ischemia. For example, the tall c-v wave of mitral regurgitation can be seen regardless of the etiology of mitral valve incompetence. Furthermore, hypervolemia will raise mean PAWP and produce more prominent a and v waves as the distended left atrium reaches steeper portions of its compliance curve. (See Chs. 15 and 17 for more detail on pressure–volume relations and mitral regurgitation.) The clinician must consider all available information in deciding whether a given change in PAP or PAWP signifies ischemia or some other condition. One might ask: are there other ancillary clues, like ST-segment changes on the ECG? Are there accompanying hemodynamic changes that suggest an alternative explanation for the PAP changes, or have these occurred in the absence of such changes? *One could even ask whether the change in PAWP is cause or effect?* An abnormal elevation in wedge pressure may reflect altered left ventricular function *resulting from ischemia*, or the elevated wedge pressure may *result in ischemia* because of the increased left ventricular wall stress and the decreased gradient for coronary perfusion during diastole. In either case, the elevated PAWP is undesirable, and use of the pulmonary artery catheter alerts the clinician to these untoward changes.

HEMODYNAMIC PATTERNS OF ISCHEMIA: IS THERE AN ISCHEMIC CASCADE?

Perioperative myocardial ischemia may be recognized on the bedside monitor when it produces ECG abnormalities (Ch. 11) or various hemodynamic abnormalities, particularly those seen in the PAWP trace described above. In addition, left ventricular regional wall motion abnormalities detected with transesophageal echocardiography will provide supplemental clues to the presence of myocardial ischemia.[11,23,29,44,47] Unfortunately, when these various monitoring techniques are compared with one another, or with other methods for detecting ischemia, such as measurement of coronary sinus lactate production,[16] *poor*

agreement among methods is the rule.[11,16,22] Why is this the case?

None of our current methods for detecting perioperative myocardial ischemia are perfectly sensitive or specific. Just as ECG detection of ischemia has various limitations and confounding influences (see Ch. 11), hemodynamic methods for diagnosing ischemia have a number of associated problems. Although patients with left ventricular ischemia are likely to have a higher mean PAWP than those without ischemia, these differences are small and may be difficult to detect clinically.[47] Furthermore, clear quantitative threshold values for mean wedge pressure or a and v wave peak pressures that are diagnostic of ischemic have not been identified,[47] perhaps owing to the wide variation in these pressures in normal subjects. In other words, unlike the threshold value for ST-segment depression applied during ECG monitoring for ischemia that has been well validated and widely accepted (0.1 mV horizontal ST-segment depression), no comparable quantitative value exists for an ischemic wedge pressure. Different values have been used by various authors: wedge pressure a wave of 15 mmHg, or v wave of 20 mmHg,[19,20] mean wedge pressure increase of 7 mmHg,[1] and wedge pressure a and v wave peak pressures at least 5 mmHg above mean wedge pressure.[16] Still, no quantitative standard exists for this measurement. Consequently, the best approach is to *integrate* the hemodynamic information with other monitored values, looking for clues in the ECG, hemodynamic traces, and echocardiogram if it is available. When a marked change in PAWP and waveform morphology are noted in combination with other evidence suggestive of ischemia, including symptoms of angina pectoris in the awake patient, *the wedge pressure provides a valuable piece of the puzzle of perioperative ischemia* (Fig. 12.13).

Quite apart from these considerations, hemodynamic monitoring may appear unreliable for detecting perioperative ischemia because ischemia in this setting may be multifactorial and thus will not produce the classic *cascade of ischemic events* described in other settings.[17,34,48,52] For example, myocardial ischemia during coronary angioplasty balloon inflation predictably results in sequential changes in the vast majority of patients: regional systolic wall motion abnormalities seen with echocardiography, *followed by* ST-segment changes seen with ECG, *followed by* symptoms of angina pectoris.[17,52] In contrast to this situation, which is the result of pure *reduced supply ischemia*, rapid atrial pacing alters myocardial oxygen *demand*, and abnormalities of left ventricular diastolic function and LVEDP predominate over changes in global systolic function.[33]

Unlike these controlled situations in which myocardial ischemia is elicited by a single clear mechanism, perioperative myocardial ischemia has many causes, some reducing myocardial oxygen supply and others raising oxygen demand. It is not surprising, therefore, that in any individual case, the one most revealing monitor may be either the ECG, the hemodynamic waveforms, or the echocardiogram. As a practical matter and perhaps of equal importance, the clinician may *first notice* an abnormality from *any one* of the available monitors.[3] This should then trigger a rapid review of the other monitored information, all of which should be considered along with the patient's history in an *integrated* fashion before arriving at the diagnosis of myocardial ischemia.[3,51]

RIGHT VENTRICULAR ISCHEMIA

Although less commonly clinically manifest than left ventricular ischemia, right ventricular ischemia and infarction produce characteristic hemodynamic patterns that are discernible on the bedside monitor.[7,13,14,18,26,46] Just as the PAWP is elevated and the waveform displays prominent a and v waves in patients with left ventricular ischemia, the central venous pressure (CVP) will be increased (Fig. 12.14), and this venous pressure waveform may display abnormalities in a and v wave morphology in patients with right ventricular ischemia. Right ventricular diastolic dysfunction leads to elevated CVP and can produce a prominent a wave (Fig. 12.15).[30,31] Furthermore, right ventricular dilatation and systolic dysfunction may contribute to functional tricuspid valve regurgitation and produce a tall c-v wave in the venous pressure trace.[46] The CVP in right ventricular infarction is described as having an *M* or *W* configuration, which refers to the tall a and v waves and steep x and y descents (Fig. 12.15).[13,26,30,31] Moreover, CVP is elevated out of proportion to the wedge pressure and is often higher than the latter (Figs. 12.14 and 12.16).

Since right ventricular infarction generally accompanies infarction of the inferior wall of the left ventricle, the ECG will often show the characteristic pattern of Q waves and ST elevation in leads II, III, and aVF (Figs. 12.14 and 12.16) (see also Ch. 11). The diagnosis of right ventricular ischemia or infarction is best made when these ECG clues are considered in conjunction with the characteristic CVP abnormality. If right atrial infarction accompanies right ventricular infarction, the CVP a wave will be reduced, owing to the loss of normal right atrial contractile function.[13] This subtle morphologic change may portend a poorer prognosis after right ventricular infarction.[13] Other hemodynamic clues to right ventricular ischemia and infarction include bradycardia, atrioventricular conduction block (see Fig. 11.9), and reduced ventricular stroke volume and cardiac output.[26]

Severe pulmonary artery hypertension also may result in secondary right ventricular ischemia and dysfunction and produce an increase in CVP. This condition is readily distinguished from *primary* right ventricular dysfunction, since the PAP and pulmonary vascular resistance will be normal in the latter. The distinction is important, since treatment of primary right ventricular dysfunction is focused on preload augmentation and inotropic support of the right ventricle, while treatment of right ventricular dysfunction coexisting with pulmonary hypertension generally will include efforts to reduce PAP.[41]

Illustrations for
Myocardial Ischemia

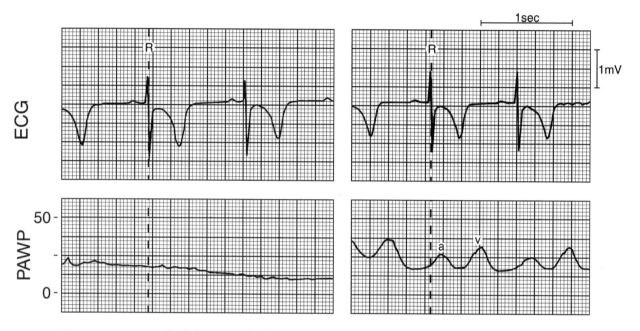

Figure 12.1 Diastolic left ventricular dysfunction accompanying myocardial ischemia reflected by an abnormal pulmonary artery wedge pressure (PAWP) trace. Initial mean PAWP is 10 mmHg, and the wedge waveform does not display any prominent pressure peaks (*left panels*). (Note that mean PAWP is recorded as 10 mmHg, not 20 mmHg, because this is the end-expiratory pressure value recorded from a patient receiving positive pressure mechanical ventilation.) Onset of myocardial ischemia causes a marked increase in mean PAWP (23 mmHg) and a change in waveform morphology, with prominent a waves (27 mmHg) and v waves (32 mmHg) now seen (*right panels*). ECG changes of myocardial ischemia are not evident, although the abnormal ST segments and inverted T waves present at baseline confound the ECG diagnosis of ischemia.

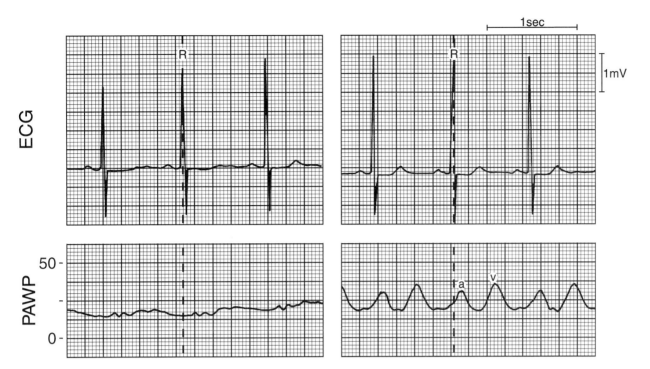

Figure 12.2 Diastolic left ventricular dysfunction accompanying myocardial ischemia reflected by an abnormal pulmonary artery wedge pressure (PAWP) trace. The increase in mean PAWP from 17 mmHg (*left panels*) to 26 mmHg (*right panels*) is less dramatic than in the previous example (Fig. 12.1), but the striking change in waveform morphology is seen again here. The ECG trace is less useful for diagnosing ischemia in this patient because of coexisting left ventricular hypertrophy caused by aortic valve stenosis.

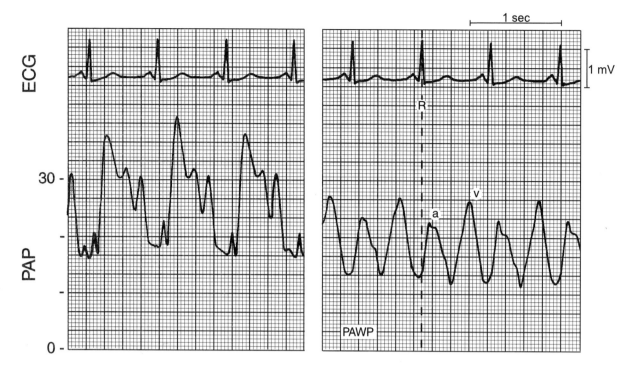

Figure 12.3 Myocardial ischemia often produces a more striking change in morphology of the pulmonary artery wedge pressure trace (PAWP) than in the pulmonary artery pressure (PAP) trace. These waveforms are recorded from a patient with known coronary artery disease following induction of general anesthesia and difficult tracheal intubation. Although PAP is elevated (37/16 mmHg), the most abnormal features seen in these traces are the tall a and v waves observed in the PAWP waveform (23 and 26 mmHg, respectively). Two additional important features may be noted in these traces. First, prominent PAWP a and v waves can be seen distorting the unwedged PAP trace. Second, pulmonary artery diastolic pressure (16 mmHg) is a good estimate for mean PAWP but underestimates left ventricular end-diastolic pressure. In this patient with diastolic dysfunction, left ventricular end-diastolic pressure is best estimated by the PAWP a wave pressure peak, 23 mmHg in this example. (See Chs. 4 and 6 for more detail.)

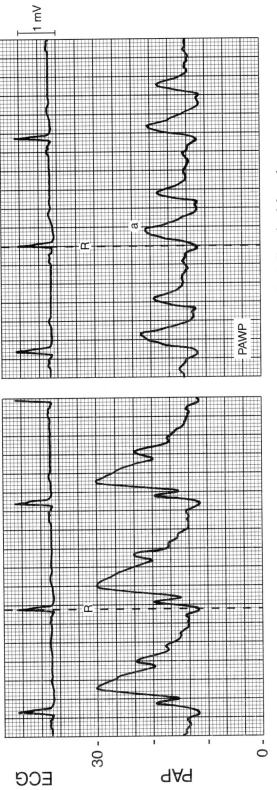

Figure 12.4 A prominent pulmonary artery wedge pressure (PAWP) a wave is the hallmark of diastolic left ventricular dysfunction in myocardial ischemia. In these traces recorded from a 75-year-old patient undergoing coronary artery bypass surgery, pulmonary artery pressure is relatively normal (30/11 mmHg), mean PAWP is slightly elevated (15 mmHg), but the PAWP morphology shows a markedly abnormal a wave (21 mmHg), which reflects the pathologic elevation in left ventricular end-diastolic pressure. See text for more detail.

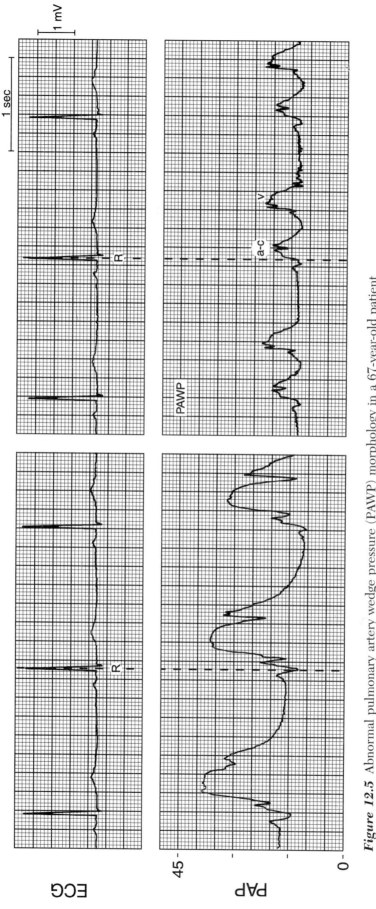

Figure 12.5 Abnormal pulmonary artery wedge pressure (PAWP) morphology in a 67-year-old patient with severe coronary artery disease. Prominent a-c and v waves are noted in the PAWP trace (20 and 22 mmHg, respectively), while the pulmonary artery pressure (PAP) recorded at end-expiration (third beat, *left panel*) is essentially normal (32/11 mmHg). The tall PAWP a-c wave reflects increased left ventricular end-diastolic pressure seen in patients with diastolic dysfunction resulting from coronary artery disease. This patient's cardiac catheterization report is shown in Fig. 12.6. See text for more detail.

```
┌─────────────────────────────────────────────────────────────┐
│              Preliminary Cath Report                          │
│                                                               │
│                                                               │
│  1. Hemodynamics                         (Normal Values)      │
│       RA      6/5/4    mmHg   a/v/m         (0-8)   mmHg       │
│       RV      18/6     mmHg   s/d         (15-30/0-8) mmHg     │
│       PA      18/9/11  mmHg   s/d/m      (15-30/4-12) mmHg     │
│       PAW     15/9/7   mmHg   a/v/m         (1-10)  mmHg       │
│       LV      140/15   mmHg   s/d       (100-140/3-12) mmHg    │
│       Art     140/65/95 mmHg  s/d/m     (70-105/60-90) mmHg    │
│       CO/CI   5.5    L/min 2.7  L/min/m²  (---/2.5-4.2)        │
│       SVR     1323      dynes-sec-cm-5     (770-1500)          │
│       PVR     58        dynes-sec-cm-5      (20-120)           │
│                                                               │
│                                                               │
│  2. Angiography                                               │
│       • LAD graft patent                                      │
│       • Ramus graft occluded                                  │
│       • PDA graft occluded                                    │
│                                                               │
│       • LAD occluded after S1                                 │
│       • RCA mid 50%, PDA 90%                                  │
│       • IMA without disease                                   │
│                                                               │
│                                                               │
│       • EF 72%, Anterior HK                                   │
│                                                               │
│  FELLOW:_____ ATTENDING:_____              │
│  Date:_____        Date:_____            │
└─────────────────────────────────────────────────────────────┘
```

Figure 12.6 Cardiac catheterization (Cath) report from the patient whose hemodynamic traces are shown in Fig. 12.5. Severe coronary artery disease is present, left ventricular systolic function as estimated by ejection fraction (EF) is normal, and diastolic dysfunction is suggested by the increased left ventricular (LV) end-diastolic pressure and pulmonary artery wedge (PAW) pressure a wave peak pressure (both 15 mmHg). Also note that *mean PAW pressure (7 mmHg) underestimates LV end-diastolic pressure (15 mmHg).* See text for more detail. RA, right atrium; RV, right ventricle; PA, pulmonary artery; Art, systemic arterial; CO/CI, cardiac output/cardiac index; SVR, systemic vascular resistance; PVR, pulmonary vascular resistance; a/v/m, a wave/v wave/mean; s/d, systolic/diastolic; s/d/m, systolic/diastolic/mean; LAD, left anterior descending; PDA, posterior descending artery; S1, first septal branch; RCA, right coronary artery; IMA, internal mammary artery; HK, hypokinesia.

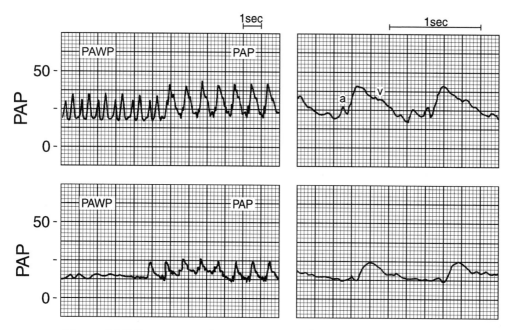

Figure 12.7 Prominent pulmonary artery wedge pressure (PAWP) a and v waves may be suspected initially by observing a distorted unwedged pulmonary artery pressure (PAP) trace. (*Top panels*) An elevated PAWP (mean 25 mmHg) with prominent a and v waves (31 and 35 mmHg, respectively) and an abnormal PAP trace. These tall wedge pressure a and v waves are noted in the unwedged PAP trace (*top right panel*). (*Bottom panels*) A nearly normal PAWP (mean 14 mmHg) without distinct phasic components and a normal PAP (24/12 mmHg) with normal morphology. See text for more detail.

Figure 12.8 Induced myocardial ischemia during repeat coronary artery bypass graft surgery manifested as left ventricular systolic dysfunction. (*A*) Operative procedure performed in a 57-year-old man who underwent single-vessel coronary artery grafting through a left thoracotomy without cardiopulmonary bypass support. A previously placed patent saphenous vein graft (SVG) to the second obtuse marginal (OM 2) coronary artery was clamped transiently to facilitate placement of a new SVG to the diseased first obtuse marginal (OM 1) coronary artery. (*B*) Hemodynamic changes during this episode of obligatory transient myocardial ischemia. At the time of vein graft occlusion (*arrow 1*), arterial blood pressure (ART) declines rapidly from 120 mmHg to 90 mmHg over 3 minutes. A transesophageal echocardiogram performed at the same time showed a new wall motion abnormality—inferior wall akinesia. Pulmonary artery pressure (PAP) changes more slowly, with the pulmonary artery diastolic pressure increasing from 12 to 15 mmHg over 6 minutes. *This pattern is typical of supply ischemia insofar as manifestations of systolic left ventricular dysfunction (arterial hypotension and wall motion abnormalities) are more pronounced than signs of diastolic dysfunction (increased pulmonary artery diastolic pressure).* (*C*) ECG complexes from leads, I, II, and V_1 recorded during this period of ischemia (*arrow 2* in Fig. B). Transmural ischemia of the inferior wall of the left ventricle is evidenced by the 2.3 mm ST-segment elevation in lead II and the ST-segment trend line, which shows progressive ST deviation over the previous few minutes.

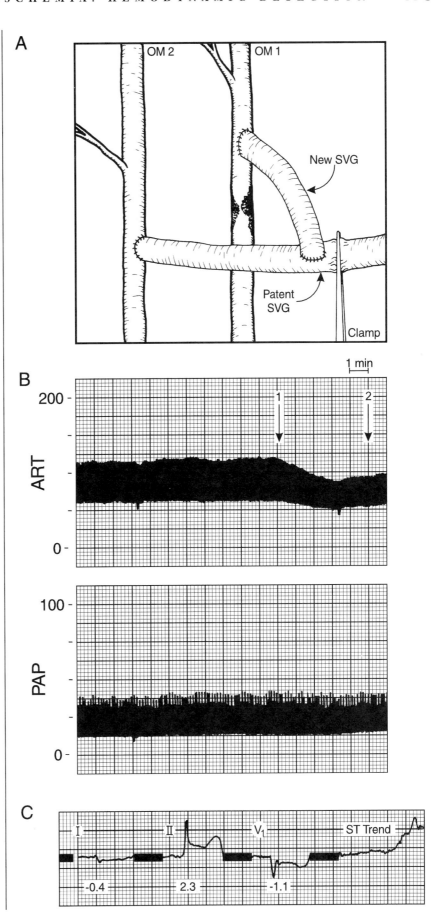

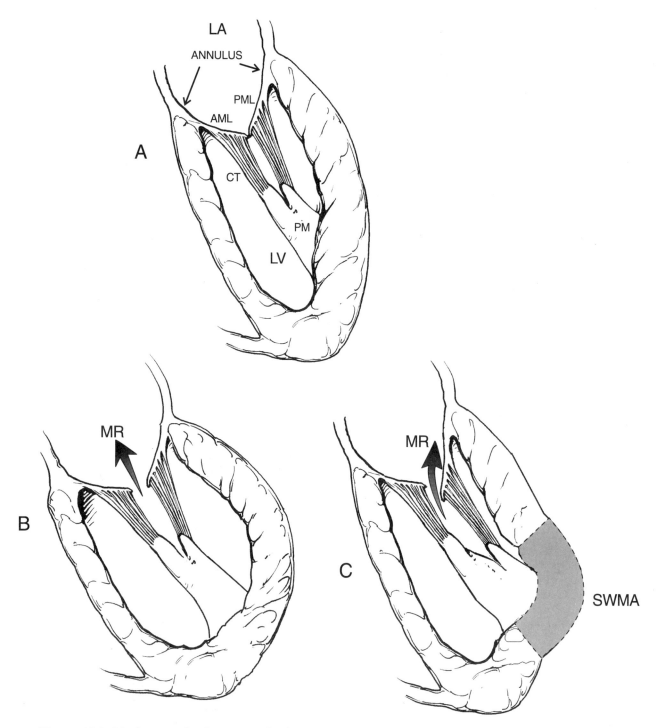

Figure 12.9 Mechanism of ischemic mitral valve regurgitation (MR). (*A*) The normal mitral valve consists of two leaflets, the anterior mitral leaflet (AML) and the posterior mitral leaflet (PML), attached to a fibrous annulus at the junction of the left atrium (LA) and left ventricle (LV), and supported by chordae tendinae (CT) attached to papillary muscles (PM), which arise from the ventricular myocardium. (*B*) Ventricular enlargement associated with LV systolic dysfunction alters normal ventricular geometry, produces annular dilatation, and results in MR from failure of leaflet coaptation. (*C*) Mitral regurgitation may also result from restricted leaflet motion because an underlying LV segmental wall motion abnormality (SWMA) effectively tethers the affected mitral leaflet through its chordal attachments. This type of MR is often termed *papillary muscle ischemia*. See text for more detail.

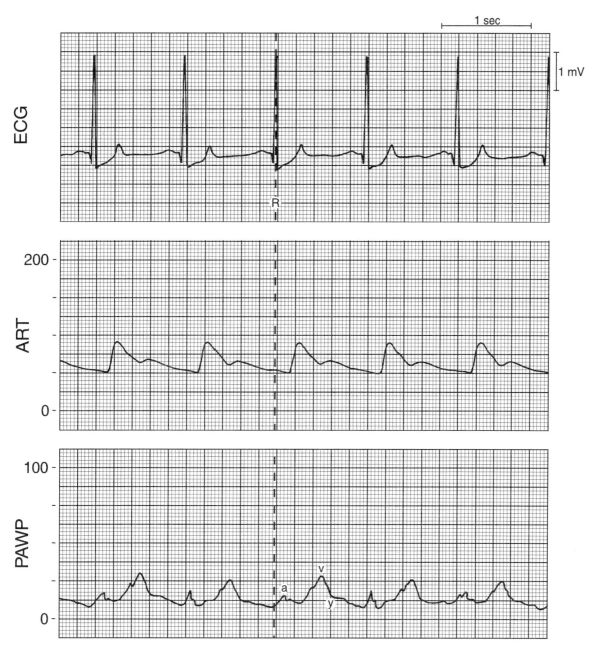

Figure 12.10 Ischemic mitral valve regurgitation produces a tall regurgitant c-v wave in the pulmonary artery wedge pressure (PAWP) trace. Note that the x descent is obscured in the broad holosystolic c-v wave (v 27 mmHg), which dominates the PAWP waveform. Other stigmata of myocardial ischemia in these traces include the ECG ST-segment depression and the systemic arterial (ART) hypotension. See text for more detail.

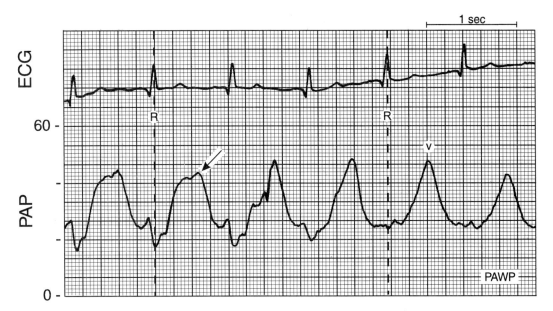

Figure 12.11 Severe mitral valve regurgitation caused by myocardial ischemia manifesting as an abnormal pulmonary artery pressure (PAP) waveform morphology. The bifid, or double-peaked, appearance of the PAP waveform is abnormal, and the second peak (*arrow*) represents the giant regurgitant v wave (v 48 mmHg), which is clearly identified in the pulmonary artery wedge pressure trace (last three beats). See text for more detail.

Figure 12.12 Severe mitral valve regurgitation causing a sudden change in pulmonary artery pressure (PAP). In this example, when the patient's legs are elevated for skin preparation prior to coronary artery bypass surgery (*arrow, left panels*), the change in systolic PAP from 32 to 50 mmHg is striking compared to the minor change in diastolic PAP. The cause of this abnormality in PAP is revealed by examining the pulmonary artery wedge pressure (PAWP) waveform, which displays a huge systolic v wave resulting from mitral regurgitation (*right panels*). Autotransfusion produced by leg elevation leads to mitral valve regurgitation in this instance. Since systemic arterial (ART) hypotension accompanies this episode, it is unlikely that the valvular regurgitation in this instance is caused by excessive left ventricular afterload. Instead, myocardial ischemia or excessive left ventricular preload is more likely to be responsible.

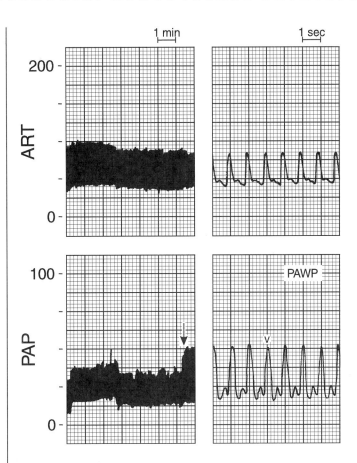

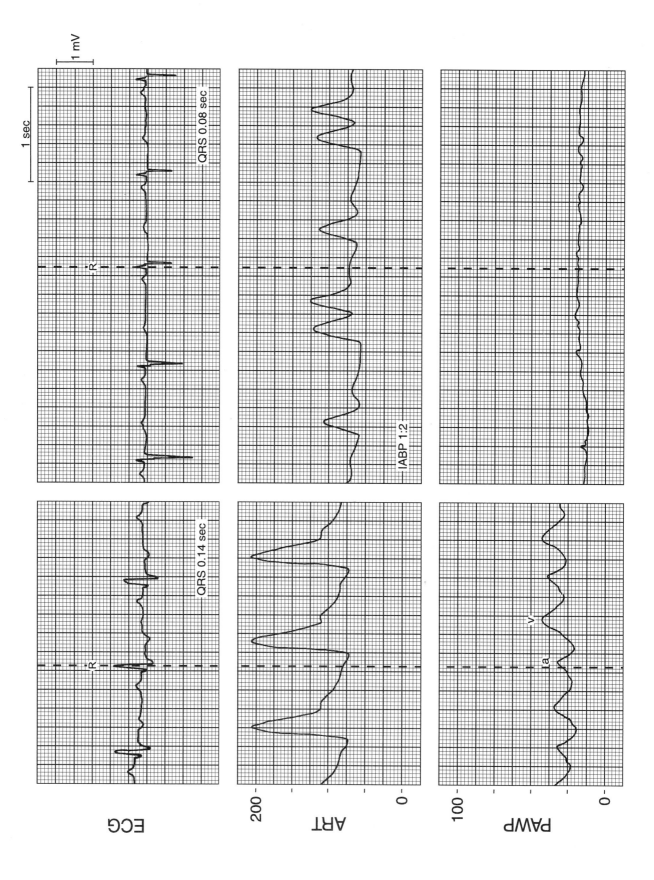

Figure 12.13 Pulmonary artery wedge pressure (PAWP) as a clue to myocardial ischemia. Abnormal PAWP (a 32 mmHg, v 42 mmHg, mean 30 mmHg) occurs in the setting of new left bundle branch block (ECG QRS duration 0.14 seconds) and systemic arterial (ART) hypertension (*left panels*). Treatment with nitroglycerin and placement of an intraaortic balloon pump (IABP 1:2 assist interval) leads to resolution of the ECG conduction abnormality (ECG QRS duration 0.08 seconds) and restoration of a more normal PAWP (mean 18 mmHg), which no longer displays pathologic waveform components. See text for more detail.

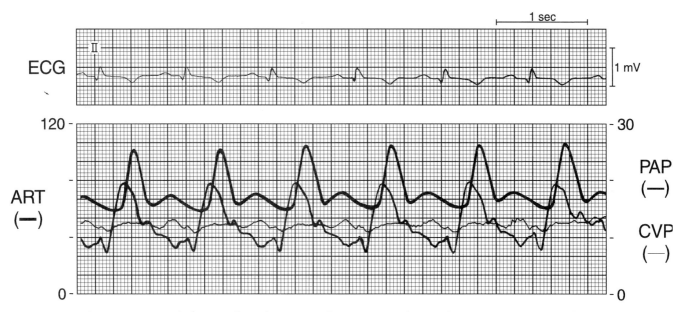

Figure 12.14 Right ventricular infarction produces increased central venous pressure (CVP). In this example, CVP (12 mmHg) is higher than diastolic pulmonary artery pressure (PAP, 7 mmHg). Other abnormalities seen in this example include Q waves in ECG lead II and systemic arterial (ART) hypotension. These traces are recorded from a patient who has both inferior left ventricular and right ventricular infarction. However, this pattern suggests that the right ventricular infarction is clinically most important, since CVP is significantly elevated while PAP is low (19/7 mmHg), a pattern that points to right ventricular failure as the limiting feature in this altered hemodynamic state. See text for more detail.

Figure 12.15 Right ventricular ischemia and infarction produce increased central venous pressure (CVP), and the waveform displays tall a and v waves and steep x and y descents, resulting in an *M* or *W* morphology. These traces are recorded from a patient who has both inferior left ventricular and right ventricular infarction. The marked increase in CVP (16 mmHg) is out of proportion to the increase in pulmonary artery wedge pressure (PAWP, 18 mmHg). Note that the lead V5 ECG is unrevealing in this instance and that mild systemic arterial (ART) hypotension (105/55 mmHg) accompanies this condition. See text for more detail. (Modified from Mark,[30] with permission.)

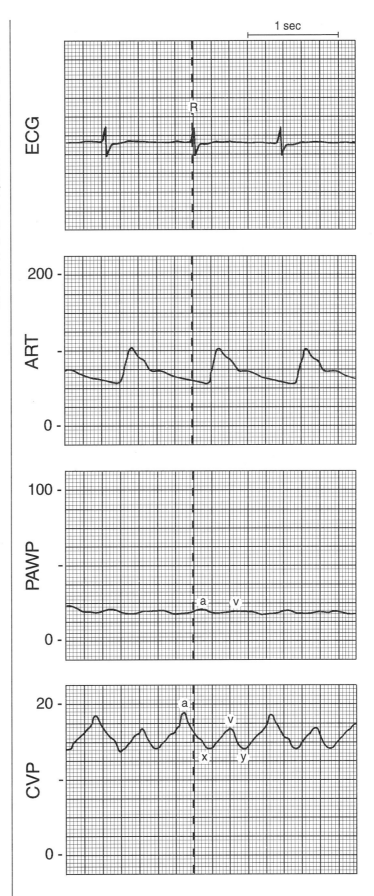

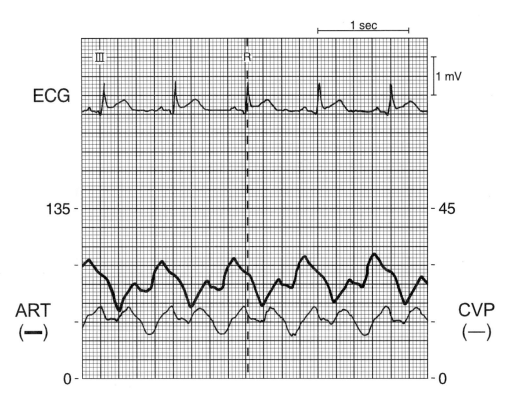

Figure 12.16 Markedly elevated central venous pressure (CVP) produced by right ventricular ischemia and infarction. These traces are recorded from a 52-year-old woman who had acute thrombotic occlusion of her right coronary artery diagnosed by cardiac catheterization. The resulting right ventricular and inferior wall left ventricular infarction produce the features noted here: ECG lead III Q waves and 1 mm ST-segment elevation, disproportionate increase in CVP (15 mmHg, M morphology) compared to pulmonary artery wedge pressure (7 mmHg, tracing not shown), and systemic arterial (ART) hypotension (mean 78 mmHg) despite 1:1 intraaortic balloon counterpulsation, which produces the tall diastolic pressure peak in the ART waveform. See text for more detail.

References

1. Attia RR, Murphy JD, Snider M, et al. Myocardial ischemia due to infrarenal aortic cross-clamping during aortic surgery in patients with severe coronary artery disease. Circulation 1976; 53:961–4

2. Bashein G, Ivey TD. Con: a pulmonary artery catheter is not indicated for all coronary artery surgery. J Cardiothorac Anesth 1987;1:362–5

3. Bergquist BD, Bellows WH, Leung JM. Transesophageal echocardiography in myocardial revascularization: II. Influence on intraoperative decision making. Anesth Analg 1996;82:1139–45

4. Bourdillon PD, Lorell BH, Mirsky I, et al. Increased regional myocardial stiffness of the left ventricle during pacing-induced angina in man. Circulation 1983;67:316–23

5. Cahalan MK. Pro: transesophageal echocardiography is the "gold standard" for detection of myocardial ischemia. J Cardiothorac Anesth 1989;3:369–71

6. Chaitman B. Exercise stress testing. In: Braunwald E, ed. Heart Disease. A Textbook of Cardiovascular Medicine (4th ed). Philadelphia, WB Saunders, 1992:161–79

7. Cohn JN, Guiha NH, Broder M, Limas CJ. Right ventricular infarction. Clinical and hemodynamic features. Am J Cardiol 1974;33:209–14

8. Dodek A, Kassebaum DG, Bristow JD. Pulmonary edema in coronary-artery disease without cardiomegaly. Paradox of the stiff heart. N Engl J Med 1972;286:1347–50

9. Dwyer EM. Left ventricular pressure-volume alterations and regional disorders of contraction during myocardial ischemia induced by atrial pacing. Circulation 1970;42:1111–22

10. Eisenberg MJ, London MJ, Leung JM, et al. Monitoring for myocardial ischemia during noncardiac surgery. A technology assessment of transesophageal echocardiography and 12-lead electrocardiography. JAMA 1992;268:210–16

11. Ellis JE, Shah MN, Briller JE, et al. A comparison of methods for the detection of myocardial ischemia during noncardiac surgery: automated ST-segment analysis systems, electrocardiography, and transesophageal echocardiography. Anesth Analg 1992; 75:764–72

12. Falicov RE, Resnekov L. Relationship of the pulmonary artery end-diastolic pressure to the left ventricular end-diastolic and mean filling pressures in patients with and without left ventricular dysfunction. Circulation 1970;42:65–73

13. Goldstein JA, Barzilai B, Rosamond TL, et al. Determinants of hemodynamic compromise with severe right ventricular infarction. Circulation 1990;82:359–68

14. Greenberg MA, Gitler B. Left ventricular rupture in a patient with coexisting right ventricular infarction. N Engl J Med 1983;309:539–42

15. Grossman W. Diastolic dysfunction in congestive heart failure. N Engl J Med 1991;325:1557–64

16. Häggmark S, Hohner P, Ostman M, et al. Comparison of hemodynamic, electrocardiographic, mechanical, and metabolic indicators of intraoperative myocardial ischemia in vascular surgical patients with coronary artery disease. Anesthesiology 1989;70:19–25

17. Hauser AM, Gangadharan V, Ramos RG, et al. Sequence of mechanical, electrocardiographic and clinical effects of repeated coronary artery occlusion in human beings: echocardiographic observations during coronary angioplasty. J Am Coll Cardiol 1985; 5:193–7

18. Isner JM. Right ventricular myocardial infarction. JAMA 1988;259:712–8

19. Kaplan JA, Wells PH. Early diagnosis of myocardial ischemia using the pulmonary arterial catheter. Anesth Analg 1981;60:789–93

20. Kaplan JA. Indications for pulmonary arterial catheterization. Anesth Analg 1982;61:477–9

21. Keats AS. Adventures in perioperative myocardial ischemia. Tex Heart Inst J 1993;20:5–11

22. Koolen JJ, Visser CA, Reichert LA, et al. Improved monitoring of myocardial ischemia during major vascular surgery using transoesophageal echocardiography. Eur Heart J 1992;13: 1028–33

23. Leung JM, O'Kelly B, Browner WS, et al. Prognostic importance of postbypass regional wall-motion abnormalities in patients undergoing coronary artery bypass graft surgery. Anesthesiology 1989;71:16–25

24. Leung JM, O'Kelly BF, Mangano DT. Study of Perioperative Ischemia. Relationship of regional wall motion abnormalities to hemodynamic indices of myocardial oxygen supply and demand in patients undergoing CABG surgery. Anesthesiology 1990;73:802–14

25. Longabaugh JP, Sheikh KH, Bengtson JR, et al. Diagnosis and management of ischemic mitral regurgitation with the use of transesophageal echocardiography. Coron Artery Dis 1992;3:377–81

26. Lorell B, Leinbach RC, Pohost GM, et al. Right ventricular infarction. Clinical diagnosis and differentiation from cardiac tamponade and pericardial constriction. Am J Cardiol 1979; 43:465–71

27. Lowenstein E. Perianesthetic ischemic episodes cause myocardial infarction in humans—a hypothesis confirmed. Anesthesiology 1985;62:103–6

28. Mangano DT, Browner WS, Hollenberg M, et al. Association of perioperative myocardial ischemia with cardiac morbidity and mortality in men undergoing noncardiac surgery. N Engl J Med 1990;323:1781–8

29. Mangano DT. Perioperative cardiac morbidity. Anesthesiology 1990;72:153–84

30. Mark JB. Central venous pressure monitoring: clinical insights beyond the numbers. J Cardiothorac Vasc Anesth 1991; 5:163–73

31. Mark JB. Getting the most from your central venous pressure catheter. In: Barash PG, ed. ASA Refresher Courses in Anesthe-

siology (Vol 23). Philadelphia: Lippincott-Raven, 1995:157–75

32. McCloskey G, Barash PG. Con: transesophageal echocardiography is not the "gold standard" for detection of myocardial ischemia. J Cardiothorac Anesth 1989;3:372–4

33. McLaurin LP, Rolett EL, Grossman W. Impaired left ventricular relaxation during pacing-induced ischemia. Am J Cardiol 1973;32:751–7

34. Nesto RW, Kowalchuk GJ. The ischemic cascade: temporal sequence of hemodynamic, electrocardiographic and symptomatic expressions of ischemia. Am J Cardiol 1987;59:23C–30C

35. Raby KE, Goldman L, Creager MA, et al. Correlation between preoperative ischemia and major cardiac events after peripheral vascular surgery. N Engl J Med 1989;321:1296–1300

36. Rahimtoola SH, Loeb HS, Ehsani A, et al. Relationship of pulmonary artery to left ventricular diastolic pressures in acute myocardial infarction. Circulation 1972;46:283–90

37. Rao TLK, Jacobs KH, El-Etr AA. Reinfarction following anesthesia in patients with myocardial infarction. Anesthesiology 1983;59:499–505

38. Roizen MF, Berger DL, Gabel RA, et al. Practice guidelines for pulmonary artery catheterization. A report by the American Society of Anesthesiologists task force on pulmonary artery catheterization. Anesthesiology 1993;78:380–94

39. Sabbah HN, Rosman H, Kono T, et al. On the mechanism of functional mitral regurgitation. Am J Cardiol 1993;72:1074–6

40. Sanchez R, Wee M. Perioperative myocardial ischemia: early diagnosis using the pulmonary artery catheter. J Cardiothorac Vasc Anesth 1991;5:604–7

41. Sibbald WJ, Driedger AA. Right ventricular function in acute disease states: pathophysiologic considerations. Crit Care Med 1983;5:339–45

42. Slogoff S, Keats AS. Does perioperative myocardial ischemia lead to postoperative myocardial infarction? Anesthesiology 1985; 62:107–14

43. Slogoff S, Keats AS. Further observations on perioperative myocardial ischemia. Anesthesiology 1986;65:539–42

44. Smith JS, Cahalan MK, Benefiel DJ, et al. Intraoperative detection of myocardial ischemia in high-risk patients. Circulation 1985;72:1015–21

45. Stott DK, Marpole DGF, Bristow JD, et al. The role of left atrial transport in aortic and mitral stenosis. Circulation 1970; 41:1031–41

46. Trager MA, Feinberg BI, Kaplan JA. Right ventricular ischemia diagnosed by an esophageal electrocardiogram and right atrial pressure tracing. J Cardiothorac Anesth 1987;1:123–5

47. van Daele MERM, Sutherland GR, Mitchell MM, et al. Do changes in pulmonary capillary wedge pressure adequately reflect myocardial ischemia during anesthesia: a correlative preoperative hemodynamic, electrocardiographic, and transesophageal echocardiographic study. Circulation 1990;81:865–71

48. Watanabe S, Buffington CW. Speed and sensitivity of mechanical versus electrographic indicators to mild or moderate myocardial ischemia in the pig. Anesthesiology 1994;80:582–94

49. Waters DD, da Luz P, Wyatt HL, et al. Early changes in regional and global left ventricular function induced by graded reductions in regional coronary perfusion. Am J Cardiol 1977; 39:537–43

50. Weintraub AC, Barash PG. Pro: A pulmonary artery catheter is indicated in all patients for coronary artery surgery. J Cardiothorc Anesth 1987;1:358–361

51. Wickey GS, Larach DR, Keifer JC, et al. Combined interpretation of transesophageal echocardiography, electrocardiography, and pulmonary artery wedge waveform to detect myocardial ischemia. J Cardiothorac Anesth 1990;4:102–4

52. Wohlgelernter D, Jaffe CC, Cabin HS, et al. Silent ischemia during coronary occlusion produced by ballon inflation: relation to

CHAPTER THIRTEEN *Monitoring Heart Rate*

The most common application of ECG monitoring in the perioperative period is the continuous measurement of heart rate. Often taken for granted, rapid estimation of the heart rate by examining the ECG trace on the bedside monitor provides invaluable information to the clinician trying to make prompt decisions about the patient's hemodynamic condition. Current monitors use multiple ECG leads to sense cardiac electrical activity.[4] This redundancy aids detection of the R wave and improves the accuracy of heart rate measurement. As a result, a single *noisy* lead, or one in which the R waves are of very low amplitude, will not prevent the monitor from calculating heart rate properly (Fig. 13.1).

While accurate detection of the QRS complex is the starting point for all ECG monitoring systems to measure heart rate, subsequent signal processing may vary considerably from monitor to monitor. The digital value displayed for heart rate is generated from an algorithm designed to count and average a certain number of beats and then display a number that is updated every 5 to 15 seconds.[1] As a result, acute but transient changes in heart rate may have little impact on the displayed digital value. For example, consider a brief 4 second episode of complete heart block, which interrupts slow sinus rhythm (Fig. 13.2). Depending on the algorithms employed by the monitor, the digital value for heart rate may show only a slight reduction from the baseline value. In this instance, the heart rate of 49 beats/min displayed by the monitor fails to alert the user of the dangerous transient bradyarrhythmia (Fig. 13.2). Although the monitor could update the digital value for heart rate after each beat, thereby reporting the instantaneous R-R interval, this would result in numbers flashing on the display screen, changing with each heart beat, owing to the normal physiologic beat-to-beat variability in heart rate. Instead, the displayed digital value for heart rate (and for all the direct pressure measurements as well) is derived by the monitor using a *moving average filter*. In more sophisticated monitors, this filter weights the most recent values more heavily than older values in deriving the average value for the digital display. Regardless of the type of measuring algorithm used by the monitor, real-time data must be obtained by observing the monitor screen and the analog ECG trace.

Occasionally, the clinician must check electrode attachment, increase monitor gain control, or select alternate leads for ECG monitoring in order to facilitate heart rate measurement. Some monitors even allow manual adjustment of the threshold or sensitivity for R wave detection. Despite these measures, inaccurate heart rates may be displayed by the monitor when the ECG trace is distorted by patient movement or other influences that create electrical interference. In the operating room, this frequently occurs when the electrosurgical unit is in use. *Visual inspection of the ECG trace should* always *be used to confirm the numeric value for heart rate displayed on the monitor.* Spurious values are recognized quickly, and true heart rate can be estimated by noting the R-R interval when the ECG trace reappears briefly on the monitor screen. In addition, the arterial pressure trace or the pulse oximeter plethysmograph helps confirm the pulse rate in these instances (Fig. 13.3).

Electrical interference seen in the ECG trace may arise from a number of sources in addition to the electrosurgical unit. Power line noise appears as a 60 Hz artifact. It may be eliminated by selecting narrower bandpass ECG filters, including a 60 Hz notch filter (see Fig. 10.12). Fortunately, this type of power line electrical artifact rarely prevents accurate ECG measurement of heart rate, and use of narrow bandpass ECG filters should not be required routinely, thereby avoiding the problem of artifactual ST-segment distortion that accompanies use of these filters. (See Ch. 10, Figs. 10.9 through 10.12, for more detail.) Other artifacts result from muscle twitching and fasciculations, as well as a variety of medical devices, including lithotripsy machines and fluid warmers. A particularly vexing ECG artifact, which precludes accurate ECG interpretation of heart rate, rhythm, or ST-segment shifts, has been reported to arise during cardiopulmonary bypass (Fig. 13.4).[2,3] This artifact has a frequency of 1 to 4 Hz, an amplitude as high as 5 mV peak to peak, and appears to be caused by a piezoelectric effect or static electricity generated by the action of the pump roller head on the plastic bypass tubing under conditions of low ambient temperature and humidity.[2] Although the *true* cardiac rhythm can be determined during bypass by direct inspection of the heart in most cases, it may be difficult to be certain that asystole, rather than fine ventricular fibrillation, has been achieved after administration of cardioplegia. Recommendations to maintain operating room temperature above 20°C and relative humidity above 50 percent may help eliminate this artifact.[2] However, multilead ECG monitoring, observation of other displayed hemodynamic waveforms, and direct cardiac inspection will aid recognition of this source of ECG interference. (Also see Ch. 14). If this artifact remains a problem, abrupt reduction of the blood flow rate on cardiopulmonary bypass should simultaneously reduce the frequency of the artifactual electrical signal as the pump arterial roller head revolution rate is decreased. Similarly, absence of any cardiac electrical activity (asystole) may be documented by transiently turning the pump off for a few seconds and examining the ECG under these conditions.

Several quick methods are available to estimate heart rate from an ECG paper trace recorded on millimeter ruled paper at the standard recording speed of 25 mm/sec. First, heart rate equals 1,500 divided by the number of small (1 mm) boxes between adjacent R waves. Second, heart rate may be calculated in any patient by counting the number of

R waves seen in 15 large (5 mm) boxes (3 seconds) and multiplying by 20. Third, one can estimate heart rate by counting the number of large (5 mm) boxes separating adjacent R waves and using the following approximation: a two-box separation equals 150 beats/min, a three-box separation equals 100 beats/min, a four-box separation equals 75 beats/min, a five-box separation equals 60 beats/min, and a six-box separation equals 50 beats/min. Note that all of these methods simply estimate the true heart rate that would be recorded over 1 minute, and they are not accurate when heart rhythm is irregular. Under these circumstances, at least 5 to 10 R-R intervals should be measured and an average heart rate calculated.

Paced rhythms often produce problems for the ECG measurement of heart rate. When tall pacing spikes are present, the monitor may misinterpret these high-amplitude signals as R waves and miscalculate the heart rate (Figs. 13.5 and 13.6). Tall T waves may produce the same artifact when the monitor mistakenly *double counts* these T waves along with the R waves. These problems may be ameliorated by decreasing ECG gain, adjusting R wave detection sensitivity, or changing the ECG lead to one with a reduced pacing spike or T wave amplitude. When temporary pacing is being employed, decreasing current output from the external pulse generator or changing from *unipolar* pacing to *bipolar* pacing will markedly reduce pacing spike amplitude recorded by the surface ECG.

PULSE RATE OR HEART RATE?

Although the preceding discussion has focused on methods to estimate heart rate from the ECG trace, it might be argued that monitoring pulse rate is more important than monitoring heart rate, in terms of hemodynamic assessment in the perioperative period. By definition, the distinction between the two centers on whether a given electrical depolarization and systolic contraction of the heart (*heart rate*) results in a palpable peripheral arterial pulsation (*pulse rate*). *Pulse deficit* describes the extent to which the pulse rate is less than the heart rate. This is typically seen in patients with atrial fibrillation, where short R-R intervals compromise cardiac filling during diastole, result-

ing in a reduced stroke volume and an imperceptible arterial pulse (Fig. 13.7). The most extreme example of a pulse deficit is electrical-mechanical dissociation (EMD, or pulseless electrical activity, PEA), seen in patients with cardiac tamponade, extreme hypovolemia, and other conditions in which cardiac contraction does not generate a palpable peripheral pulse.

Most monitors report heart rate and pulse rate separately. The former is measured from the ECG trace, and the latter is determined by a pulse source, which is generally selectable by the user. For example, the pulse oximeter plethysmograph trace will provide a suitable pulse measurement source for most patients except those with severe arterial occlusive disease or those with marked peripheral vasoconstriction. When direct arterial pressure measurement is in place, this pressure waveform serves as a reliable pulse source. As emphasized above, this is particularly useful in distinguishing artifactual ECG signals and erroneous heart rates (Fig. 13.3) from important real cardiac events (Fig. 13.2). On occasion, however, the arterial pressure trace may be misleading when nonsystolic arterial pulsations are detected by the monitor and counted separately. This is noted most often in patients being treated with intraaortic balloon counterpulsation, where the pressure pulse resulting from balloon inflation during diastole is detected by the monitor and results in a factitiously high pulse rate (Fig. 13.8). Some monitors have a *smart balloon pump* setting, which obviates this problem (as well as the accompanying problem of erroneously displaying the augmented diastolic peak pressure as the systolic blood pressure). Alternatively, a reliable pulse rate can be monitored by selecting another source for the pulse signal, like the pulmonary artery pressure waveform, which is undisturbed by balloon pump action. Other arterial pressure waveforms that have a bisferiens, double-peaked morphology, such as those arising in patients with aortic valve regurgitation, may produce a similar artifactual pulse rate measurement. (See Ch. 17 for more detail.)

In summary, pulse rate monitoring and heart rate monitoring complement each other. As with all numeric information displayed on the bedside monitor, *check the analog ECG and pressure waveforms to ensure the veracity of the numbers on the screen.*

Illustrations for Monitoring Heart Rate

Figure 13.1 Multilead ECG monitoring improves R wave detection for heart rate measurement. Low-amplitude R waves in leads I and II may not be recognized and counted by the monitor, but the R wave in lead V_5 is tall enough to be detected and allow an accurate heart rate of 100 beats/min to be measured.

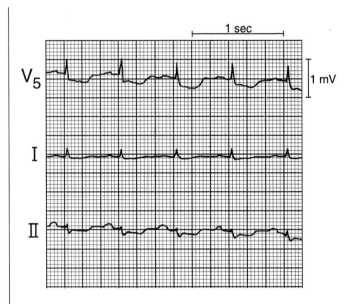

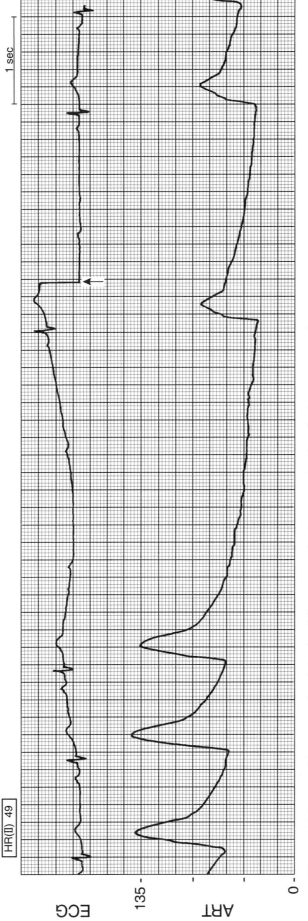

Figure 13.2 Digital heart rate (HR) display fails to warn of a dangerous bradyarrhythmia. Direct observation of the ECG and arterial blood pressure (ART) traces reveals complete heart block and a 4-second period of asystole, while the digital display reports a HR of 49 beats/min recorded from ECG lead II. Note that the ECG filter corrects the baseline drift (*arrow*) so that the trace remains on the monitor screen or paper recording. See text for more detail.

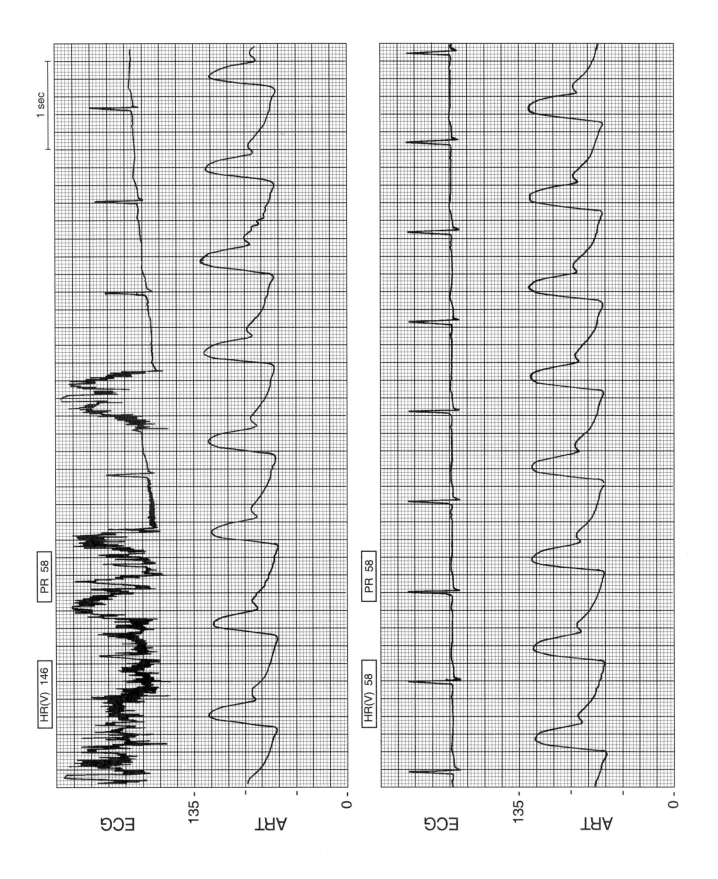

Figure 13.3 Electrical ECG artifact created by the electrosurgical unit distorts the ECG waveform and generates an artifactual value for heart rate (HR) derived from ECG lead V$_5$ (HR[V]146). (*Top panel*) The true HR can be estimated by noting the R-R interval of the three ECG complexes that appear briefly at the end of the recording. The HR is confirmed by observing the arterial blood pressure (ART) waveform and the pulse rate (PR) digital display that is generated from this arterial waveform (PR 58). (*Bottom panel*) As expected, HR and PR measurements are identical once the ECG artifact disappears.

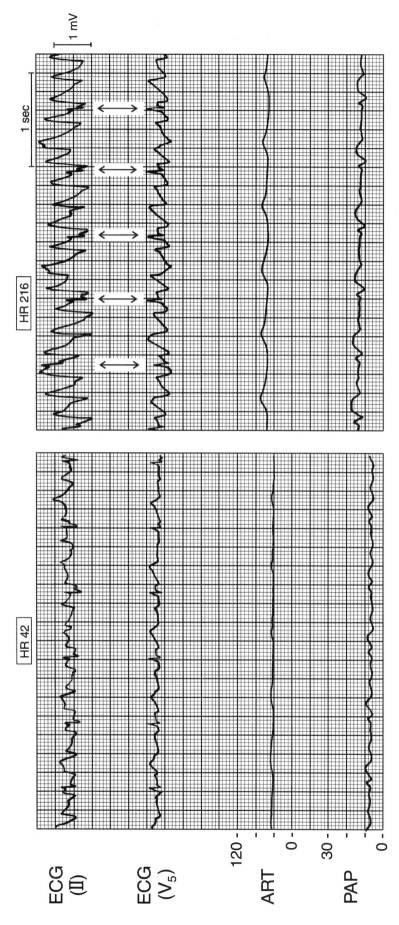

Figure 13.4 Electrical ECG artifact created by the cardiopulmonary bypass pump. (*Left panel*) Small R waves are seen in ECG leads II and V$_5$, but these are not of sufficient amplitude to allow accurate heart rate (HR) measurement by the monitor. The ECG trace reveals a HR of 88 beats/min, while the digital display shows HR to be 42 beats/min. Small but observable pulsations seen in the arterial blood pressure (ART) and pulmonary artery pressure (PAP) traces confirm the HR of 88 beats/min. (*Right panel*) The ECG artifact worsens later during bypass. The ECG R waves (*arrows*) are nearly totally obscured by the artifactual electrical signal, and an erroneous value for HR is derived from the ECG for the digital display (HR 216). With the patient now on partial bypass, the larger ART and PAP pulsations identify the pulse rate and guide the search for R waves in the distorted ECG waveforms. See text for more detail.

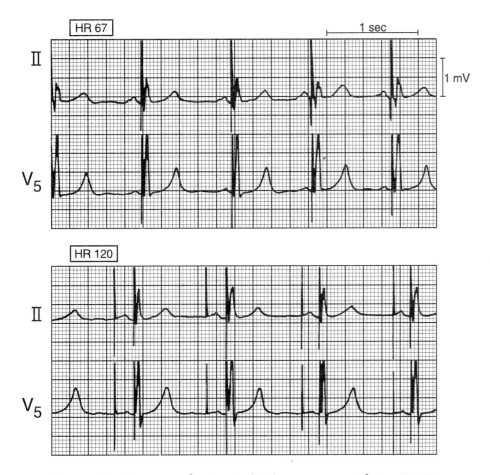

Figure 13.5 Erroneous heart rate (HR) measurement during DDD mode cardiac pacing. (*Top panel*) Native atrial P waves are sensed and ventricular pacing follows. The monitor display for HR is accurate (HR 67), since the ventricular pacing spikes are not counted separate from the R waves by the monitor. (*Bottom panel*) Atrioventricular (AV) sequential pacing is initiated at a rate of 60 beats/min with an AV interval of 200 msec. The tall atrial pacing spikes are misinterpreted by the monitor as R waves and result in an erroneous value for HR measurement (HR 120). Note the slight variability to the R-R interval in the top panel when the DDD pacer is functioning in the atrial sensing mode and thus responding to the normal physiologic variation in sinus rate.

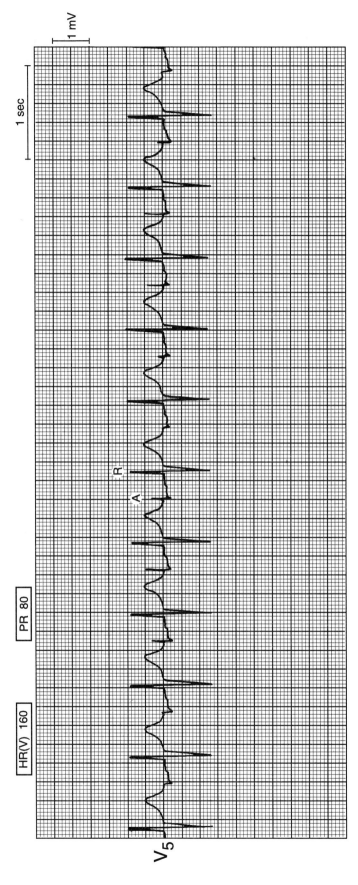

Figure 13.6 Erroneous heart rate (HR) measurement during atrial (A) cardiac pacing. The A pacing spikes are counted by the monitor in addition to the ECG R waves, resulting in an artifactual doubling of the HR measured from ECG lead V₅ (HR[V] 160) compared to the pulse rate (PR 80) measured from the pulse oximeter plethysmograph.

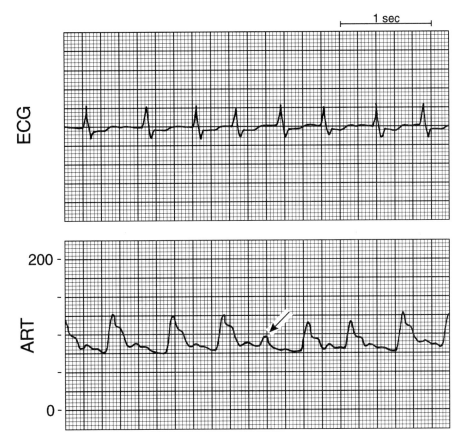

Figure 13.7 Pulse deficit in atrial fibrillation. The short R-R interval between the third and fourth ECG complexes reduces the time for diastolic filling and results in decreased stroke volume and arterial blood pressure (ART). If this diminished ART pulsation (*arrow*) is not perceptible as a peripheral pulse, then a pulse deficit exists and pulse rate will be less than heart rate.

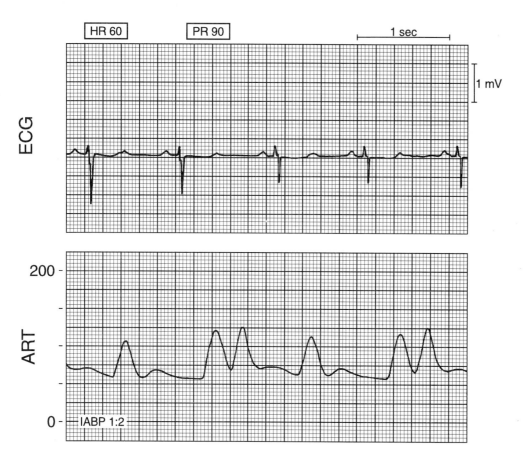

Figure 13.8 Erroneous pulse rate (PR) measurement during intraaortic balloon pump (IABP) counterpulsation. The IABP assist ratio is 1:2, as evident from the augmented diastolic arterial blood pressure (ART) seen on alternate beats. The ECG clearly reveals the heart rate (HR) to be 60 beats/min. The monitor miscalculates the PR because the diastolic ART pulsations generated by the IABP are erroneously counted in addition to the normal systolic arterial pulsations (PR 90). See text for more detail.

References

1. Block FE. What is heart rate, anyway? J Clin Monit 1994; 10:366–70

2. Khambatta HJ, Stone JG, Wald A, Mongero LB. Electrocardiographic artifacts during cardiopulmonary bypass. Anesth Analg 1990;71:88–91

3. Metz S. ECG artifacts during cardiopulmonary bypass—an alternative method. Anesth Analg 1991;72:715–6

4. Weinfurt PT. Electrocardiographic monitoring: an overview. J Clin Monit 1990;6:132–8

CHAPTER FOURTEEN Arrhythmias

AN INTEGRATED ECG AND HEMODYNAMIC APPROACH

Bedside ECG monitoring for detection of arrhythmias has become a standard of care in operating rooms and intensive care units.[2,9,16] In these settings, a wide variety of arrhythmias and conduction abnormalities can be diagnosed from the ECG trace displayed on the monitor. In some cases, however, the diagnosis remains unclear, and since the ECG can reveal only the electrical activity of the heart, the hemodynamic consequences of a given ECG abnormality are never immediately evident.[8] Indeed, the ECG may provide a false sense of security and appear relatively normal despite severe coexisting hemodynamic compromise, as in electrical-mechanical dissociation (EMD, also termed pulseless electrical activity [PEA]).

During the perioperative period, patients with advanced cardiac disease often have additional hemodynamic monitoring, including direct arterial blood pressure, pulmonary artery pressure (PAP), or central venous pressure (CVP). These additional pressure traces displayed on the bedside monitor provide unique and timely diagnostic information. First, the hemodynamic impact of an abnormal ECG trace will be evident at once. Second, and equally important, the hemodynamic waveforms may provide the *initial clues* that cardiac conduction or rhythm problems are present. This is the hallmark of *integrated monitoring*, combining information from all the traces on the bedside monitor to arrive quickly at the proper diagnosis. Rather than provide a review of cardiac arrhythmias and conduction disturbances, which are well described in many other standard texts,[18,19] this chapter emphasizes an approach to arrhythmia detection using the bedside monitor that takes advantage of the supplemental hemodynamic data available on the monitor screen. The message that ECG monitoring complements hemodynamic monitoring and vice versa can be seen most vividly by considering arrhythmias that alter normal atrioventricular synchrony.

ATRIAL FIBRILLATION AND FLUTTER

The most common cause of disturbed atrioventricular synchrony is atrial fibrillation, where the normal end-diastolic atrial contribution to ventricular filling is lost. Inspection of the accompanying CVP trace is often confusing, because this trace generally displays two pressure peaks in each cardiac cycle (Fig. 14.1), similar to the pattern seen in normal sinus rhythm. However, unlike sinus rhythm, where the two most prominent pressure peaks are the a and v waves (see Ch. 2, Fig. 2.3), the two peaks seen in the venous waveform in atrial fibrillation are the c and v waves.[6,7] The a wave has disappeared, owing to the loss of normal atrial contraction. Furthermore, the c wave is more prominent than usual. This occurs because atrial volume at end-diastole remains abnormally high in the absence of atrial contraction, and the subsequent isovolumic ventricular contraction, which dis-

places the tricuspid valve toward the right atrium, creates a taller early systolic pressure wave, the prominent c wave. The integrated ECG, arterial pressure, and CVP recordings (Fig. 14.1) highlight several other pertinent hemodynamic aspects of atrial fibrillation. Pressure wave morphologies change as the ECG R-R interval changes, owing to variations in chamber filling and contractile state that occur as heart rate varies.[12] Short R-R intervals limit time for ventricular filling in diastole and lead to marked reductions in stroke volume and blood pressure, a common problem in patients with atrial fibrillation and a rapid ventricular response. Finally, it may be argued that the arrhythmia is not easily recognized from the ECG trace alone, especially since small P waves often go undetected and large portions of the ECG trace appear to have a regular rate (Fig. 14.1). However, the irregularity of the cardiac cycle is highlighted by both the arterial and venous pressure traces. In other words, *the hemodynamic waveforms may provide the first clues to the onset of the arrhythmia.*

In addition to the c and v waves normally seen in the venous pressure trace in patients with atrial fibrillation, other small amplitude pressure waves may be identified that reflect the underlying atrial mechanical activity. These *fibrillation/flutter waves* appear superimposed on the predominant c and v waves and identify the cardiac rhythm disturbance (Figs. 14.2 and 14.3).[6,7] Note that c wave onset in Figure 14.3 appears delayed relative to the ECG R wave (compare Figs. 14.2 and 14.3). This observation demands an explanation and focuses attention back on the ECG trace, which reveals a wide QRS complex. This patient has right bundle branch block, which retards contraction of the right ventricle and results in a delayed c wave in the venous pressure trace.

ATRIOVENTRICULAR DISSOCIATION

During general anesthesia, particularly when nitrous oxide or other potent inhaled anesthetics are employed, loss of normal atrioventricular synchrony commonly occurs. Although it is often called *junctional rhythm*,[1,4,11] this arrhythmia is most accurately described as *isorhythmic atrioventricular dissociation*.[13–15] In both instances, there is a single supraventricular site of origin for ventricular pacing, but in junctional rhythm, there is retrograde conduction to the atria from this *single* pacing site, while in isorhythmic atrioventricular dissociation, a *second* supraventricular pacing site controls atrial depolarization at approximately the same rate as the ventricular rate (*isorhythmic or isochronic*). Although normal atrioventricular synchrony is lost in both situations, the two arrhythmias have slightly different hemodynamic signatures.

Quick observation of the ECG trace alone may not clearly reveal the absence of sinus rhythm, particularly when P wave amplitude is small (Fig. 14.4A) and the heart rate is essentially unchanged from the normal sinus rate. Evidence for atrioventricular dissociation, with P waves marching through the QRS complex, may not be recognized, because the P waves remain hidden within the greater amplitude QRS (Fig. 14.4B). Here again, the hemodynamic traces aid the diagnosis by calling attention to the onset of the arrhythmia. When there is loss of normal atrioventricular synchrony, and atrial contraction occurs during ventricular systole, a tall *cannon a wave* (or *cannon wave*) is inscribed in the CVP trace (Fig. 14.5).[6,7] This cannon wave is caused by atrial contraction against a closed tricuspid valve during systole. Note also that systemic arterial hypotension results when the normal end-diastolic atrial kick is lost and diastolic filling of the ventricle is compromised. Whereas atrial contraction normally provides up to 15 per cent of left ventricular end-diastolic pressure and volume, patients with ventricular hypertrophy and other causes of increased diastolic stiffness may be much more dependent upon a properly timed atrial contraction to augment ventricular preload. In such patients, the atrial contribution to ventricular filling may reach 40 percent or more of the total end-diastolic volume and pressure.[17] Such patients are critically dependent upon normal atrioventricular synchrony, and onset of junctional rhythm or atrioventricular dissociation causes abrupt and profound arterial hypotension (Fig. 14.6).[7] Often, the earliest and clearest clues to this arrhythmia are not discovered in the ECG trace but rather in changes in morphology of the venous waveform and arterial blood pressure (Figs. 14.5 and 14.6).

Cannon a waves that appear in early ventricular systole are superimposed on the normal venous pressure c wave and produce a composite wave of large amplitude (Fig. 14.5). When atrial depolarization and contraction occur in mid- to late ventricular systole, the cannon a waves may appear after the c wave (Fig. 14.7). In fact, in isorhythmic atrioventricular dissociation, cannon a waves may be observed before, during, or after the c wave, as the temporal relation between atrial and ventricular contraction varies slightly (Fig. 14.8). In contrast, the position of the cannon waves in the cardiac cycle will not vary in junctional rhythm where there is a fixed relation between ventricular and atrial contraction resulting from retrograde conduction of the junctional beat to the atrium. Finally, it should be noted that cannon a waves will be evident in any venous waveform, including the pulmonary artery wedge pressure or left atrial pressure (LAP) traces (Fig. 14.9). In each of these examples, the abnormal venous waveform focuses attention back on the ECG and aids the prompt diagnosis of atrioventricular dysynchrony. Differences in CVP contour and timing of atrial and ventricular contraction have been used in the nonoperative setting as well to distinguish atrioventricular nodal re-entrant tachycardia from supraventricular tachycardia caused by circus movement through an accessory pathway.[3]

ARTIFACT RECOGNITION

Because arrhythmias may cause sudden, marked hemodynamic changes, the onset of these changes should trigger a closer examination of the ECG trace to confirm the diagnosis. On occasion, a striking hemodynamic abnormality may be an isolated finding and prove to be artifactual in nature. For example, the clinician must recognize when a pressure transducer falls well below the level of the patient's heart and causes spurious elevation in the pressure reading or when a pressure recording is damped because of air or blood clot in the fluid-filled tubing (see Ch. 9, Figs. 9.3 and 9.21).

In contrast to these easily recognizable monitoring problems, some artifacts noted on the bedside monitor closely resemble pathophysiologic waveforms. At first glance, the intermittent tall, wide beats in Figure 14.10 resemble short runs of slow ventricular tachycardia. The arterial blood pressure is stable, however, and closer examination of the ECG shows a regular rhythm with P waves preceding each QRS complex. The changing QRS morphology is caused by cardiac axis changes over the respiratory cycle in a patient with left bundle branch block. In this example, the stable, regular arterial pressure trace underscores the artifactual nature of the arrhythmia.

When the bedside monitor displays multiple pressure traces along with the ECG, additional clues help the clinician distinguish fact from artifact. *It is rare to have an arrhythmia or other hemodynamic event alter a single monitored value.* Although one might detect the abnormality first in any single trace on the monitor screen, further scrutiny of the other traces is required to confirm the diagnostic pattern. As noted above, cannon a waves in the CVP trace may be the initial and most striking observation in a patient with junctional rhythm (Fig. 14.5), but the accompanying arterial hypotension and ECG abnormality confirm the diagnosis (Figs. 14.5 and 14.6). In contrast, "cannon waves" in the venous pressure trace that occur without changes in the arterial pressure or ECG traces must have a different etiology. In this example (Fig. 14.11), the tall early systolic waves seen in the CVP trace must be artifactual in nature, since the ECG clearly shows the rhythm to be sinus. Here the CVP is recorded from the proximal port of a pulmonary artery catheter. This recording site, located 30 cm from the tip of the catheter, was positioned at the level of the tricuspid valve and recorded right ventricular pressures in early systole. When the catheter was withdrawn several centimeters, the artifactual CVP trace disappeared, although junctional rhythm accompanied by true cannon a waves developed later in this patient (Fig. 14.11).

With practice, one can learn to suspect artifactual recordings in slow trend recordings, where the individual waveforms are not even seen. In this example (Fig. 14.12), the tall

CVP waves occur without any change in arterial pressure or ECG recordings. These waves occur approximately six times each minute and reflect the influence of the positive pressure respiratory cycle displacing the CVP recording port into the right ventricle, similar to the previous example (Fig. 14.11) (compare Figs. 14.11 and 14.12 with 14.5 and 14.6). All of these examples serve to highlight the importance of *integrated monitoring*.

PACING AND ATRIOVENTRICULAR SYNCHRONY

When electrical pacing of the heart is contemplated either to treat bradycardia or restore normal atrioventricular synchrony, the hemodynamic traces provide clear evidence of the success or failure of pacing to achieve the desired goals. Although the ECG trace alone might suggest the need for pacing, the hemodynamic condition of the patient is the ultimate determinant of the need for this form of therapy. For example, first degree heart block generally has little hemodynamic impact, and one might not suspect there is a need for atrioventricular sequential pacing from observing the ECG trace alone (Fig. 14.13). However, when the PR interval is prolonged markedly, particularly in a patient who is dependent on the end-diastolic atrial kick to provide adequate cardiac filling and stroke volume, atrioventricular sequential pacing with a normal PR interval may have a striking impact on the hemodynamic condition of the patient.[10] In this example (Fig. 14.14), first degree heart block accompanies atrial pacing and is poorly tolerated from a circulatory standpoint. The PR (or AV) interval is greater than 400 msec, more than twice the normal value. Atrial contraction occurs during the end of the previous systolic cycle, thereby inscribing a cannon wave in the CVP trace. Of greater importance, atrial contraction does not provide effective end-diastolic loading of the ventricle, resulting in a low stroke volume, cardiac output, and arterial blood pressure. Atrioventricular pacing at the same rate but with a normal PR interval (200 msec) restores the arterial pressure by improving ventricular filling and boosting cardiac output more than 50 percent. The CVP trace returns to a more normal morphology and helps underscore the hemodynamic improvement.

By focusing on the arterial and venous pressure waveforms, the clinician can determine rapidly when attempts at atrial, ventricular, and atrioventricular sequential pacing are effective. Although the ECG should provide definitive evidence for successful pacing, the ECG trace may be very difficult to interpret intraoperatively, owing to inherent difficulties recognizing pacing spikes and their association with P waves or QRS complexes, especially in the electrically noisy operating room environment. Ventricular pacing commonly produces a cannon wave in the CVP trace, since

there is often retrograde atrial conduction of the electrical depolarization initiated in the ventricle, which causes atrial contraction against a closed tricuspid valve during systole. When atrioventricular sequential pacing is initiated in this example (Fig. 14.15), the arterial and venous pressure waveforms remain unchanged and confirm the fact that atrioventricular synchrony has not been restored. Although this fact is readily seen from the hemodynamic traces, the ECG is misleading because it shows clear atrial pacing spikes but does not reveal that these spikes have failed to provide atrial capture.

In contrast, effective atrioventricular sequential pacing should alter both the CVP and arterial pressure waveforms, the former by obliterating the systolic cannon waves and the latter by increasing the blood pressure (Fig. 14.16). Like the CVP trace, a wedge pressure or LAP trace will prove similarly useful for identifying cannon waves during pacing (Fig. 14.17).

These cannon waves may have a fixed position in the cardiac cycle if there is retrograde conduction and capture of the atrium with each ventricular paced beat (Figs. 14.15 and 14.16). Alternatively, atrial contractions that occur with no fixed relation to the ventricular cycle will produce a *chaotic venous waveform* of varying morphology (Figs. 14.17 and 14.18), depending on whether atrial contraction occurs during systole when the tricuspid valve is closed, or during diastole when the tricuspid valve is open.[6,7] Variable timing of atrial contraction will also produce a varying arterial waveform, as ventricular loading conditions and stroke output change with each beat (Fig. 14.18).

In summary, hemodynamic waveforms, particularly CVP waveforms, provide unique insights about atrioventricular synchrony during cardiac pacing. Cannon waves resulting from systolic atrial contraction against a closed tricuspid valve underscore the presence of atrioventricular dysynchrony, whether caused by a primary arrhythmia (Fig. 14.19)[5] or by electrical pacing (Figs. 14.15 to 14.18). The ECG displayed on the bedside monitor may be hard to decipher, especially in the presence of electrical interference produced by the electrosurgical unit (Fig. 14.20A). The clinician should suspect pacing failure by noting new irregularities in the hemodynamic waveforms, which identify loss of atrioventricular synchrony and failure of the pacemaker to capture the chamber as intended (Fig. 14.20).

ATRIOVENTRICULAR DYSYNCHRONY DURING CARDIOPULMONARY BYPASS

Unusual hemodynamic waveforms are seen occasionally during cardiopulmonary bypass, and their proper interpretation depends upon reviewing all the information from the bedside monitor. After initiation of bypass and induction of systemic hypothermia, ventricular fibrillation often develops during cardiac manipulation (Fig. 14.21). The systemic arterial pulse pressure vanishes as left ventricular ejection ceases (see also Ch. 7, Fig. 7.1). Why then does the CVP trace sometimes show small regular waves, when the rhythm is ventricular fibrillation (Fig. 14.21)? This is another, albeit unusual, example of atrioventricular dissociation, where ventricular fibrillation coexists with atrial sinus rhythm. Small regular atrial pressure waves are seen in the CVP trace. PAP waves result from these atrial contractions, as the fibrillating right ventricle serves as a passive conduit in this instance. Since continued atrial electrical activity is a sign of inadequate cardioplegic arrest of the atrium, atrial contractile dysfunction may be present after bypass if this persistent atrial electrical activity is not recognized and treated. Presumably, the same atrial contraction phenomenon is occurring on the left side of the circulation, although systemic arterial pressure waves resulting from left atrial contraction are less evident in the higher pressure arterial circuit (Fig. 14.21).

Cyclic CVP waves of small amplitude also may be produced by an automated infusion pump, which administers fluid in a pulsatile fashion into a monitored venous pressure line. However, these pulsations are generally too small in magnitude to produce an increase in PAP, and they would never be seen in an LAP trace.

Another curious venous pressure phenomenon seen occasionally during cardiopulmonary bypass arises from the sump action of the venous return line, which collapses the compliant right atrium rhythmically every few seconds. This produces a sudden sharp decrease in CVP. As venous return from the vena cavae fills the collapsed right atrium, this chamber pops open again, CVP returns to its baseline value, and venous return to the pump is restored. Every second or two, the entire cycle repeats itself, thus producing these curious rhythmic venous pressure waves.

Illustrations for Arrhythmias

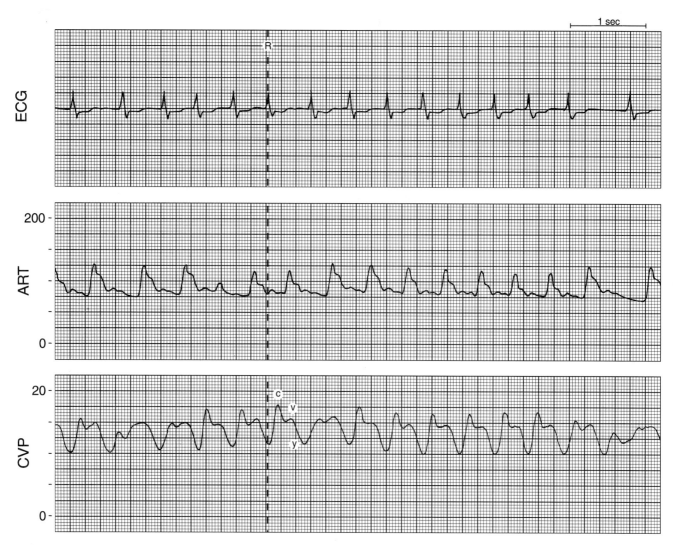

Figure 14.1 Atrial fibrillation obliterates the central venous pressure (CVP) a wave, augments the c wave, and preserves the v wave and y descent. The variable ECG R-R interval in atrial fibrillation produces changes in both the CVP and arterial blood pressure (ART) traces. See text for more detail. (Modified from Mark,[6] with permission.)

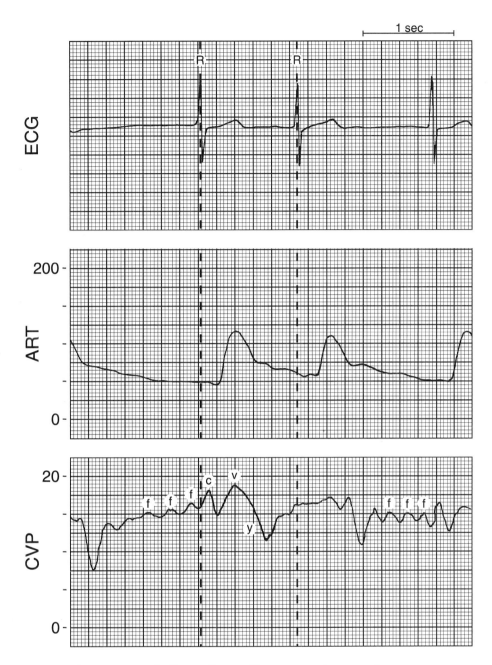

Figure 14.2 Fibrillation/flutter (f) waves in the central venous pressure (CVP) trace reveal the underlying atrial arrhythmia. The CVP c and v waves are noted, along with the dominant y descent. The arterial blood pressure (ART) waveform is also shown. See text for more detail. (Modified from Mark,[6] with permission.)

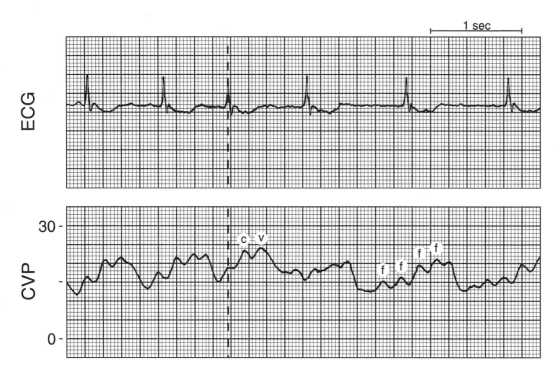

Figure 14.3 Fibrillation/flutter (f) waves in the central venous pressure (CVP) trace reveal the underlying atrial arrhythmia. The CVP c and v waves are seen, along with the dominant y descent, which follows the v wave in early diastole. Note that the c wave appears delayed relative to the ECG R wave because right bundle branch block delays onset of right ventricular contraction. Compare with Fig. 14.2. See text for more detail.

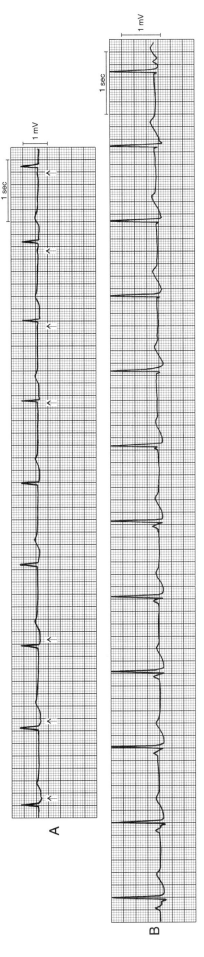

Figure 14.4 Isorhythmic atrioventricular dissociation. (A) At standard ECG gain, P waves (arrows) are difficult to identify, and this arrhythmia may go unnoticed. Although atrial and ventricular rates are nearly identical (isorhythmic), the atrial rate (48 beats/min) is slightly faster than the ventricular rate (46 beats/min). This accounts for the observation that the P wave follows the R wave at the beginning of the trace and emerges before the R wave eight beats later, at the end of the trace. (B) Increased ECG gain to 16 mm/mV helps identify P waves and diagnose this arrhythmia in another patient. In this case, the atrial rate (48 beats/min) is slightly slower than the ventricular rate (50 beats/min), and thus the P waves appear before the R waves at the beginning of the trace and progressively march through the QRS, highlighting the dissociation of atrial and ventricular pacemakers. Note that the P wave is hidden within the QRS complex in the 8th through 11th beats.

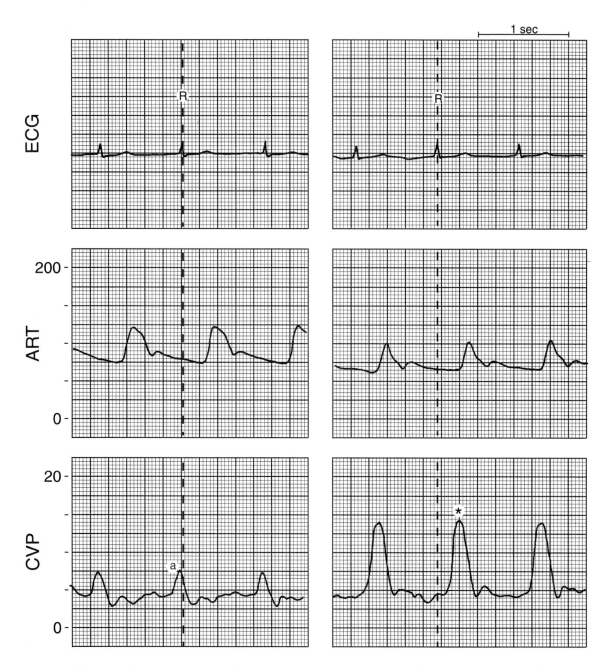

Figure 14.5 Cannon waves (°) in the central venous pressure (CVP) trace are the hallmark of junctional rhythm or atrioventricular dissociation. (*Left panels*) The ECG, arterial blood pressure (ART), and CVP during normal sinus rhythm. (*Right panels*) With onset of junctional rhythm, atrial contraction against a closed tricuspid valve during systole produces a tall cannon wave (°) in the CVP trace and results in arterial hypotension, owing to loss of normal end-diastolic atrial contribution to ventricular filling. Compare the CVP cannon wave (°) to the normal CVP a wave (a) in terms of timing and amplitude. Note that the ECG traces do not help distinguish these conditions, because the P waves are too small to be seen in the top left panel, and they are buried within the QRS complex in the top right panel. See text for more detail. (Modified from Mark,[6] with permission.)

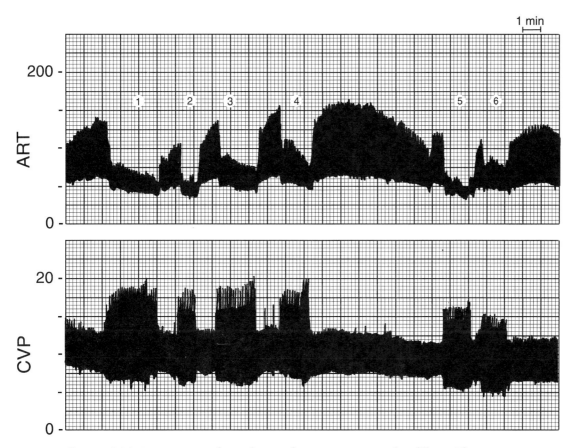

Figure 14.6 Importance of atrial contribution to ventricular filling. These traces were recorded from a patient with aortic stenosis and severe left ventricular hypertrophy. During each numbered interval (1 to 6), a sudden marked decrease in arterial blood pressure (ART) is accompanied by the appearance of cannon waves in the central venous pressure (CVP) trace. The CVP recording helps determine the cause of hemodynamic instability and graphically illustrates that loss of atrioventricular synchrony may produce profound arterial hypotension in patients with diastolic left ventricular dysfunction. In this case, ART changes more than 50 mmHg in less than 20 seconds. See text for more detail. (Modified from Mark,[7] with permission.)

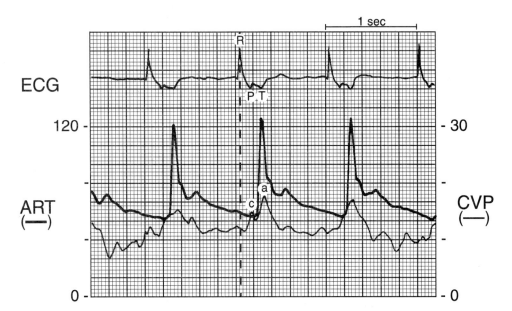

Figure 14.7 During junctional rhythm, central venous pressure (CVP) cannon a waves (a) may appear in mid- to late systole following the normal CVP c wave (c). Note the abnormal P wave in the ECG, which is not concealed within the QRS complex, but instead appears between the ECG R and T waves and distorts the ST-segment. Arterial blood pressure (ART) is low (122/54 mmHg, mean 71 mmHg), and the ART waveform is narrow, reflecting the reduced left ventricular stroke volume that accompanies this arrhythmia.

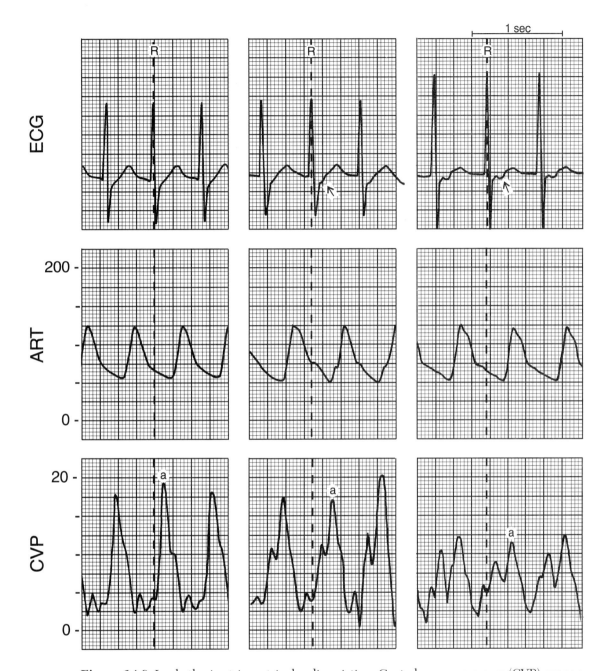

Figure 14.8 Isorhythmic atrioventricular dissociation. Central venous pressure (CVP) cannon a waves (a) appear in early systole (*left panels*), mid-systole (*middle panels*), or late systole (*right panels*) as the temporal relation between atrial and ventricular contraction changes slightly in this arrhythmia. The corresponding variable timing of atrial and ventricular electrical activity is seen in the ECG. Initially, the P wave is hidden within the QRS complex (*left panels*), then it is observed in mid-systole (*middle panels*), and finally it is seen during late systole (*right panels*) distorting the ST-segment. Although the CVP waveform changes as the precise timing of atrial and ventricular contraction shift slightly, the arterial blood pressure (ART) waveform does not change significantly, because atrial contraction never occurs in diastole when it would contribute to ventricular filling. Compare left, middle, and right panels.

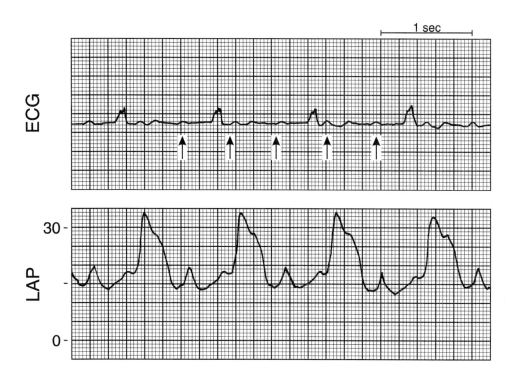

Figure 14.9 Venous cannon waves recorded in a left atrial pressure (LAP) trace during 2:1 atrioventricular block and left bundle branch block. The tall cannon waves alternate with normal LAP a waves, depending on whether the atrial contraction occurs in systole (against a closed mitral valve) or in diastole, when there is no impairment of atrial emptying.

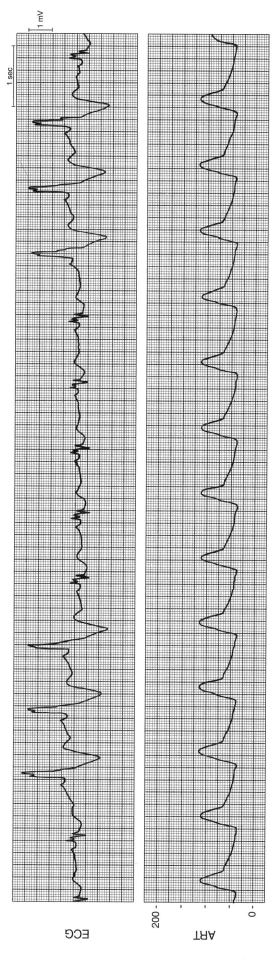

Figure 14.10 Artifactual rhythm change. Casual observation of the ECG trace suggests a rhythm disturbance, with wide QRS complexes that resemble ventricular ectopic beats. However, arterial blood pressure (ART) remains stable (115/40 mmHg) throughout the recording. Closer scrutiny of the ECG reveals a regular rhythm with P waves preceding each QRS complex. The changing QRS morphology is caused by a cardiac axis shift during the respiratory cycle in this patient with underlying left bundle branch block. The ART trace underscores the absence of arrhythmia in this case.

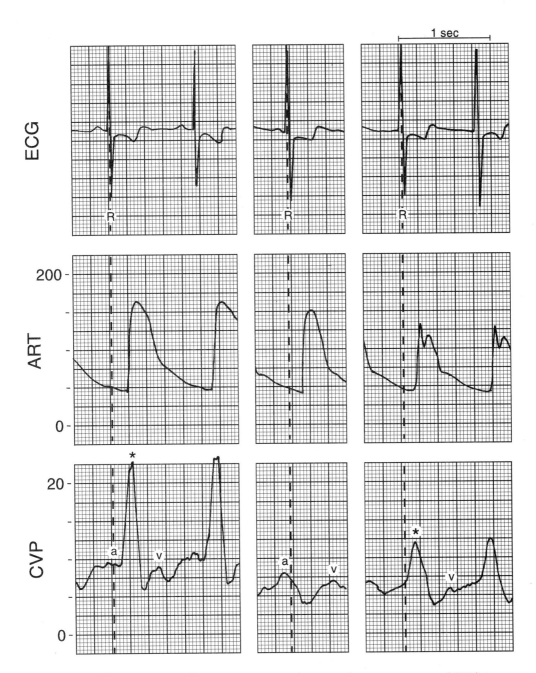

Figure 14.11 *Pseudo-cannon waves* in the central venous pressure (CVP) waveform. (*Left panels*) The tall early systolic CVP wave (*, *left panels*) is artifactual, since the ECG clearly shows the rhythm to be sinus. The CVP in this case is recorded from the proximal port of a pulmonary artery catheter. This recording port is positioned near the level of the tricuspid valve and is recording right ventricular pressure in early systole. After the catheter is withdrawn 5 cm, a CVP trace with normal a and v waves is recorded (*middle panels*). Later, true cannon waves appear in the CVP trace (*, *right panels*) when junctional rhythm develops. The accompanying changes in both the ECG morphology and the arterial blood pressure (ART) waveform confirm the presence of the arrhythmia.

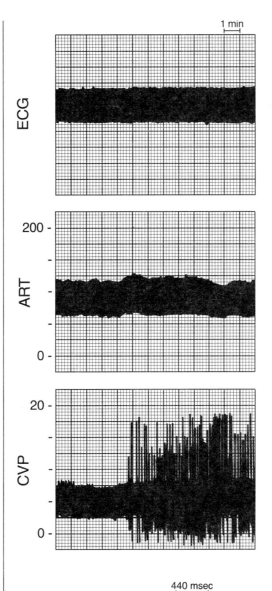

Figure 14.12 *Pseudo-cannon waves* in the central venous pressure (CVP) waveform. Tall venous pressure waves appear approximately six times each minute and are not accompanied by changes in the ECG or arterial blood pressure (ART) recordings, raising the suspicion of a measurement artifact. As in Fig. 14.11, the CVP in this case is recorded from the proximal port of a pulmonary artery catheter. With each positive pressure respiratory cycle, the recording port is displaced transiently into the right ventricle and thus records right ventricular systolic pressure rather than CVP.

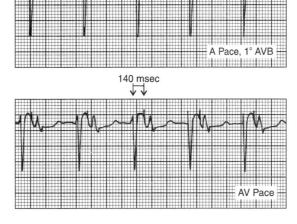

Figure 14.13 The ECG does not reveal the hemodynamic consequences of different modes of pacing. (*Top panel*) Atrial pacing and severe first degree atrioventricular block (A Pace, 1° AVB) with a PR interval of 440 msec. (*Bottom panel*) Atrioventricular sequential pacing (AV Pace) with a normal PR interval of 140 msec. Although the ventricular rate (83 beats/min) is identical and atrioventricular synchrony is maintained in both recordings, institution of sequential pacing produces a marked increase in blood pressure in this example. Clearly, additional hemodynamic data help determine the efficacy of different modes of pacing. Compare with Fig. 14.14. See text for more detail.

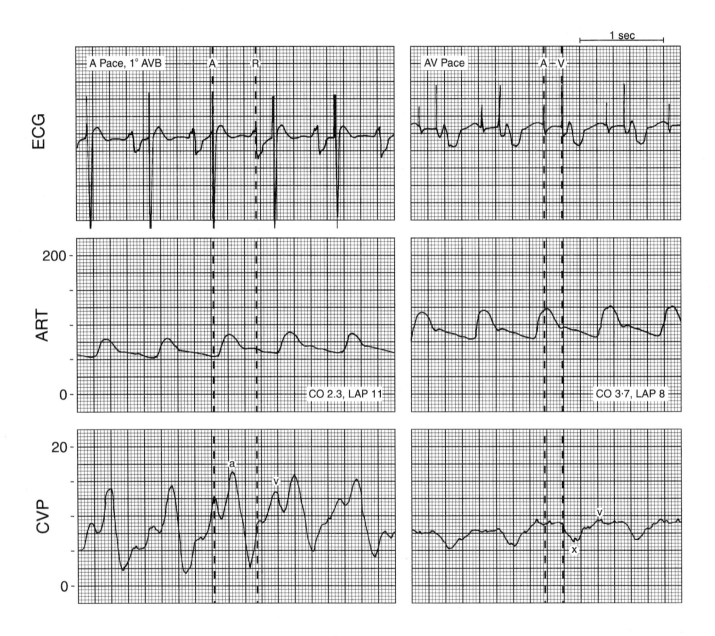

Figure 14.14 Benefits of atrioventricular sequential pacing (AV Pace) during severe first degree atrioventricular block (1° AVB). The left panels show atrial pacing (A Pace) and first degree AVB with a 480-msec interval between the atrial pacing spike (A) and the ECG R wave (R). This AV interval is so long that atrial contraction occurs during the previous systolic cycle and inscribes a cannon wave (a) in the central venous pressure (CVP) trace. The normal CVP v wave (v) is identified and highlights the abnormal temporal relationship between atrial and ventricular events during the cardiac cycle. Owing to ineffective timing of atrial contraction, left ventricular filling is compromised and results in low cardiac output (CO 2.3 L/min) and arterial blood pressure (ART, 85/55 mmHg). The right panels show the hemodynamic improvement that occurs with atrioventricular sequential pacing. Despite pacing at the same ventricular rate (80 beats/min), restoration of a normal PR or AV interval (200 msec) increases CO (3.7 L/min) and ART (125/80 mmHg). Note that the improved CO and ART occur despite a reduction in mean left atrial pressure (LAP 11 mmHg during atrial pacing [*left panels*], LAP 8 mmHg during atrioventricular pacing [*right panels*]), because properly timed atrial contraction at end-diastole effectively boosts left ventricular preload and eliminates venous cannon waves caused by poorly timed atrial contraction during ventricular systole. In addition, the improved hemodynamic condition during atrioventricular pacing is highlighted by the CVP waveform, which shows resolution of the cannon waves and results in lower mean pressure and more normal waveform morphology (x descent and v wave). This complicated example emphasizes the value of integrated monitoring and the wealth of information available through careful scrutiny of all the monitored waveforms.

The critical observer also may have noted changes in the atrial pacing spike amplitudes in the left and right ECG panels. All of these recordings were made in the operating room during periods of temporary epicardial pacing. Unipolar pacing employs a single active electrode attached to the surface of the paced cardiac chamber and a second ground electrode attached at a remote site on the skin. Because of the long current path created by this electrode configuration, unipolar pacing produces a tall amplitude pacing spike on the surface ECG. In contrast, bipolar pacing requires that both the active and ground electrodes be attached to the paced chamber. Because of this different pacing lead configuration, a shorter current path is produced, and bipolar pacing results in smaller pacing spikes on the surface ECG. In this example, initial atrial pacing was unipolar (*left ECG panel*), and subsequent atrioventricular pacing was bipolar, both atrial bipolar and ventricular bipolar (*right ECG panel*).

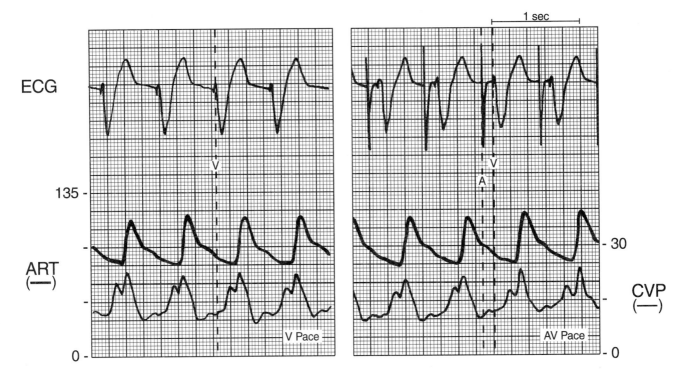

Figure 14.15 Failed atrial capture during pacing. (*Left panel*) The ECG shows ventricular pacing (V Pace) at a rate of 91 beats/min, along with the accompanying arterial blood pressure (ART) and central venous pressure (CVP) waveforms. The CVP trace reveals cannon waves that occur during ventricular pacing when there is retrograde conduction of the ventricular impulse to the atrium, which causes atrial contraction during systole. (*Right panel*) The ECG shows evidence of atrioventricular sequential pacing (AV Pace) at the same rate (91 beats/min) with a normal PR or AV interval (120 msec). However, the ineffectiveness of the atrioventricular pacing is underscored by the absence of hemodynamic changes in the ART or CVP traces. Despite the fact that the ECG suggests atrioventricular pacing, the atrial pacing spike has failed to capture the atrium and provide properly timed end-diastolic atrial contraction. Compare with Fig. 14.16.

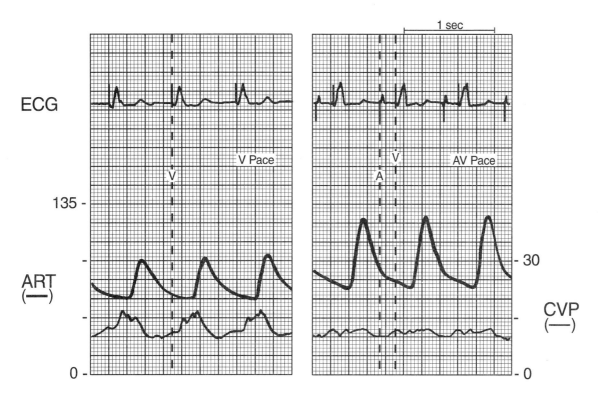

Figure 14.16 Successful atrial capture during pacing. (*Left panel*) The ECG shows ventricular pacing (V Pace) at a rate of 86 beats/min, along with the accompanying arterial blood pressure (ART) and central venous pressure (CVP) waveforms. The CVP trace reveals cannon waves that occur during ventricular pacing when there is retrograde conduction of the ventricular impulse to the atrium, which causes atrial contraction during systole. (*Right panel*) The ECG shows evidence of atrioventricular sequential pacing (AV Pace) at the same rate (86 beats/min) with a normal PR or AV interval (160 msec). Clear changes occur in the accompanying hemodynamic traces when atrioventricular pacing is instituted. The CVP cannon waves are eliminated, and there is a marked increase in ART from 93/60 mmHg during ventricular pacing to 124/68 mmHg during atrioventricular sequential pacing. Successful atrial capture during sequential pacing restores normal atrioventricular synchrony and leads to hemodynamic improvement. Compare with Fig. 14.15.

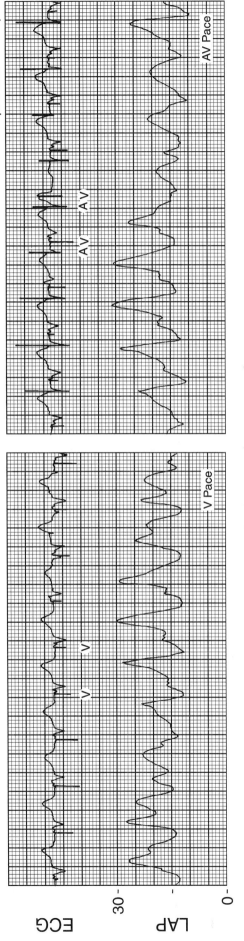

Figure 14.17 Failed atrial capture during pacing. (*Left panel*) The ECG shows ventricular pacing (V Pace, 125 beats/min) with two ventricular pacing spikes highlighted (V). Like the central venous pressure waveform, a left atrial pressure (LAP) waveform may reveal cannon waves during ventricular pacing. Atrial contraction occurs without any fixed relation to the ventricular cycle, resulting in a variable, chaotic appearing LAP waveform. (*Right panel*) Attempted atrioventricular sequential pacing (AV Pace, 125 beats/min) with the atrial and ventricular pacing spikes highlighted in the middle of the trace (A, V, AV interval 110 msec). Despite the fact that the ECG suggests atrioventricular pacing, the atrial pacing spike has failed to capture the atrium and restore atrioventricular synchrony. This fact is underscored by the absence of change in the LAP waveform, which still demonstrates cannon waves. In this example, the left-sided venous pressure waveform serves the same purpose as the central venous pressure waveform in demonstrating absence of atrioventricular synchrony.

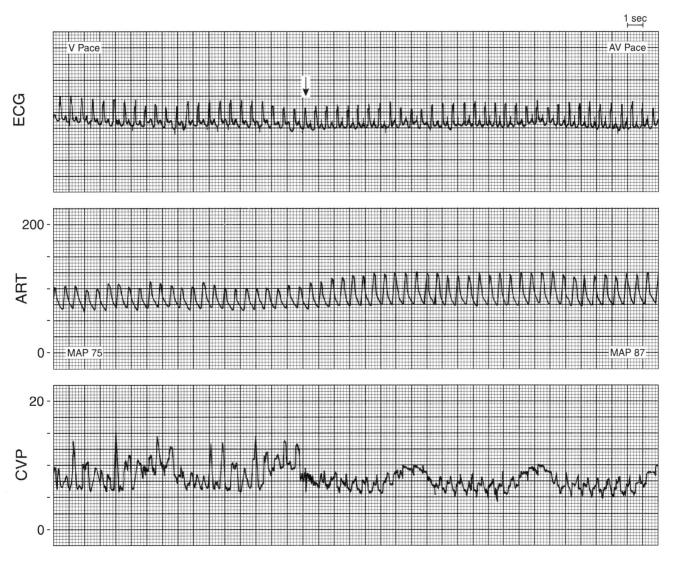

Figure 14.18 Restoration of atrioventricular synchrony during pacing is revealed by the hemodynamic waveforms. Although it is difficult to see the details in the ECG in this slow speed recording, the left side of the panel shows ventricular pacing (V Pace), which changes to atrioventricular sequential pacing (AV Pace) after 16 seconds (arrow). The accompanying hemodynamic traces highlight the changes that occur with effective restoration of atrioventricular synchrony. During ventricular pacing, there is no fixed relation between the timing of atrial and ventricular contraction, and both the arterial blood pressure (ART) and the central venous pressure (CVP) vary from beat to beat, depending on whether atrial contraction occurs during ventricular diastole or ventricular systole. When normal atrioventricular synchrony is reestablished during sequential pacing, the cannon waves disappear from the CVP trace and the beat to beat variability of the ART waveform resolves. Furthermore, effective atrial loading of the ventricle is highlighted by the increase in blood pressure from a mean arterial pressure (MAP) of 75 mmHg to a MAP of 87 mmHg. (Note that some phasic variation in both the ART and CVP waveforms remains during atrioventricular sequential pacing because of the cyclic effects of positive pressure mechanical ventilation.) (Modified from Mark,[6] with permission.)

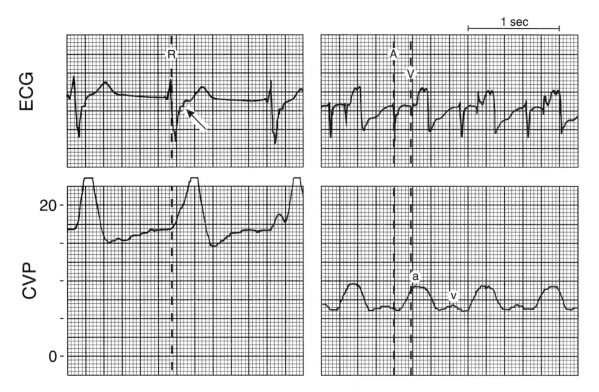

Figure 14.19 The central venous pressure (CVP) waveform as a clue to the presence of normal atrioventricular synchrony. (*Left panels*) Junctional rhythm (56 beats/min) with a retrograde P wave distorting the ST-segment in the ECG (arrow) and a giant cannon wave in the CVP trace. Restoration of normal atrioventricular synchrony is achieved with atrioventricular sequential pacing (A, V, 83 beats/min, AV interval 170 msec, *right panels*) and is reflected clearly by the CVP waveform, which now displays normal a and v waves. (Modified from Mark,[5] with permission.)

Figure 14.20 The hemodynamic waveforms provide clues to the presence of atrioventricular synchrony during attempted cardiac pacing. (A) Electrical interference produced by the electrosurgical unit in the operating room precludes ECG interpretation, although pacing spikes at a rate of 88 beats/min are visible. The marked irregularity of both the arterial blood pressure (ART) and central venous pressure (CVP) waveforms highlights the absence of atrioventricular synchrony. Note that the fifth beat is a ventricular premature beat, rather than a paced beat. (B) Ventricular pacing at 88 beats/min results in the typical variability in both ART and CVP waveforms, depending on the relative timing of atrial and ventricular contraction. Note that the third beat has the highest blood pressure and lowest CVP, because of the fortuitous timing of atrial contraction at end-diastole, immediately prior to the ventricular pacing spike and the onset of ventricular systole. (C) Attempted atrioventricular sequential pacing (88 beats/min, AV interval 140 msec) is unsuccessful. The atrial and ventricular pacing spikes seen in the ECG bear no relationship to the underlying electrical activity, which is detectable as small amplitude QRS complexes. Again, even if the ECG is difficult to interpret, the marked beat to beat variability in both ART and CVP waveforms highlights the absence of atrioventricular synchrony. (D) Successful atrioventricular sequential pacing (88 beats/min, AV interval 140 msec). The ART and CVP waveforms are regular and normal in morphology. Venous cannon waves have disappeared, and blood pressure is higher than in the other panels. These examples were all recorded in the operating room over a period of several minutes, and they serve as an example of how the hemodynamic waveforms are a vital component of integrated monitoring that help to decipher confusing ECG traces.

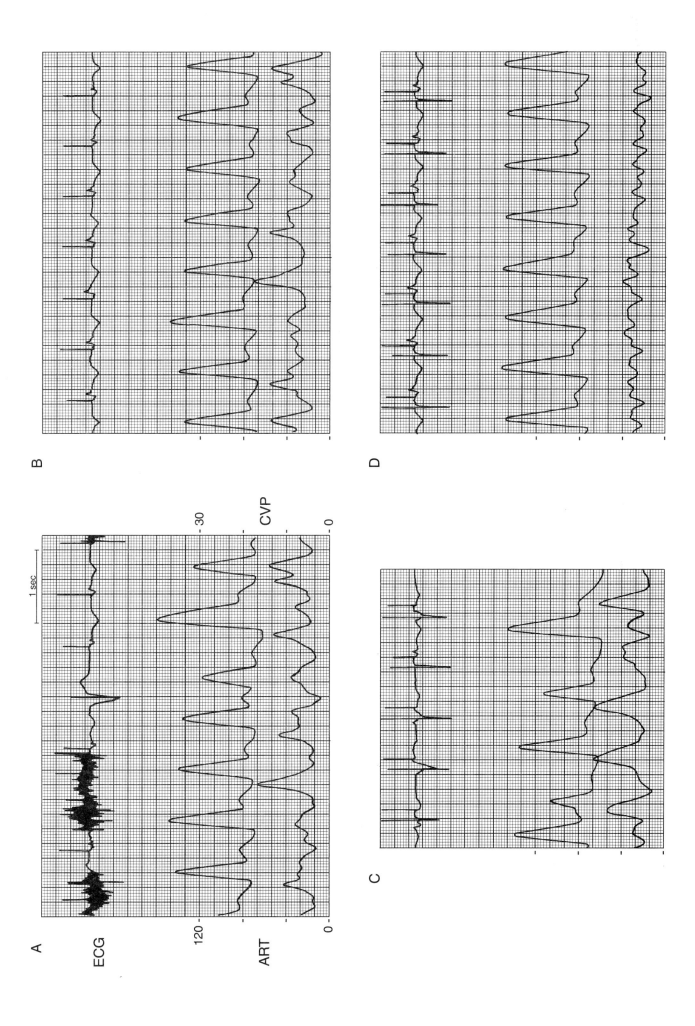

Figure 14.21 An unusual example of unsynchronized atrial and ventricular activity during cardiopulmonary bypass. (*Left panels*) A slow speed recording of the ECG, arterial blood pressure (ART), pulmonary artery pressure (PAP), and central venous pressure (CVP). The ECG shows ventricular fibrillation, but regular small amplitude pulsations are seen in the PAP and CVP traces. A standard speed recording (*right panels*) shows regular 2 to 3 mmHg pressure pulsations at a rate of 86 beats/min in the PAP and CVP waveforms. Direct inspection of the heart in this case reveals that a regular atrial rhythm (or perhaps even sinus rhythm) coexists with ventricular fibrillation. Atrial contraction generates small pressure waves (a) in the CVP trace, and these pressure waves are transmitted to the pulmonary artery after a delay of approximately 120 msec. See text for more detail.

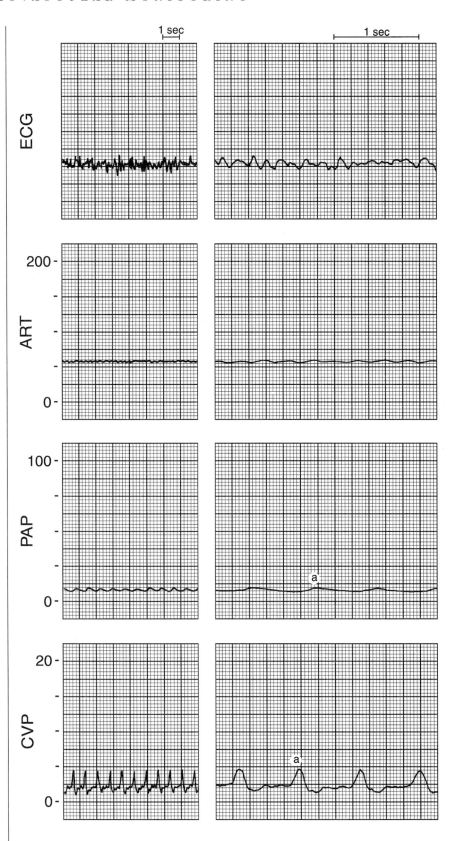

References

1. Boba A. Significant effects on the blood pressure of an apparently trivial atrial dysrhythmia. Anesthesiology 1978;48:282–3

2. Eichhorn JH, Cooper JB, Cullen DJ, et al. Standards for patient monitoring during anesthesia at Harvard Medical School. JAMA 1986;256:1017–20

3. Gürsoy S, Steurer G, Brugada J, et al. Brief report: the hemodynamic mechanism of pounding in the neck in atrioventricular nodal reentrant tachycardia. N Engl J Med 1992;327:772–4

4. Laver MB, Turndorf H. Atrial activity and systemic blood pressure during anesthesia in man. Circulation 1963;28:63–71

5. Mark JB. Systolic venous waves cause spurious signs of arterial hemoglobin desaturation. Anesthesiology 1989;71:158–60

6. Mark JB. Central venous pressure monitoring: clinical insights beyond the numbers. J Cardiothorac Vasc Anesth 1991;5:163–73

7. Mark JB. Getting the most from your central venous pressure catheter. In: Barash PG, ed. ASA Refresher Courses in Anesthesiology (vol 23). Philadelphia: Lippincott–Raven, 1995: 157–75

8. Mazzia VDB, Ellis CH, Siegel H, Hershey SG. The electrocardiograph as a monitor of cardiac function in the operating room. JAMA 1966;198:123–7

9. Mirvis DM, Berson AS, Goldberger AL, et al. Instrumentation and practice standards for electrocardiographic monitoring in special care units. Circulation 1989;79:464–71

10. Nishimura RA, Symanski JD, Hurrell DG, et al. Dual-chamber pacing for cardiomyopathies: a 1996 perspective. Mayo Clin Proc 1996;71:1077–87

11. Roizen MF, Plummer GO, Lichtor JL. Nitrous oxide and dysrhythmias. Anesthesiology 1987;66:427–31

12. Schlant RC, Sonnenblick EH. Normal physiology of the cardiovascular system. In: Schlant RC, Alexander RW, ed. The Heart Arteries and Veins. New York: McGraw-Hill, 1994:126

13. Schubart AF, Marriott HJL, Gorten RJ. Isorhythmic dissociation. Am J Med 1958;24:209–14

14. Sethna DH, Deboer GE, Millar RA. Observations on "junctional rhythms" during anaesthesia. Br J Anaesth 1984;56:924–5

15. Sosis M, Cooper PS, Herr G. The diagnosis of "junctional rhythms" with halogenated anesthetics. Anesthesiology 1985; 63:233–4

16. Standards for basic anesthesia monitoring. In: ASA Standards, Guidelines and Statements. Park Ridge, II: American Society of Anesthesiologists, 1993:4–5

17. Stott DK, Marpole DGF, Bristow JD, et al. The role of left atrial transport in aortic and mitral stenosis. Circulation 1970; 41:1031–41

18. Thys DM, Kaplan JA. The ECG in Anesthesia and Critical Care. New York: Churchill Livingstone, 1987

19. Wagner GS. Marriott's Practical Electrocardiography (9th ed). Baltimore, MD: Williams & Wilkins, 1994

CHAPTER FIFTEEN *Pressure–Volume Relations, Transmural Pressure, and Preload*

The Frank-Starling principle states that the force of cardiac contraction is directly proportional to end-diastolic muscle fiber length at any given level of intrinsic contractility or inotropy.[23,31] This muscle fiber length, or *preload*, is proportional to end-diastolic chamber *volume*. While it would be ideal to monitor cardiac chamber volumes continuously in critically ill patients, we rely instead on hemodynamic monitoring of cardiac filling *pressures* to estimate left or right ventricular preload. Unfortunately, changes in filling pressure do not always correspond to proportional changes in filling volume, and on occasion, *diastolic pressure and volume can change in opposite directions.*[5,8,9,15,30]

This chapter explores the relation between filling pressures and volumes and introduces the concept of transmural pressure. The reader should be forewarned that this chapter is a bit different from others in this book, since it contains no waveform recordings. Instead, the following discussion focuses on principles that are fundamental for understanding cardiac preload and that provide an intuitive framework to help the clinician recognize when cardiac filling pressure measurements may be misleading.

DIASTOLIC PRESSURE–VOLUME RELATIONS

When we use left ventricular end-diastolic pressure (LVEDP) or wedge pressure as a surrogate for left ventricular end-diastolic volume, we make an assumption that these two variables change in the same direction and in direct proportion to one another. Unfortunately, this is not the case, because the pressure–volume relation in cardiac muscle is not linear, but curvilinear (Fig. 15.1).[22,24,26,30] As a result, one cannot assume that a given measured change in central venous pressure (CVP) or pulmonary artery wedge pressure (PAWP) will result in a proportional change in right or left ventricular preload.[1] When the ventricle is operating along the *flat* portion of the diastolic filling curve, a modest increase in filling pressure produces a substantial increase in filling volume or preload, while the same increase in filling pressure has little impact on preload when the ventricle is operating on the *steep* portion of this curve (Fig. 15.1). An even more confusing situation arises when the diastolic pressure–volume relation of the ventricle changes, for example, with the onset of myocardial ischemia (Fig. 15.2).[16,18,21,25,26] Rather than move along the same diastolic pressure–volume curve, the ventricle has now shifted to a different curve with a new shape. In this situation. *a measured increase in filling pressure may be associated with a decrease in filling volume and vice versa* (Fig. 15.2).[8,15] (See also Ch. 6.)

Note that this diastolic pressure–volume curve represents one limb of a pressure–volume loop that describes the rela-

tion between these two variables for the left (or right) ventricle during an entire cardiac cycle (Fig. 15.3). In this instance we are concerned with the diastolic filling portion of the loop, which has a curvilinear morphology and a progressively steeper slope at higher volumes. Pressure–volume curves and loops have been used to describe the operation of both the right and left ventricles. For the current discussion, it may be easiest to think about left ventricular volume and pressure alone, but the principles apply equally well to an analysis of the right side of the heart.

It is easy to appreciate that the relation between a given change in ventricular volume and the corresponding change in filling pressure depends on the portion of the pressure–volume curve over which the patient's heart is currently operating. In addition to the operating position on a given diastolic pressure–volume curve, the shape of the curve will also determine the relationship between pressure and volume (Fig. 15.4). Commonly termed *ventricular compliance*,[11,12,23,31] this change in pressure for a given change in volume is actually the reciprocal of compliance. Alternative terms often applied to this pressure–volume relation include *ventricular elastance, distensibility* or *stiffness* ($\Delta P/\Delta V$). It follows that a patient with an abnormally stiff left ventricle will have a greater change in end-diastolic pressure for any given change in end-diastolic volume, and the converse is true for a patient with an abnormally compliant ventricle (Fig. 15.4). Diastolic dysfunction resulting in an abnormal increase in left ventricular stiffness occurs in patients with impaired ventricular relaxation (myocardial ischemia),[13,14,16,21,25] those with ventricular hypertrophy (systemic hypertension, aortic stenosis, hypertrophic cardiomyopathy),[25,28] and those with other myopathic processes (fibrosis from myocardial infarction, amyloidosis, restrictive cardiomyopathy).[17,27] In contrast, chronic left ventricular dilation resulting from valvular regurgitation, shunts, or cardiomyopathy may produce a ventricle with increased compliance.[30]

A number of factors contribute to the left ventricular diastolic pressure–volume relationship. Intrinsic properties of the ventricle, such as the passive mechanical properties of cardiac muscle, chamber geometry, relaxation, and a variety of other factors all play an important role. In addition, external forces exerted by the pericardium, right ventricle, coronary vasculature, and pleural pressure will further influence the left ventricular pressure–volume relationship in diastole (see below). A full discussion of these factors and their role in left ventricular diastolic function is beyond the scope of this chapter and can be found in a number of other sources.[4,11,12,18,22,24,25,27] The important message to keep in mind in light of these considerations is that it may be misleading to equate cardiac filling pressures with filling volumes when patients are functioning over wide ranges of their diastolic pressure–volume curve or under conditions where diastolic stiffness is abnormal or changing.

CENTRAL VENOUS PRESSURE AS A MEASURE OF LEFT VENTRICULAR PRELOAD

Although one of the primary reasons for monitoring cardiac filling pressures is to estimate left ventricular preload, accurate determination of myocardial fiber length or end-diastolic chamber volume remains an elusive goal in clinical practice. While transesophageal echocardiography has brought continous monitoring of left ventricular volume (or cross-sectional area) a step closer,[2] the accuracy of this technique applied in real-time remains suboptimal.[3] Consequently, LVEDP remains the gold standard pressure estimate for left ventricular preload. Under most circumstances, left atrial pressure, PAWP, and pulmonary artery diastolic pressure are used as alternatives to LVEDP, despite the limitations of these measurements. The farther we move upstream from direct measurement of LVEDP, the more likely it is that confounding influences alter the relation between that measure and LVEDP (Fig. 15.5).[23,30] (See Ch. 6.)

This problem is particularly evident when CVP is chosen to estimate left ventricular preload.[6] The diastolic pressure–volume curves for the left and right ventricles are different even in healthy individuals, with the former being stiffer or less complaint (Fig. 15.6). For the same change in left or right ventricular volume, the change in left ventricular pressure will be much greater than the corresponding change in right ventricular pressure (Fig. 15.6). As a result, the issue is not whether there is a *correlation* between a change in CVP and PAWP, because in most cases, changes in CVP, PAWP, and pulmonary artery diastolic pressure all occur in the same direction.[20] Instead, the real question is whether small changes in CVP are *clinically detectable*, since they often coexist with larger changes in PAWP simply because the right and left ventricles have different diastolic pressure–volume curves (Fig. 15.6).[19]

Use of CVP to estimate left ventricular preload is associated with additional interpretive problems, owing to the fact that the right and left ventricles share a common septal wall and are both constrained by the surrounding pericardium. As a consequence, the diastolic pressure–volume relation of the left ventricle is influenced directly by right ventricular diastolic volume and pressure. These confounding influences are termed *ventricular interdependence* and *pericardial constraint* and suggest that alterations in right ventricular filling volume or pressure may change the left ventricular diastolic pressure–volume relation.[1,24,27,30] For example, acute pulmonary artery hypertension may cause an increase in right ventricular end-diastolic volume and pressure, shift the ventricular septum leftward, and produce a higher LVEDP but a smaller left ventricular end-diastolic volume, simply because of this shift in the left ventricular pressure–volume relation to a steeper, stiffer curve (Fig. 15.7). In view of these considerations, reliance on CVP to estimate left ventricular preload is often misleading in critically ill patients.

TRANSMURAL PRESSURE

In general, when we describe any intravascular pressure, the numeric value assigned is referenced to atmospheric pressure. Indeed, the first step in pressure transducer setup is to *zero* the transducer by exposing it to atmospheric pressure and assigning this pressure a value of zero by pressing the *zero pressure* button on the attached monitor. (See also Ch. 9.) Thus, a left atrial pressure of 10 mmHg is 10 mmHg higher than ambient atmospheric pressure. Does this pressure value accurately represent the distending force across the left atrial (and left ventricular) wall at end-diastole?

To answer this question, we need to consider *transmural pressure*. The cardiac chambers are all contained within the pericardium and the thorax. Clearly, changes in pressure in the structures surrounding the heart will influence pressures recorded within the heart. *Transmural pressure is the difference between chamber pressure and juxtacardiac or pericardial pressure.* Ventricular preload, end-diastolic volume, or fiber length are determined by this transmural pressure.[23,30] It is easy to imagine that the same diastolic filling pressure (referenced to atmospheric pressure) can be associated with markedly different transmural pressures and chamber volumes, depending on whether the juxtacardiac pressure is high or low (Fig. 15.8). Although the juxtacardiac pressure can be ignored under some circumstances, marked alterations in pleural and pericardial pressures occur commonly and must be considered when any cardiac filling pressure is interpreted. (See Ch. 16.)

In summary, *transmural pressure is* always *the pressure of physiologic interest.* Our clinical focus on intravascular pressures referenced to ambient atmospheric pressure results from our inability to measure juxtacardiac pressure easily and accurately. Nonetheless, one must always consider that the measured central vascular pressure may be a poor estimate of transmural pressure, under conditions of altered pericardial or intrathoracic pressure.

IS PRELOAD OPTIMAL? USE OF THE FLUID CHALLENGE

This chapter has highlighted the fact that reliance on central vascular pressures as estimates of left ventricular preload must be undertaken with caution. The curvilinear nature of the left ventricular pressure–volume relation, the need to consider transmural pressure as the relevant distending pressure, and the confounding influences of ventricular interdependence and pericardial constraint all combine to make it extremely difficult to answer the question: is the filling pressure telling us what we want to know about left ventricular preload? When the PAWP is used as an index of preload, we make assumptions about diastolic stiffness (Fig. 15.4) and juxtacardiac pressure (Fig. 15.8) and then select a target pressure value that we consider to be optimal for a given patient. This optimal target value is determined in part by knowing the patient's preexisting cardiac disease. For example, a patient with an acute myocardial infarction may need a wedge pressure 50 percent greater than the normal upper limit of 12 mmHg.[7,10]

Achieving a left ventricular filling pressure that results in an optimal stroke volume and cardiac output may be problematic when this ventricular preload is provided at the expense of excess lung water. A delicate balance must be struck between an adequate left ventricular preload and the risk of producing hydrostatic pulmonary edema. Clearly, patients with primary pulmonary injuries must be managed at a lower wedge pressure than those with primary myocar-

dial injuries. The clinician must select a target value, then adjust intravascular volume until the therapeutic goals are realized, or adverse consequences such as pulmonary edema develop.[23]

When the wedge pressure is extremely high or low, it is easy to recognize that this value must be adjusted to avoid pulmonary edema or improve cardiac output. However, things are rarely so clear in critically ill patients, and the target value for optimal wedge pressure is uncertain and usually empirically derived. Under these circumstances, a rapid fluid challenge is useful. For example, 250 ml of crystalloid solution is given rapidly intravenously over 15 minutes, and the change in PAWP is measured. If the baseline wedge pressure is high or if a severe pulmonary capillary injury is known to preexist, a reduced volume is chosen for infusion.[23,29,30] Small increases in wedge pressure following the fluid challenge (e.g., less than 3 mmHg) suggest that the ventricle is operating on the flat portion of its diastolic filling curve, while large increases in wedge pressure (e.g., 7 mmHg or greater) suggest that the steep portion of the curve has been reached and that little further increase in stroke volume and cardiac output can be achieved without a substantial risk of producing hydrostatic pulmonary edema (Fig. 15.1).[23,30]

Illustrations for Pressure–Volume Relations, Transmural Pressure, and Preload

Figure 15.1 The pressure–volume relation of cardiac muscle is not linear (*top panel*), but, rather, curvilinear (*bottom panel*), thereby confounding interpretation of cardiac filling pressures. (*Top panel*) A *linear relation* between pressure and volume. For the same change in measured pressure ($\Delta P_1 = \Delta P_2$) there will be an identical corresponding change in volume ($\Delta V_1 = \Delta V_2$), regardless of the baseline level of volume and pressure. For example, a 5 mmHg increase in measured pressure (ΔP_1, ΔP_2) corresponds to the same 20 ml increase in chamber volume (ΔV_1, ΔV_2), regardless of whether these changes occur between points A and B or between points C and D. (*Bottom panel*) The *curvilinear relation* that exists in cardiac muscle. In this situation, the same change in measured pressure ($\Delta P_1 = \Delta P_2$) is associated with a markedly different change in volume ($\Delta V_1 \neq \Delta V_2$). In this case, a 2 mmHg increase in measured pressure (ΔP_1, ΔP_2) corresponds to either a large, 42-ml increase in chamber volume (ΔV_1) or a small, 3 ml increase in chamber volume (ΔV_2), depending on whether the heart muscle is working over the *flat* (point A to point B) or the *steep* (point C to point D) portion of its pressure–volume curve, respectively. Here, a small increase in measured cardiac filling pressure may belie a large increase in end-diastolic volume or preload. See text for more detail.

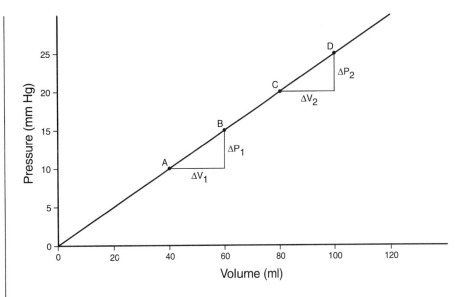

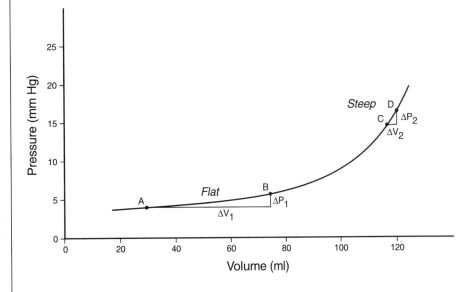

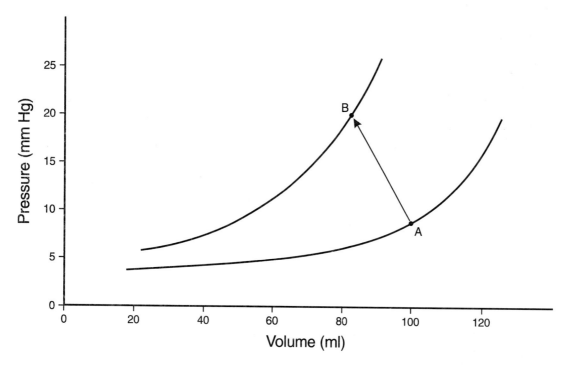

Figure 15.2 A shift in the ventricular diastolic pressure–volume relation confounds interpretation of cardiac filling pressures. In general, one assumes that an increase in measured filling pressure reflects an increase in ventricular volume. However, with the onset of ventricular diastolic dysfunction, shift of the pressure–volume relation up and to the left invalidates this assumption. In this example, an *increase* in measured filling pressure from 9 mmHg (point A) to 20 mmHg (point B) is associated with a *decrease* in left ventricular volume from 100 ml (point A) to 80 ml (point B), because of the concomitant change in ventricular diastolic function. See text for more detail.

Figure 15.3 The diastolic pressure–volume curve depicted in Figs. 15.1 and 15.2 represents one of the four limbs of a ventricular pressure–volume loop. This curve forms the *diastolic filling* limb of the loop, represented by the bold curve (limb 1, points D to A). The other three limbs include *isovolumic systolic contraction* (limb 2, points A to B), *systolic ejection* (limb 3, points B to C), and *isovolumic diastolic relaxation* (limb 4, points C to D). In this model, point A is end-diastole and shows normal end-diastolic pressure (9 mmHg) and normal end-diastolic volume (100 ml). See text for more detail.

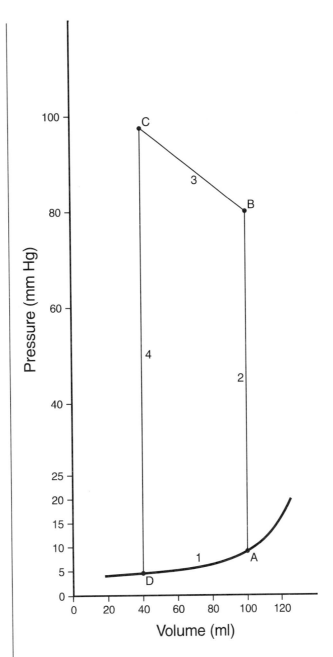

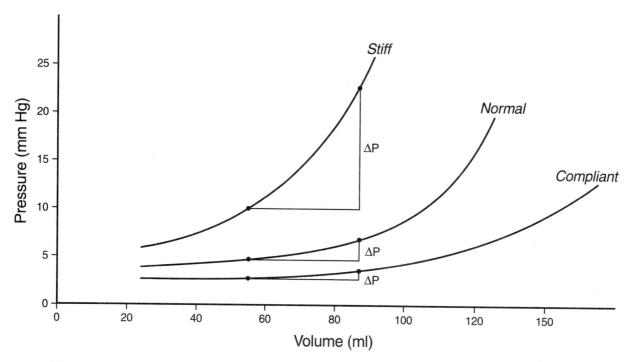

Figure 15.4 The shape of the ventricular diastolic pressure–volume curve determines the relation between a given change in measured pressure and the corresponding change in ventricular volume. In this example, for the same change in ventricular volume from 55 to 85 ml, the change in measured filling pressure (ΔP) will be 12, 2, or 1 mmHg, depending on whether the ventricle is *stiff, normal,* or *compliant,* respectively. See text for more detail.

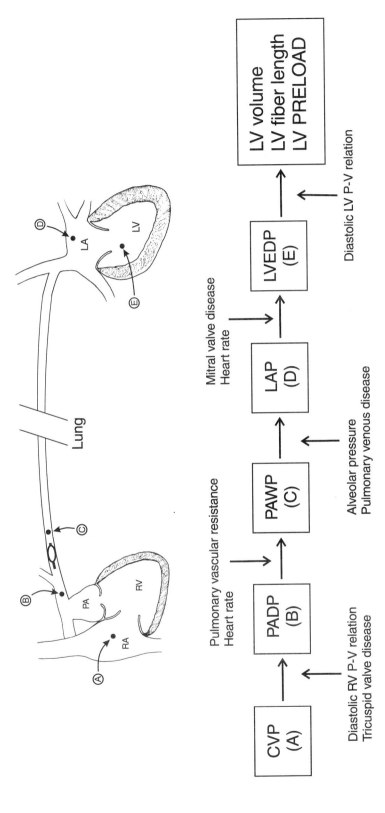

Figure 15.5 Pressure measurement surrogates for left ventricular (LV) preload and the common major confounding physiologic factors. Left ventricular end-diastolic pressure (LVEDP, measurement point E) provides the most accurate pressure estimate for preload. The diastolic LV pressure–volume (P-V) curve describes the relation between LVEDP and LV volume, fiber length, or preload. As one moves farther upstream from direct measurement of LVEDP (measurement points A, B, C, and D), many additional physiologic and anatomic factors may alter the ability of these measurements to predict LV preload accurately. RA, right atrium; RV right ventricle; PA, pulmonary artery; LA, left atrium; CVP, central venous pressure PADP, pulmonary artery diastolic pressure; PAWP, pulmonary artery wedge pressure; LAP, left atrial pressure. (See Ch. 6 for a complete discussion of the relation between LVEDP, PAWP, and PADP.)

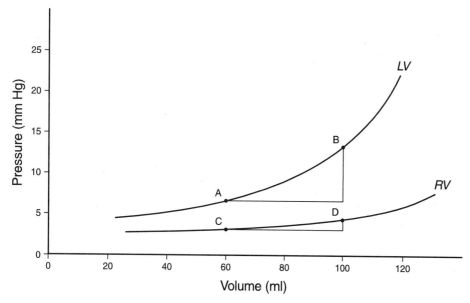

Figure 15.6 Because the left ventricle (LV) and the right ventricle (RV) have different diastolic pressure–volume curves, the same volume change from 60 to 100 ml will produce a larger change in LV pressure (6 mmHg, point A to point B) than the corresponding change in RV pressure (1 mmHg, point C to point D). In this situation, the accompanying change in pulmonary artery wedge pressure, which reflects LV filling pressure, would be readily detectable, while the corresponding change in central venous pressure, which reflects RV filling pressure, would be very small and might be overlooked easily during routine hemodynamic monitoring. See text for more detail.

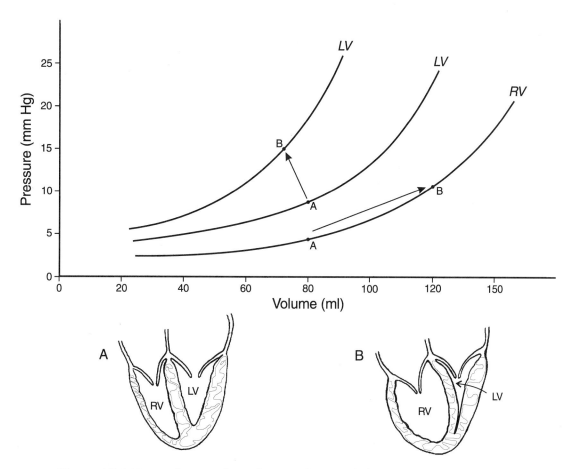

Figure 15.7 Ventricular interdependence and pericardial constraint contribute to the limitations of using right ventricular (RV) filling pressure as an estimate of left ventricular (LV) preload. Point A represents normal baseline conditions for ventricular filling volumes and pressures at end-diastole (LV: 80 ml, 8 mmHg; RV: 80 ml, 4 mmHg). Onset of acute pulmonary hypertension reduces RV ejection, and as the RV attempts to restore its stroke output, RV end-diastolic volume and pressure increase (point B, RV: 120 ml, 10 mmHg). These anatomic changes lead to an effective reduction in LV diastolic compliance, shifting the LV diastolic pressure–volume curve up and to the left, and increasing LV end-diastolic pressure (15 mmHg) despite a decrease in LV end-diastolic volume (72 ml). See text for more detail.

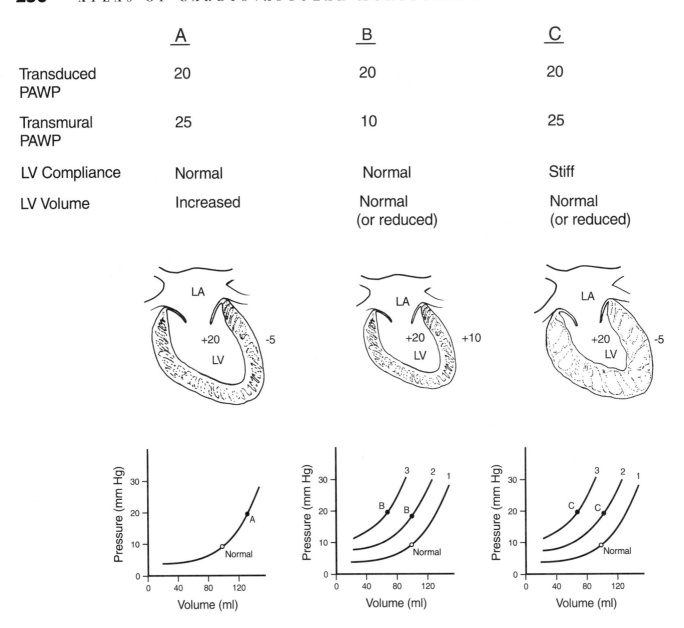

	A	B	C
Transduced PAWP	20	20	20
Transmural PAWP	25	10	25
LV Compliance	Normal	Normal	Stiff
LV Volume	Increased	Normal (or reduced)	Normal (or reduced)

Figure 15.8 The limitation of using pulmonary artery wedge pressure (PAWP) as an estimate of left ventricular (LV) preload is illustrated by considering the three different conditions that may result in an elevated PAWP of 20 mmHg, as measured with a standard pressure transducer referenced to atmospheric pressure. Despite the *same transduced PAWP* in all three conditions, *transmural PAWP varies* because it is influenced by juxtacardiac pressure. Furthermore, *LV volume or preload varies* because it is influenced by both transmural PAWP and LV compliance. Cartoons of the LV and left atrium (LA) represent the three different conditions leading to a transduced PAWP of 20 mmHg. Pressure–volume curves that describe the relation between transduced PAWP and LV volume are shown for each of these conditions. Note that the same abnormal transduced PAWP (20 mmHg) is denoted by the closed circles on each curve (points A, B, and C). Normal baseline LV end-diastolic volume and transduced PAWP (100 ml, 10 mmHg) is denoted on the curves by the open circles. (*Condition A*) *Hypervolemia.* Transmural PAWP is *increased* (+20 – [–5] = 25 mmHg) and LV volume is *increased* (point A, 130 ml). (*Condition B*) *Increased juxtacardiac or pericardial pressure.* Transmural PAWP is *decreased* (+20 – [+10] = 10 mmHg) and LV volume is *normal* (point B, curve 2, 100 ml) or *decreased* (point B, curve 3, 75 ml). (*Condition C*) *Increased chamber stiffness.* Transmural PAWP is *increased* (+20 – [–5] = 25 mmHg) and LV volume is *normal* (point C, curve 2, 100 ml) or *decreased* (point C, curve 3, 75 ml).

References

1. Alderman EL, Glantz SA. Acute hemodynamic interventions shift the diastolic pressure-volume curve in man. Circulation 1976;54:662–71

2. Bergquist BD, Bellows WH, Leung JM. Transesophageal echocardiography in myocardial revascularization: II. Influence on intraoperative decision making. Anesth Analg 1996;82:1139–45

3. Bergquist BD, Leung JM, Bellows WH. Transesophageal echocardiography in myocardial revascularization: I. Accuracy of intraoperative real-time interpretation. Anesth Analg 1996;82:1132–8

4. Brutsaert DL, Sys SU. Relaxation and diastole of the heart. Physiol Rev 1989;69:1228–315

5. Calvin JE, Driedger AA, Sibbald WJ. Does the pulmonary capillary wedge pressure predict left ventricular preload in critically ill patients? Crit Care Med 1981;9:437–43

6. Cohn JN, Tristani FE, Khatri IM. Relationship between left and right ventricular function. J Clin Invest 1969;48:2008–18

7. Crexells C, Chatterjee K, Forrester JS, et al. Optimal level of filling pressure in the left side of the heart in acute myocardial infarction. N Engl J Med 1973;289:1263–6

8. Dwyer EM. Left ventricular pressure-volume alterations and regional disorders of contraction during myocardial ischemia induced by atrial pacing. Circulation 1970;42:1111–22

9. Ellis RJ, Mangano DT, VanDyke DC. Relationship of wedge pressure to end-diastolic volume in patients undergoing myocardial revascularization. J Thorac Cardiovasc Surg 1979;78:605–13

10. Forrester JS, Diamond G, McHugh TJ, Swan HJC. Filling pressures in the right and left sides of the heart in acute myocardial infarction. A reappraisal of central-venous-pressure monitoring. N Engl J Med 1971;235:190–3

11. Gaasch WH, Levine HJ, Quinones MA, Alexander JK. Left ventricular compliance: mechanisms and clinical implications. Am J Cardiol 1976;38:645–53

12. Grossman W, McLaurin LP. Diastolic properties of the left ventricle. Ann Intern Med 1976;84:316–26

13. Grossman W. Why is left ventricular diastolic pressure increased during angina pectoris? J Am Coll Cardiol 1985;5:607–8

14. Grossman W. Diastolic dysfunction in congestive heart failure. Engl J Med 1991;325:1557–64

15. Hansen RM, Viquerat CE, Matthay MA, et al. Poor correlation between pulmonary arterial wedge pressure and left ventricular end-diastolic volume after coronary artery bypass graft surgery. Anesthesiology 1986;64:764–70

16. Kramer DC, Oka Y, Yellin EL. Post-ischemic diastolic function: pursuing a cautious path from laboratory to operating room. J Cardiothorac Vasc Anesth 1994;8:609–10

17. Kushwaha SS, Fallon JT, Fuster V. Restrictive cardiomyopathy. N Engl J Med 1997;336:267–76

18. Labovitz AJ, Pearson AC. Evaluation of left ventricular diastolic function: clinical relevance and recent Doppler echocardiographic insights. Am Heart J 1987;114:836–51

19. Lowenstein E, Teplick R. To (PA) catheterize or not to (PA) catheterize—that is the question. Anesthesiology 1980;53:361–3

20. Mangano DT. Monitoring pulmonary arterial pressure in coronary-artery disease. Anesthesiology 1980;53:364–70

21. Marsch SCU, Dalmas S, Philbin DM, et al. Post-ischemic diastolic dysfunction. J Cardiothorac Vasc Anesth 1994;8:611–7

22. Nishimura RA, Housmans PR, Hatle LK, Tajik AJ. Assessment of diastolic function of the heart: background and current applications of Doppler echocardiography. Part I. Physiologic and pathophysiologic features. Mayo Clin Proc 1989;64:71–81

23. O'Quin R, Marini JJ. Pulmonary artery occlusion pressure: clinical physiology, measurement, and interpretation. Am Rev Respir Dis 1983;128:319–26

24. Pagel PS, Grossman W, Haering JM, Warltier DC. Left ventricular diastolic function in the normal and diseased heart. Perspectives for the anesthesiologist (first of two parts). Anesthesiology 1993;79:836–54

25. Pagel PS, Grossman W, Haering JM, Warltier DC. Left ventricular diastolic function in the normal and diseased heart. Perspectives for the anesthesiologist (second of two parts). Anesthesiology 1993;79:1104–20

26. Pantely GA, Bristow JD. Ischemic cardiomyopathy. Prog Cardiovasc Dis 1984;27:95–114

27. Shah PM, Pai RG. Diastolic heart failure. Curr Probl Cardiol 1992;(December):787–845

28. Shepherd RFJ, Zachariah PK, Shub C. Hypertension and left ventricular diastolic function. Mayo Clin Proc 1989;64:1521–32

29. Teplick RS. Measuring central vascular pressures: a surprisingly complex problem. Anesthesiology 1987;67:289–91

30. Tuman KJ, Carroll GC, Ivankovich AD. Pitfalls in interpretation of pulmonary artery catheter data. J Cardiothorac Anesth 1989;3:625–41

31. Wiedemann HP, Matthay MA, Matthay RA. Cardiovascular-pulmonary monitoring in the intensive care unit (part 1). Chest 1984;85:537–49

CHAPTER SIXTEEN *Respiratory– Circulatory Interactions*

INTERPRETING CENTRAL VASCULAR PRESSURES DURING THE RESPIRATORY CYCLE: AVERAGE OR END-EXPIRATORY PRESSURE?

The primary goal in monitoring central vascular pressures is to estimate cardiac filling volume or preload. Although it is clear that transmural pressure is the physiologically relevant measure of filling pressure, in daily practice, we measure and report central vascular pressures referenced to ambient atmospheric pressure and generally ignore the potentially confounding influence of intrathoracic (pleural) or juxtacardiac (pericardial) pressure (also see Ch. 15). This does not present a problem in interpretation as long as the juxtacardiac pressure is constant and nearly equal to atmospheric pressure. Under these conditions, the measured cardiac filling pressures remain accurate indicators of transmural filling pressures and in turn reflect filling volumes. As a practical matter, this is the case during quiet spontaneous respiration. However, when intrathoracic pressure becomes markedly negative during forceful spontaneous inspiration, or markedly positive as occurs during the inspiratory phase of a positive pressure breath, the central vascular pressures measured referenced to atmospheric pressure may show significant decreases (Fig. 16.1) or increases (Fig. 16.2) during the respiratory cycle.[12,13] What is the best method to measure and report cardiac filling pressures under these conditions?

Figure 16.1 shows central vascular pressures recorded from a patient who is *breathing spontaneously but forcefully*. During inspiration, pulmonary artery diastolic pressure (PADP) falls from 22 to 10 mmHg. One approach to central vascular pressure measurement in this patient is to take the *average* value recorded over the respiratory cycle, somewhere between 22 and 10 mmHg. The value reported in the monitor digital display, 18 mmHg in this case, is not a simple average but, rather, a time-weighted average, which reflects the greater influence of the higher pressure values that are present for more time during each respiratory cycle. An alternative method for recording the PADP is to make the measurement at *end-expiration*, giving a value of 22 mmHg in this case. Note that the central venous pressure (CVP) shows similar cyclic variation throughout the respiratory cycle in this recording.

Figure 16.2 shows the CVP recorded from a patient receiving *positive pressure ventilation*. In contrast to the previous example, inspiration causes an increase in the CVP measured relative to atmospheric pressure. Again, we could record the *average* value for CVP taken over the respiratory cycle (10 mmHg) or the *end-expiratory* value (8 mmHg).

When central vascular pressures vary in a phasic manner during the respiratory cycle, measuring and reporting the pressures at end-expiration will obviate the confounding influence of markedly negative or positive excursions in intrapleural pressure. At end-expiration, measured and transmural central vascular pressures will be almost identical, regardless of whether the patient is breathing spontaneously or receiving positive pressure ventilation. Since end-expiratory central vascular pressure values most closely approximate transmural pressure values, they provide the most accurate estimate of central vascular volumes.[17,28]

Focusing on end-expiratory rather than average values for central vascular pressures is clearly important in the patient receiving positive pressure mechanical ventilation, since inspiration always produces a significant increase in pleural pressure, which will be transmitted in part to the CVP (Fig. 16.2), PADP (Fig. 16.3), or pulmonary artery wedge pressure (PAWP) (Fig. 16.4). Measuring end-expiratory values may be equally important for the patient breathing spontaneously. Although quiet, unobstructed breathing causes slight decreases in intrathoracic pressure during inspiration, which in turn produce minor decreases in central vascular pressure (Fig. 16.5), forceful breathing in a dyspneic patient or one with partial airway obstruction produces a dramatic, large inspiratory reduction in intrathoracic pressure; this becomes manifest as a large decrease in the recorded CVP, PADP, and PAWP (Figs. 16.1, 16.6, and 16.7).[12] Just as in the case of positive pressure ventilation, recording central vascular pressures at end-expiration in patients breathing spontaneously will avoid the confounding influence of altered intrathoracic pressure that occurs during inspiration. Once again, measured and transmural pressures will be nearly identical when they are recorded at end-expiration.

DETECTING PRESSURES AT END-EXPIRATION

Careful observation of analog pressure waveforms on a calibrated monitor screen or paper tracing is critical for detecting end-expiratory central vascular pressure values (also see Ch. 1). Digital displays are largely inaccurate, since sampling and averaging algorithms cannot account for the variability introduced by arrhythmias and altered breathing patterns. Although a variety of methods have been described that attempt to detect end-expiratory pressure values,[1,2,4,6,9,14] none seem as accurate and reliable as visual observation of the analog waveform.[28] Even when the less pulsatile central vascular pressures (CVP, PAWP) are measured, the phasic variations in the pressure traces produced during the *cardiac cycle* (e.g., a, c, and v waves) may be distorted or misinterpreted by algorithms aimed at detecting pressure fluctuations introduced by the *respiratory cycle*.[28]

Despite potential problems with relying on digital values, some authors have suggested that measurement of CVP and PAWP can be aided by choosing either the *systolic* or *diastolic* numeric display values on the monitor.[16] In theory, the *systolic* digital values measure the *highest* pressures and therefore might estimate end-expiratory pressure values better in patients breathing spontaneously, since the spuriously low inspiratory values for central vascular pressures would not be chosen for the *systolic* display. Conversely, the *diastolic* digital values measure the *lowest* pressures and would approximate end-expiratory pressures best in patients receiving positive pressure ventilation because the factitiously high inspiratory central vascular pressures would not be selected for the *diastolic* display. This method is not fully reliable, in large part because prominent cardiac pulsations create additional pressure peaks and troughs that may be selected erroneously by the monitor and presented as systolic or diastolic digital values. For example, in Figure 16.6, mean CVP varies between 16 and 8 mmHg, but the a wave peak reaches a high value of 21 mmHg, and the x descent nadir reaches a low value of 2 mmHg. These extreme values, 21 and 2 mmHg, might be selected improperly as the systolic or diastolic values, respectively, rather than a value closer to 16 or 8 mmHg.

In addition to observing the analog pressure waveform on a calibrated display, *prior knowledge of the respiratory pattern* aids accurate identification of end-expiratory pressures. The lower values for CVP and pulmonary artery pressure (PAP) are end-expiratory values in patients receiving positive pressure ventilation (Figs. 16.2 to 16.4), while the higher values are end-expiratory in patients breathing spontaneously (Figs. 16.1, 16.5 to 16.7). Thus, by knowing whether the patient is breathing spontaneously or receiving positive pressure ventilation, the clinician can identify the end-expiratory portions of the traces quickly and arrive at a good estimate for the central vascular pressure.

These bedside estimates are made best when a *slow speed tracing* is available, either on the monitor screen or a paper chart recording. Instead of the standard tracing speed of 25 mm/sec (Figs. 16.3, bottom panel, and 16.4, bottom panel), which offers optimal resolution of waveform details, slower tracings recorded at 10 mm/sec (Figs. 16.3, top panel; 16.4, top panel; and 16.7) or 5 mm/sec (Figs. 16.1, 16.2, 16.5, and 16.6) better highlight the phasic variation in central vascular pressure, since pressure recordings measured over several respiratory cycles are visualized at once.

Two additional clues for identifying the end-expiratory portion of the pressure trace deserve brief mention. In patients who are not tachypneic or being mechanically ventilated at rapid rates (e.g., greater than 20 breaths/min), the expiratory phase of the respiratory cycle lasts longer than the inspiratory phase. (Patients receiving inverse I:E ratio positive pressure ventilation are the exception to this general rule.) As a result, one may identify expiratory pressure values with reasonable certainty by choosing the pressure values that persist for a longer proportion of the tracing duration.[6,14,28] Applying this approach, we identify an end-expiratory mean CVP value of 16 mmHg in Figure 16.6 (spontaneous ventilation) compared to a value of 8 mmHg in Figure 16.2 (positive pressure ventilation). In both instances, the respiratory rate is slow, approximately 8 breaths/min, and the expiratory pressure values predominate in the tracings.

Finally, one should recognize that *central vascular pressure values should not be less than zero in supine patients, except when these individuals are breathing spontaneously and inspire forcefully*. This circumstance typically arises in a severely dyspneic patient or one with an obstructed airway, where the patient's inspiratory effort generates large negative intrathoracic pressures that are transmitted to the heart and central vascular structures (Fig. 16.8). At a glance, one can discern the end-expiratory plateau pressures, interrupted by negative pressure excursions caused by forceful spontaneous inspiratory efforts.

END-EXPIRATORY PRESSURE VALUES: CAVEATS

Under some circumstances, appropriate identification of pressure values at the end of expiration may be more difficult than suggested by the preceding examples. Simply selecting the highest pressure values in patients breathing spontaneously or the lowest pressure values in mechanically ventilated patients becomes problematic when patients *both breathe spontaneously and receive positive pressure ventilation at the same time*. For example, during intermittent mandatory ventilation, end-expiratory central vascular pressure values are neither the highest nor the lowest values recorded by the monitor but instead lie somewhere in between these extremes (Fig. 16.9). Although a number of methods have been described to determine end-expiratory pressure values in the presence of these positive and negative intrathoracic pressure excursions, no technique appears to be as reliable as examination of the analog waveform on a calibrated monitor screen or paper trace.[6,14,28] All of the methods incorporated into bedside monitor algorithms depend on identifying the most commonly occurring pressure or pressure plateau. These pressure plateaus may be difficult to discern (Fig. 16.7 and 16.10), particularly in tachypneic patients and those with mixed positive and negative pressure swings during inspiration. Coexistence of rapid respiratory rates and slow heart rates provides the greatest challenge to automated monitor algorithms designed to identify end-expiratory central vascular pressures.

Another factor that confounds end-expiratory measurement and interpretation of cardiac filling pressures is the influence of *positive end-expiratory pressure (PEEP)*.[8] As emphasized in Chapter 6, PEEP may raise alveolar pressure sufficiently to create zone 1 or 2 conditions in the lung, so that PAWP reflects alveolar pressure rather than downstream intravascular left atrial pressure.[16,26] Of greater importance for the present discussion, *all transmural central vascular pressures will be influenced by the application of PEEP*. As PEEP raises intrathoracic, intrapleural and juxtacardiac pressures, the corresponding *transmural* pressure measurement will be reduced, while at the same time, the central vascular pressure measured relative to atmospheric pressure will be increased.[7,19,28] The extent to which PEEP (or any positive airway pressure) is transmitted to the intrapleural and juxtacardiac spaces depends on the relative compliance of the lung and chest wall. Stiff lungs (e.g., patients with acute respiratory distress syndrome) result in *less* transmission of PEEP to the thorax, while a stiff chest wall (e.g., patients with morbid obesity) results in *greater* transmission of PEEP to the thorax.[16,17] Conversely, patients with increased lung compliance (e.g., emphysema) or increased chest wall compliance (e.g., muscle paralysis) will exhibit the opposite responses to application of PEEP.

In summary, PEEP acts to reduce transmural central vascular pressures to a variable degree, depending on the mechanical properties of the lung and chest wall. These effects will be manifest during passive exhalation and will thereby influence vascular pressure measurements, including those recorded at the end of expiration. Fortunately, patients requiring the highest levels of PEEP generally have severely reduced lung compliance[27] and thus less transmission of the high end-expiratory airway pressures to the pleural space and intrathoracic vasculature. For a more detailed discussion of this topic, including a mathematical derivation of the effects of PEEP and airway pressures on vascular pressures, the reader should see other sources.[15–17,29]

While end-expiratory intrathoracic pressure should be nearly equal to atmospheric pressure unless PEEP is applied intentionally, there are two circumstances in which this may not occur. Patients who are sedated heavily or snoring may have expiratory airflow obstruction in addition to inspiratory obstruction. In this situation, dramatic cyclic variation in central vascular pressures are noted. Furthermore, airway pressure and intrathoracic pressure may not return to ambient atmospheric pressure even at end-expiration (Figs. 16.7, 16.8, 16.11, and 16.12). The end-expiratory values for these central vascular pressures may *overestimate* true transmural pressures, since expiratory airflow obstruction prevents the lungs from emptying completely, thus artificially raising intrathoracic pressure and the measured vascular pressure at end-expiration.

A similar problem may arise surreptitiously in mechanically ventilated patients who have underlying bronchospasm or chronic obstructive lung disease. This *auto-PEEP effect* is produced by air trapping behind partially obstructed airways and is more likely in patients with increased lung compliance and increased airway resistance, particularly when expiratory time is inadequate for complete lung emptying.[15,16,29] The hemodynamic effects will be similar to those seen when PEEP is applied intentionally, and end-expiratory central vascular pressures will again overestimate transmural pressures. This auto-PEEP effect may be insidious; it will not be detected by the pressure manometer in the breathing circuit, because this manometer is located downstream from the site of flow limitation. Disconnecting the patient from mechanical ventilation should allow full passive exhalation and a more valid estimate of transmural central vascular pressures. In addition, the auto-PEEP effect can be quantitated by occluding the expiratory port of the ventilator circuit just prior to delivery of the next positive pressure breath and measuring this end-expiratory airway occlusion pressure.[15,16]

AUTOMATED MEASUREMENT OF WEDGE PRESSURE

Most bedside monitors incorporate algorithms that measure PAWP automatically. In general, a slow tracing is recorded, and the computer attempts to discern the wedge pressure, first by distinguishing the wedge trace from the more pulsatile PAP waveform, and then by measuring the value for wedge pressure at end-expiration. In the example in Figure 16.13, recorded from a patient receiving positive pressure mechanical ventilation, the end-expiratory mean value for wedge pressure has been measured properly by the monitor and denoted by the horizontal line superimposed over the tracing at 20.5 mmHg. The clinician should *always verify the computer-aided measurement* by examining the placement of the horizontal cursor over the analog tracing to ensure that it is properly positioned. In another example recorded from a patient breathing spontaneously (Fig. 16.14), the initial assignment of a value for wedge pressure is erroneous, since the computer has detected mean PAP (35 mmHg) instead of wedge pressure (Fig. 16.14, top panel). The next recording from the same patient (Fig. 16.14, middle panel) is also in error, since the assigned value for the wedge pressure (15 mmHg) is not recorded at end-expiration, but is taken as an average throughout the respiratory cycle. Note also that this patient must be breathing spontaneously, since the wedge pressure trace periodically falls below zero, a sign of forceful inspiration and the accompanying reduction in intrathoracic pressure. In order to measure the wedge pressure correctly, the horizontal cursor is adjusted manually on the bedside monitor until it falls through the mean value for wedge pressure at end-expiration (28 mmHg) (Fig. 16.14, bottom panel).

POSITIVE PRESSURE VENTILATION: A CLOSER LOOK AT PRELOAD EFFECTS

The manner in which respiratory actions influence cardiac filling pressures has now been considered in some detail. We have focused on how changing intrathoracic pressure influences transmural chamber pressure and thereby alters chamber volume or preload (also see Ch. 15). We now need to consider more broadly how positive pressure mechanical ventilation influences the circulation and the interpretation of arterial pressure waveforms. Although a brief discussion of the major effects follows, the reader is referred to other sources for a more complete considera-tion of this topic.[3,10,17,18,22–24]

All of the determinants of cardiac output—preload, after-load, heart rate, and contractility—may be influenced by institution of mechanical ventilation. Unless mechanical ventilation markedly ameliorates hypoxemia or hypercar-bia, only small changes in heart rate or contractility would be expected. Instead, the major effects of mechanical ven-tilation are produced by the fluctuations in intrathoracic pressure and the resultant changes in cardiac preload and afterload.

The increase in intrathoracic pressure during a positive pressure breath *reduces right ventricular preload* because right atrial pressure rises, impairing venous return and hin-dering right ventricular filling. Although the transduced right atrial pressure or CVP increases, transmural pressure falls, thus reflecting the reduced right-sided filling. In con-trast, *left ventricular preload increases* during positive pres-sure inspiration, because blood contained in the pulmonary venous bed is squeezed out of the lungs as they inflate. Not only do the transduced indices of left ventricular preload (left atrial pressure or PAWP) increase relative to atmos-pheric pressure, but the transmural left atrial and wedge pressures also increase, reflecting the true increase in left ventricular filling (Fig. 16.15).[10,22,24] The fact that positive pressure inspiration increases both transduced CVP and PAWP, yet reduces right ventricular filling while increasing left ventricular filling, once again underscores the value of measuring all central vascular pressures at end-expiration in order to obviate these confounding interpretive issues.

The extent to which positive pressure ventilation produces these preload changes depends on the interaction of sever-al factors.[16,17] First, the change in pleural pressure during mechanical inspiration depends on the tidal volume and the compliances of both the lung and chest wall. Large tidal volumes, compliant lungs, and a stiff chest wall all act to produce a large increase in pleural pressure during inspira-tion, with corresponding significant effects on preload. Second, the intravascular volume status of the patient will determine the extent to which these pleural pressure changes alter cardiac filling. For example, hypovolemic patients will have a reduced pulmonary blood volume, and consequently, less pulmonary venous blood would be avail-able to be propelled to the left heart during lung inflation.

Positive pressure inspiration thus has opposite effects on the filling of the left and right ventricles (Fig. 16.15). The initiation of the positive pressure breath creates a transient disparity between the filling and outputs of the two ventri-cles, with left ventricular stroke volume rising and right ventricular stroke volume falling.[17,25] Later in the respira-tory cycle, reduced right ventricular stroke output *catches up* with the left ventricle, and now, left ventricular filling and output will fall below that of the right ventricle, partic-ularly with the onset of expiration, which reduces pleural pressure and restores right heart filling. Thus, positive pressure ventilation produces cyclic changes in pleural pressure, which are manifest as cyclic alterations in right and left ventricular preload and stroke output.

POSITIVE PRESSURE VENTILATION: A CLOSER LOOK AT AFTERLOAD EFFECTS

Although we commonly consider the preload changes pro-duced by positive pressure ventilation, there may be equal-ly significant alterations in both right and left ventricular afterload. Just as transmural pressure is considered to be the pressure of physiologic interest in estimating filling pressure or preload, the pressure that determines afterload is best estimated by the transmural pressure across the ven-tricular wall during systole. While changes in afterload pro-duced by positive pressure inspiration do not alter right ventricle performance significantly in most cases,[17] the same increase in pleural pressure associated with positive pressure inspiration has a consistent effect in reducing left ventricular afterload. There are two ways to think of this. First, as pleural pressure rises during positive pressure inspiration, this increased pressure is transmitted to the left ventricle and thoracic aorta, transiently raising these pres-sures above those of the extrathoracic arterial vessels, and thereby reducing the force needed to eject the left ventric-ular stroke volume, that is, a reduction in afterload. Alter-natively, one can consider that the afterload of the left ven-tricle must consider transmural pressure, and therefore, any increase in pleural pressure associated with positive pressure inspiration acts to reduce transmural left ventricular systolic pressure, that is, a reduction in afterload. Both concepts lead to the same important conclusion, that left ventricular afterload is reduced during the increase in pleural (and juxtacardiac) pressure accompanying the inspiratory phase of positive pressure mechanical ventilation.

A corollary of this point is provided by considering the effects of marked reductions in pleural pressure produced during spontaneous ventilatory efforts in patients with upper airway obstruction or severe laryngospasm or during the Müller maneuver (a forced respiratory maneuver distinguished from the Valsalva maneuver, in that the subject inspires [rather than exhales] forcefully against a closed glottis, thereby creating large negative intrapleural pressures).[3,23,24] In these circumstances, left ventricular afterload increases as transmural left ventricular systolic pressure rises dramatically, owing to the markedly negative juxtacardiac pressure produced during inspiration.

In summary, cyclic variations in pleural pressure produced during positive pressure mechanical ventilation will produce phasic alterations in right and left heart preload and left ventricular afterload. These changes are best understood by considering transmural pressures. Variations in the arterial blood pressure result from these altered loading conditions and are considered in the following section.

SYSTOLIC PRESSURE VARIATION: A CLINICAL APPLICATION OF RESPIRATORY–CIRCULATORY INTERACTION

Based on the previous description of the way in which positive pressure ventilation alters preload and afterload, one might predict that the arterial pressure waveform will reflect these cyclic changes in left ventricular stroke output.[10] Positive pressure inspiration reduces right ventricular stroke volume by decreasing right ventricular preload, while at the same time, it increases left ventricular stroke volume by augmenting left ventricular preload and reducing left ventricular afterload. Arterial blood pressure consequently increases during the onset of positive pressure inspiration. A few beats later, near the end of inspiration or early in expiration, the reduced right ventricular preload and stroke output reach the left ventricle, result in a reduced left ventricular stroke volume, and arterial blood pressure now falls.

Systolic pressure variation is the difference between the maximal and minimal values of systolic arterial pressure recorded over the respiratory cycle.[5,11,17,25] Using end-expiration as the equilibrium period for pressure measurement, the total systolic pressure variation can be divided into an

early inspiratory increase in pressure, termed Δ *up*, and a later decrease in pressure, termed Δ *down* (Fig. 16.16).[17,25] Δ Up reflects the inspiratory augmentation in left ventricular output, and Δ down reflects the impairment in systemic venous return that becomes manifest in the arterial pressure trace shortly thereafter. Normally, mechanically ventilated patients will have Δ up and Δ down of about 5 mmHg each and total systolic pressure variation of approximately 10 mmHg.[17] Note that the baseline plateau value for systolic blood pressure is recorded at end-expiration, and Δ up and Δ down are measured relative to this baseline. Even when the end-expiratory plateau is hard to discern, total systolic pressure variation can still be measured accurately by recording the difference between the highest and lowest systolic blood pressure values.

The greatest clinical utility of this concept of systolic pressure variation has focused on the early diagnosis of hypovolemia (Fig. 16.16 and 16.17).[5,17,20,25] Both in experimental animals and patients, hypovolemia has been associated with a marked exaggeration in the amount of systolic pressure variation, particularly the Δ down portion of the arterial pressure trace.[5,11,17,20,25] Some authors have suggested that the increase in systolic variation and Δ down may herald hypovolemia, even in patients in whom the arterial blood pressure is maintained near normal by compensatory arterial vasoconstriction.[17] In a heterogeneous group of intensive care patients, Marik[11] demonstrated that a large systolic pressure variation (greater than 15 mmHg) was highly predictive of a low pulmonary artery wedge pressure (less than 10 mmHg). Using echocardiography to measure left ventricular cross-sectional area as a surrogate for preload, Coriat et al found the Δ down to be an even better predictor of left ventricular preload than the wedge pressure. In this example (Fig. 16.17), intraoperative blood loss was accompanied by increased systolic pressure variation (26 mmHg) with Δ down of 17 mmHg, despite maintenance of a normal arterial blood pressure (systolic arterial pressure 122 mmHg, mean arterial pressure 88 mmHg). Rapid volume infusion reduced the systolic pressure variation to 11 mmHg with Δ down 4 mmHg. Minor changes in systolic or mean arterial blood pressure did not reveal the severity of hypovolemia, which was confirmed in this case by CVP recordings.

Just as the Δ down may reflect changes in cardiac preload, the Δ up portion of the arterial pressure trace may provide clues to the afterload dependence of the left ventricle.[17,25] As mentioned earlier, left ventricular preload augmentation and afterload reduction occur with the onset of positive pressure ventilation. Preliminary evidence suggests that a marked increase in the Δ up segment reflects the importance of afterload reduction in improving the stroke output of the failing left ventricle.[17,25] In the example in Figure 16.18, increased systolic pressure variation results from a large Δ up component and is consistent with the underlying severe impairment in left ventricular systolic function. During positive pressure inspiration, increased pleural pressure reduces transmural left ventricular pressure, markedly improves left ventricular stroke output, and raises arterial systolic pressure and pulse pressure in the failing, afterload-dependent left ventricle. The importance of positive pressure ventilation in providing such afterload reduction to the failing left ventricle has been highlighted by other authors.[21,22]

In summary, systolic pressure variation in the arterial pressure waveform has been noted as an incidental observation on the bedside monitor for a long time, but only recently has it been shown to have clear diagnostic implications. A number of studies have provided physiologic insights into its underlying mechanism.[3,10,17,22–25] The most important clinical application appears to be in using systolic pressure variation, particularly the Δ down portion, to detect latent hypovolemia in patients receiving positive pressure mechanical ventilation.[25] Although its interpretation may be confounded by the influence of changing ventilatory parameters and underlying cardiopulmonary disease, *systolic pressure variation is yet another example of how careful observation of hemodynamic waveforms provides useful clinical diagnostic insights.*

Illustrations for Respiratory–Circulatory Interactions

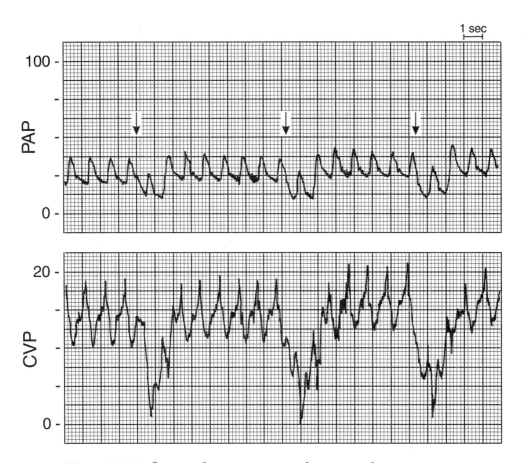

Figure 16.1 Influence of spontaneous ventilation on pulmonary artery pressure (PAP) and central venous pressure (CVP). Forceful inspiration (*arrows*) produces transient reductions in both PAP and CVP. Pulmonary artery diastolic pressure decreases from approximately 22 mmHg at end-expiration to 10 mmHg during inspiration, while mean CVP decreases from 14 mmHg at end-expiration to 4 mmHg during inspiration. Note the slow-speed recording (5 mm/sec) makes it easier to discern the phasic variation in central vascular pressures produced during the respiratory cycle. See text for more detail.

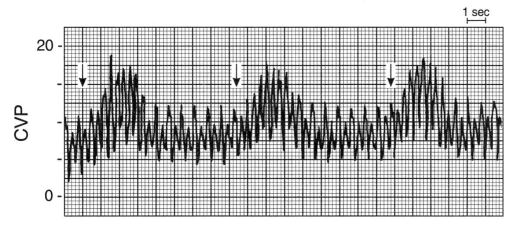

Figure 16.2 Influence of positive pressure ventilation on central venous pressure (CVP). Inspiration (*arrows*) causes mean CVP to increase from an end-expiratory value of 8 to 13 mmHg. See text for more detail. (Modified from Mark,[13] with permission.)

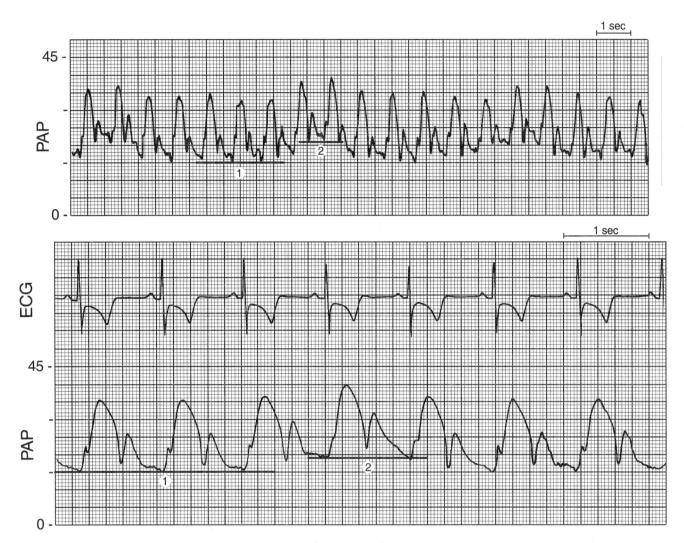

Figure 16.3 Influence of positive pressure ventilation on pulmonary artery pressure (PAP) and estimation of pulmonary artery diastolic pressure. (*Top panel*) A slow speed recording (10 mm/sec) best illustrates the phasic effects of the respiratory cycle. Pulmonary artery diastolic pressure at end-expiration is 15 mmHg (1) and increases to 21 mmHg during positive pressure inspiration (2). (*Bottom panel*) A standard speed recording (25 mm/sec) best illustrates PAP waveform details but makes it more difficult to distinguish the end-expiratory pulmonary artery diastolic pressure (15 mmHg, 1) from the inspiratory value (19 mmHg, 2). See text for more detail.

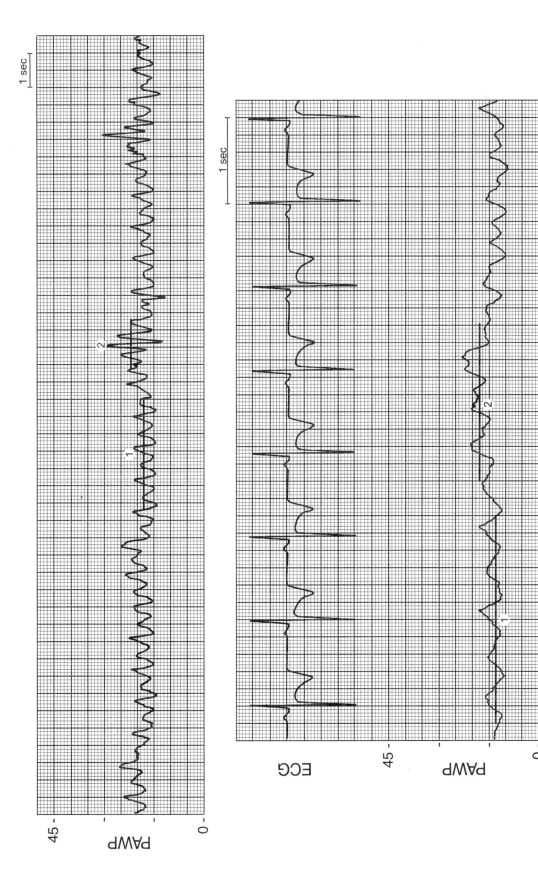

Figure 16.4 Influence of positive pressure ventilation on pulmonary artery wedge pressure (PAWP). (Top panel) A slow speed recording (10 mm/sec) best illustrates the phasic effects of the respiratory cycle. At end-expiration, PAWP is 18 mmHg (1) and increases to 22 mmHg during positive pressure inspiration (2). (Bottom panel) A standard speed recording (25 mm/sec) best illustrates PAWP waveform details (a and v waves, x and y descents), but makes it more difficult to distinguish PAWP at end-expiration (13 mmHg, 1) from PAWP during inspiration (18 mmHg, 2). Note that a similar pattern of phasic variation in central vascular pressure is produced during positive pressure ventilation, whether one is examining PAWP, pulmonary artery pressure (Fig. 16.3), or central venous pressure (Fig. 16.2). See text for more detail.

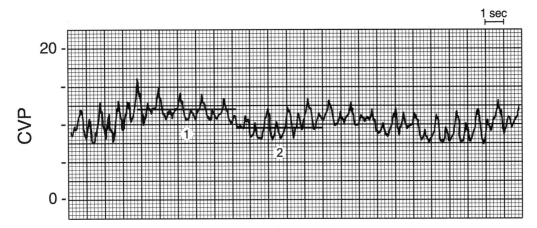

Figure 16.5 Influence of spontaneous ventilation on central venous pressure (CVP). With quiet unobstructed breathing, there is a slight decrease in CVP from its end-expiratory value of 12 mmHg (1) to 9.5 mmHg (2) during inspiration. Compare with Fig. 16.6. (Modified from Mark,[12] with permission.)

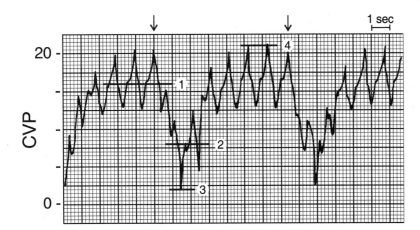

Figure 16.6 Influence of spontaneous ventilation on central venous pressure (CVP). During partial upper airway obstruction, forceful inspiration (*arrows*) produces a large sudden decrease in intrathoracic pressure, which is reflected in the CVP. Mean CVP measured at end-expiration is 16 mmHg (1) and decreases to 8 mmHg (2) during inspiration. In addition to this phasic respiratory variation in CVP, prominent cardiac pulsations produce transient pressures as low as 2 mmHg (3) and as high as 21 mmHg (4). These values may be chosen inappropriately by the monitor algorithm if the digital pressure display is set to the systolic/diastolic display mode. See text for more detail. (Modified from Mark,[12] with permission.)

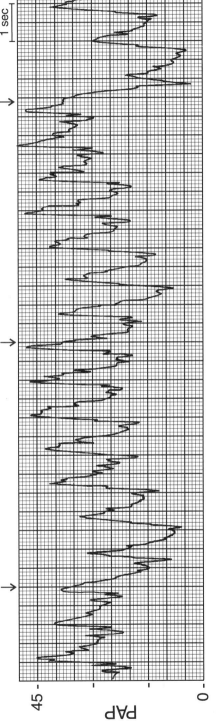

Figure 16.7 Influence of spontaneous ventilation on pulmonary artery pressure (PAP). With forceful inspiration (*arrows*), PAP decreases to a variable degree depending on the inspiratory effort and the resultant fall in intrathoracic pressure. In this example, pulmonary artery diastolic pressure decreases approximately 15, 10, and 25 mmHg, respectively, during the inspiratory phase of the three respiratory cycles shown (*arrows*). End-expiratory pulmonary artery diastolic pressure varies between 20 and 30 mmHg here, and a single value for end-expiratory pulmonary artery diastolic pressure is difficult to determine because an end-expiratory pressure plateau cannot be discerned. In addition to inspiratory airway obstruction, this patient has bronchospasm, which results in raised intrathoracic pressure at end-expiration and influences the PAP measurement. See text for more detail.

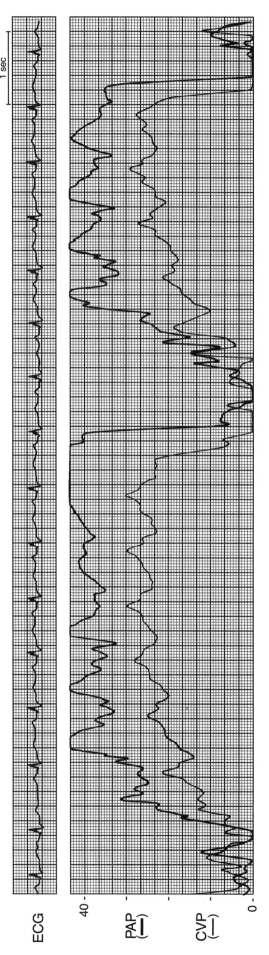

Figure 16.8 Influence of spontaneous ventilation on pulmonary artery pressure (PAP) and central venous pressure (CVP). Since the expiratory phase of the respiratory cycle generally lasts longer than the inspiratory phase, end-expiratory values for PAP and CVP can be determined by choosing those pressure values that persist for a greater proportion of the recording duration. With this principle in mind, end-expiratory values for pulmonary artery diastolic pressure (33 mmHg) and mean CVP (25 mmHg) can be estimated by inspecting these traces. Another distinct feature of the phasic variation in pressures seen here is that the central vascular pressures decrease below zero at the beginning, middle, and end of the recording (although the traces are clipped at the zero line). This is caused by a marked decrease in intrathoracic pressure, which only occurs during spontaneous ventilation and forceful inspiration. See text for more detail.

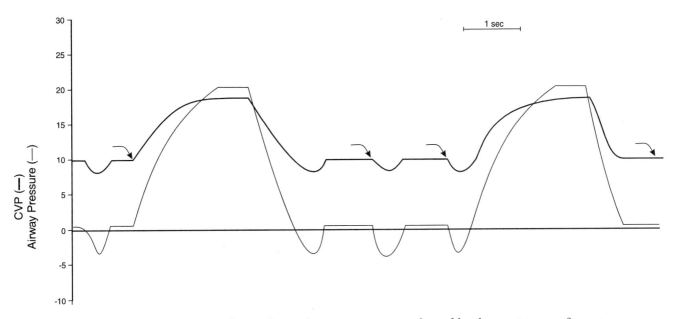

Figure 16.9 Measurement of central vascular pressures is complicated by the coexistence of spontaneous and positive pressure ventilation, as in a patient receiving intermittent mandatory ventilation. This schematic diagram plots both central venous pressure (CVP) and airway pressure against time. Two positive pressure breaths and four spontaneous breaths are noted in the airway pressure trace. During positive pressure inspirations, airway pressure increases to 20 mmHg and CVP increases to 18 mmHg, while during spontaneous inspiration, airway pressure decreases to -4 mmHg and CVP decreases to 8 mmHg. The best estimate for end-expiratory CVP is 10 mmHg and is measured at the arrows, just prior to any positive or negative excursions in airway pressure. In a real CVP trace recorded from a patient with this pattern of ventilation, superimposed cardiac pulsations would make it even more difficult to discern the end-expiratory value for CVP. In these cases, careful observation of the central vascular pressure tracing along with the knowledge of the respiratory pattern will allow a reasonable estimation of end-expiratory pressure values.

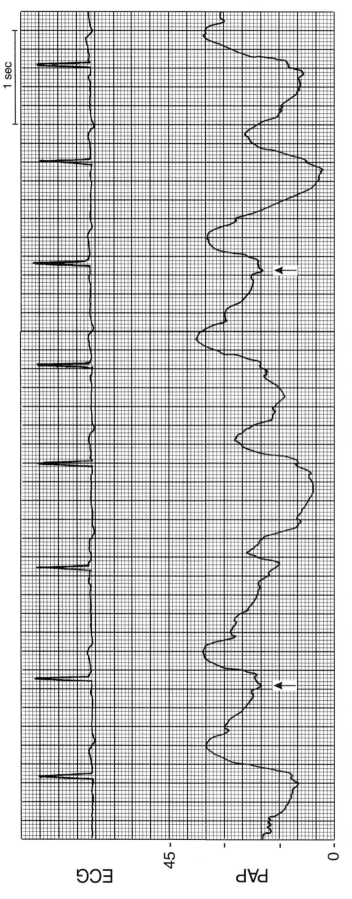

Figure 16.10 End-expiratory central vascular pressure measurement is difficult when a clear pressure plateau is not evident. In this recording of pulmonary artery pressure (PAP), no two sequential beats have the same pressure, because the heart rate is slow (58 beats/min) relative to the respiratory rate (18 breaths/min). Through careful examination of this trace, one can estimate end-expiratory pulmonary artery diastolic pressure to be 20 mmHg (*arrows*). Although manual identification of end-expiratory pressures is difficult at best, a bedside monitor algorithm will likely produce an unreliable value for end-expiratory pressure when a pressure plateau is not present.

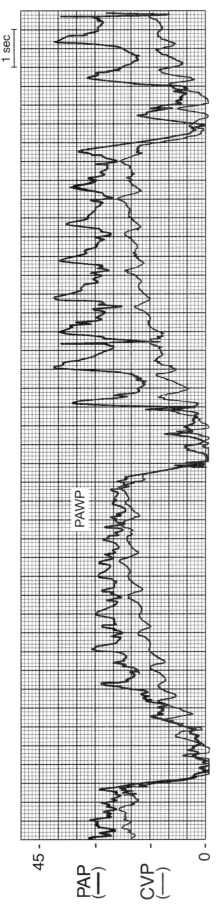

Figure 16.11 Influence of expiratory airflow obstruction during spontaneous ventilation on measurement of central vascular pressures. End-expiratory plateau values for pulmonary artery pressure (PAP), pulmonary artery wedge pressure (PAWP, left side of PAP trace), and central venous pressure (CVP) can be estimated from this recording; however, these values may overestimate true transmural filling pressures, because incomplete exhalation results in raised intrathoracic pressure at end-expiration, which will increase the measured central vascular pressure. The negative pressure excursions in PAP, PAWP, and CVP highlight the presence of forceful spontaneous inspiratory efforts during this recording. See text for more detail.

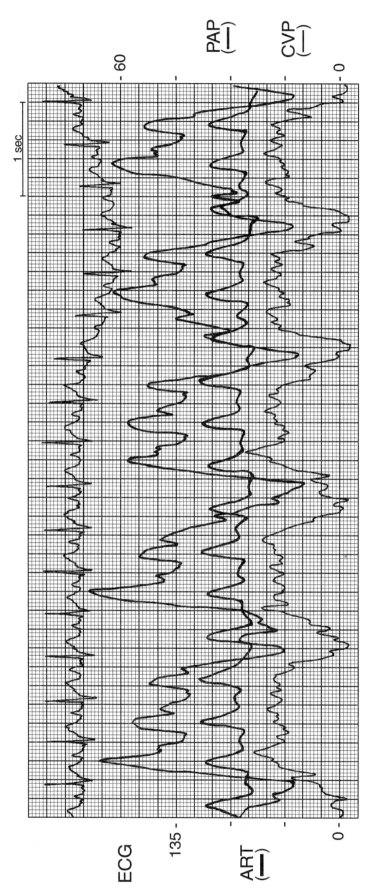

Figure 16.12 Influence of respiratory distress on recordings of arterial blood pressure (ART), pulmonary artery pressure (PAP), and central venous pressure (CVP). These traces were recorded from a 27-year-old man scheduled to undergo lung transplantation. Preoperative forced expiratory volume in 1 second was 11 percent of the predicted value, and an arterial blood gas revealed pH 7.34, partial pressure of carbon dioxide 88 mmHg, partial pressure of oxygen 64 mmHg. End-expiratory pulmonary artery diastolic pressure (42 mmHg) and CVP (17 mmHg) are markedly elevated as a consequence of the patient's underlying pulmonary disease, which caused pulmonary hypertension and cor pulmonale. These values likely overestimate true transmural filling pressures because expiratory airflow obstruction results in elevated intrathoracic pressure at end-expiration. In addition, severely increased pulmonary vascular resistance from the underlying disease process, compounded by hypercarbia, will cause the pulmonary artery diastolic pressure to overestimate wedge pressure and left atrial pressure. (See Ch. 6, Fig. 6.11.) Finally, forceful inspiratory efforts are revealed by the negative pressure excursions in the CVP trace.

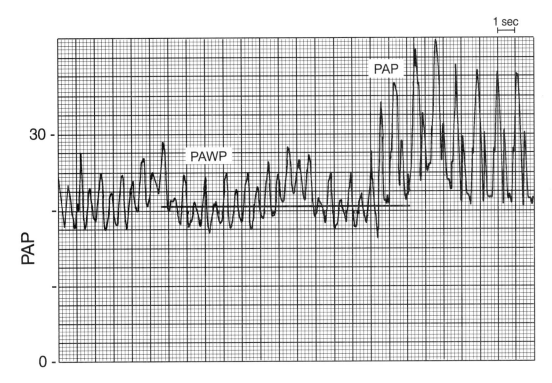

Figure 16.13 Automated computer-assisted measurement of pulmonary artery wedge pressure (PAWP). The pulmonary artery pressure (PAP) trace is displayed on the right side of the recording, and a PAWP trace with prominent a and v waves is noted on the left. The end-expiratory mean value for PAWP has been identified properly at 20.5 mmHg (*solid horizontal cursor line*). Note the phasic variation in PAWP and PAP introduced by the respiratory cycle during positive pressure ventilation.

Figure 16.14 Automated computer-assisted measurement of pulmonary artery wedge pressure. The pulmonary artery pressure (PAP) trace is displayed on the right side of the recording, and a wedge trace with prominent v wave is noted on the left. Initial automated measurement of wedge pressure (35 mmHg, *solid horizontal cursor line 1, top panel*) is erroneous, because the monitor has selected the mean PAP as the wedge pressure. The second automated measurement (15 mmHg, *solid horizontal cursor line 2, middle panel*) is erroneous as well, because the monitor has selected the wedge pressure as an average over the entire respiratory cycle. The last measurement (28 mmHg, *solid horizontal cursor line 3, bottom panel*) is correct and is performed by manual adjustment of the cursor line to measure wedge pressure at end-expiration. Note the phasic variation introduced by the respiratory cycle during spontaneous ventilation with forceful inspiration, which causes the PAP and wedge pressure to fall transiently below zero.

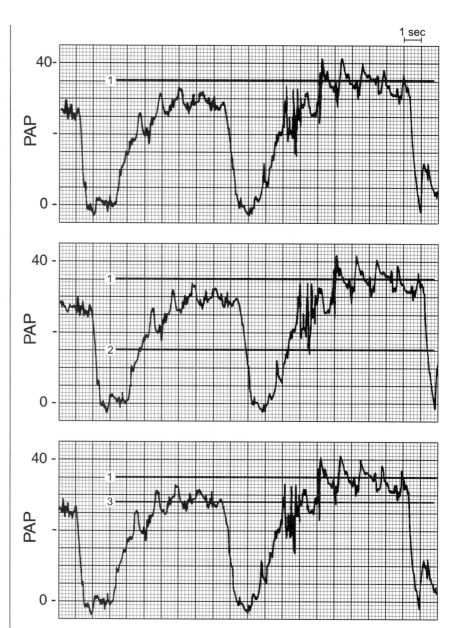

	End-Expiration ($P_{PL}=0$)			Inspiration ($P_{PL}=10$)	
	P_{TX}	P_{TM}		P_{TX}	P_{TM}
CVP (RAP)	5	5		12	2
PAWP (LAP)	10	10		22	12

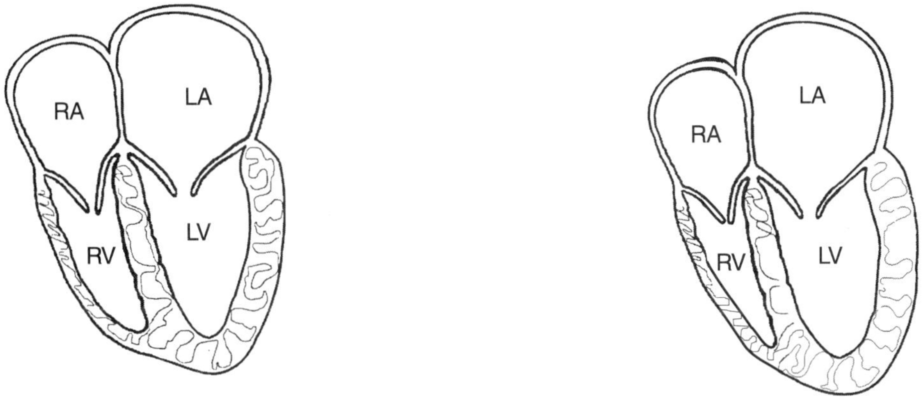

Figure 16.15 Influence of positive pressure ventilation on right and left heart filling pressures. At end-expiration, pleural pressure (P_{PL}) is approximately zero and equal to atmospheric pressure. Consequently, the transduced filling pressures (P_{TX}) and the transmural filling pressures (P_{TM}) will be equal, since $P_{TM} = P_{TX} - P_{PL}$. In this example, central venous pressure (CVP) or right atrial pressure (RAP) is 5 mmHg and pulmonary artery wedge pressure (PAWP) or left atrial pressure (LAP) is 10 mmHg. During positive pressure inspiration, P_{PL} increases to 10 mmHg and venous return to the right heart is impeded, while at the same time, venous filling of the left heart is augmented. Although both transduced CVP (12 mmHg) and transduced PAWP (22 mmHg) increase during inspiration, the transmural CVP (2 mmHg) decreases at the same time that the transmural PAWP (12 mmHg) increases. These changes in right and left heart filling during positive pressure ventilation are reflected by the changes in cardiac chamber sizes depicted in the diagrams of the heart at end-expiration and during inspiration. Right atrium, RA; right ventricle, RV; left atrium, LA; left ventricle, LV. See text for more detail.

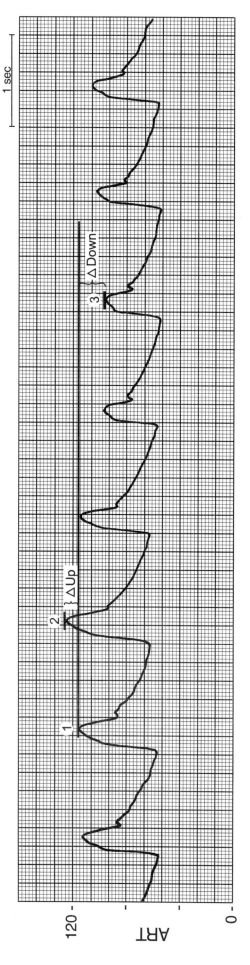

Figure 16.16 Systolic pressure variation is the difference between maximal and minimal values of systolic arterial blood pressure (ART) recorded over the respiratory cycle during positive pressure ventilation. An end-expiratory baseline value for systolic pressure is identified (116 mmHg, *solid horizontal cursor line 1*). Total systolic pressure variation consists of an early inspiratory increase in systolic pressure, termed Δ up (10.5 mmHg, *solid horizontal cursor line 2*) plus a later decrease in pressure, termed Δ down (18.5 mmHg, *solid horizontal cursor line 3*). Thus, total systolic pressure variation is 29 mmHg in this example, which is much greater than the normal value of 10 mmHg or less. The combination of a marked increase in systolic pressure variation and an exaggerated Δ down component suggests the diagnosis of hypovolemia, despite the fact that systolic blood pressure is relatively normal (116 mmHg) and compensatory tachycardia is absent (heart rate 52 beats/min). See text for more detail.

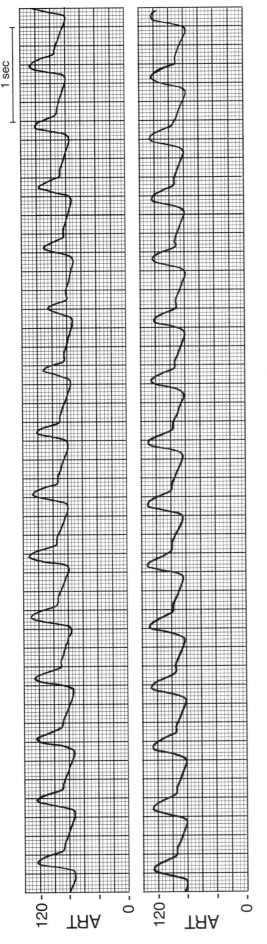

Figure 16.17 Increased systolic pressure variation as a sign of hypovolemia. Arterial blood pressure (ART) traces were recorded from a 42-year-old man during kidney-pancreas transplantation. In the top panel, baseline systolic pressure is 122 mmHg, Δ up is 9 mmHg, and Δ down is 17 mmHg, giving a total systolic pressure variation of 26 mmHg. This tracing was recorded following an occult 750 ml blood loss, and the presence of hypovolemia is suggested by the large systolic pressure variation, particularly the Δ down component. Although neither hypotension nor tachycardia are present, a central venous pressure recording confirmed this hemodynamic observation, since this pressure fell from 12 to 6 mmHg following the blood loss. In the bottom panel, following intravenous volume resuscitation, baseline systolic pressure is 125 mmHg and the total systolic pressure variation is reduced to 11 mmHg. Restoration of the central venous pressure to 11 mmHg accompanied these changes in the blood pressure waveform. In this case, minor changes in systolic or mean arterial pressure or heart rate do not reveal the severity of hypovolemia. See text for more detail.

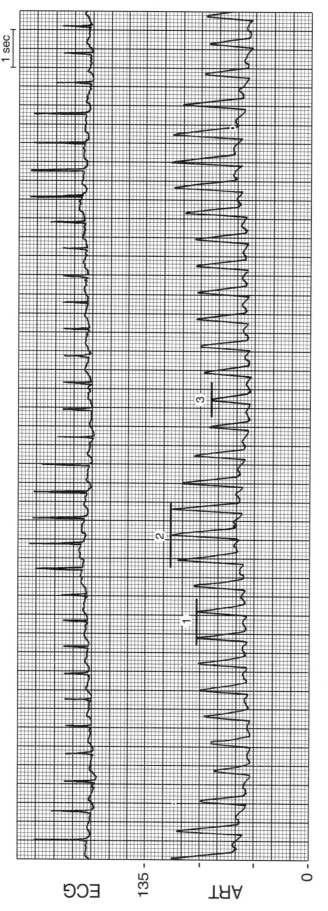

Figure 16.18 Increased systolic pressure variation as a sign of left ventricular failure. Arterial blood pressure (ART) is recorded during positive pressure ventilation in a patient with a left ventricular ejection fraction of 0.20. Baseline systolic pressure is 93 mmHg (*solid horizontal cursor line 1*), Δ up is 21 mmHg (*solid horizontal cursor line 2*), and Δ down is 7 mmHg (*solid horizontal cursor line 3*). The marked increase in the Δ up component of systolic pressure variation highlights the afterload dependence of the failing left ventricle, which increases its stroke output during positive pressure inspiration as intrathoracic pressure rises and left ventricular afterload falls. The increased Δ down component of systolic pressure variation suggests hypovolemia may be present as well. The ECG trace also demonstrates a phasic variation in R wave amplitude during the respiratory cycle, as a result of altered cardiac filling and changes in cardiac axis produced by lung inflation. (Also see Ch. 11, Figs. 11.23 and 11.24.) See text for more detail.

References

1. Bellamy PE, Mercurio P. An alternative method for coordinating pulmonary capillary wedge pressure measurements with the respiratory cycle. Crit Care Med 1986;14:733–4

2. Berryhill RE, Benumof JL, Rauscher LA. Pulmonary vascular pressure reading at the end of exhalation. Anesthesiology 1978;49:365–8

3. Buda AJ, Pinsky MR, Ingels NB, et al. Effect of intrathoracic pressure on left ventricular performance. N Engl J Med 1979;301:453–9

4. Cengiz M, Crapo RO, Gardner RM. The effect of ventilation on the accuracy of pulmonary artery and wedge pressure measurements. Crit Care Med 1983;11:502–7

5. Coriat P, Vrillon M, Perel A, et al. A comparison of systolic blood pressure variations and echocardiographic estimates of end-diastolic left ventricular size in patients after aortic surgery. Anesth Analg 1994;78:46–53

6. Ellis DM. Interpretation of beat-to-beat blood pressure values in the presence of ventilatory changes. J Clin Monit 1985;1:65–70

7. Geer RT. Interpretation of pulmonary-artery wedge pressure when PEEP is used. Anesthesiology 1977;46:383–4

8. Guyton RA, Chiavarelli M, Padgett CA, et al. The influence of positive end-expiratory pressure on intrapericardial pressure and cardiac function after coronary artery bypass surgery. J Cardiothorac Anesth 1987;1:98–107

9. Hoeksel SAAP, Blom JA, Jansen JRC, Schreuder JJ. Correction for respiration artifact in pulmonary blood pressure signals of ventilated patients. J Clin Monit 1996;12:397–403

10. Jardin F, Farcot J-C, Gueret P, et al. Cyclic changes in arterial pulse during respiratory support. Circulation 1983;68:266–74

11. Marik PE. The systolic blood pressure variation as an indicator of pulmonary capillary wedge pressure in ventilated patients. Anaesth Intensive Care 1993;21:405–8

12. Mark JB. Central venous pressure monitoring: clinical insights beyond the numbers. J Cardiothorac Vasc Anesth 1991;5:163–73

13. Mark JB. Getting the most from your central venous pressure catheter. In: Barash PG, ed. ASA Refresher Courses in Anesthesiology (vol 23). Philadelphia: Lippincott-Raven, 1995;157–75

14. Mitchell MM, Meathe EA, Jones BR, et al. Accurate, automated, continuously displayed pulmonary artery pressure measurement. Anesthesiology 1987;67:294–300

15. Nadeau S, Noble WH. Misinterpretation of pressure measurements from the pulmonary artery catheter. Can Anaesth Soc J 1986;33:352–63

16. O'Quin R, Marini JJ. Pulmonary artery occlusion pressure: clinical physiology, measurement, and interpretation. Am Rev Respir Dis 1983;128:319–26

17. Perel A, Pizov R. Cardiovascular effects of mechanical ventilation. In: Perel A, Stock MC, eds. Handbook of Mechanical Ventilatory Support. Baltimore: Williams & Wilkins, 1992:51–65

18. Pinsky MR. Cardiovascular effects of ventilatory support and withdrawal. Anesth Analg 1994;79:567–76

19. Pinsky M, Vincent J-L, De Smet J-M. Estimating left ventricular filling pressure during positive end-expiratory pressure in humans. Am Rev Respir Dis 1991;143:25–31

20. Pizov R, Segal E, Kaplan L, et al. The use of systolic pressure variation in hemodynamic monitoring during deliberate hypotension in spine surgery. J Clin Anesth 1990;2:96–100

21. Räsänen J, Howie MB. Mitral regurgitation during withdrawal of mechanical ventilatory support. J Cardiothorac Anesth 1988;2:60–3

22. Robotham JL, Cherry D, Mitzner W, et al. A re-evaluation of the hemodynamic consequences of intermittent positive pressure ventilation. Crit Care Med 1983;11:783–93

23. Robotham JL, Lixfeld W, Holland L, et al. Effects of respiration on cardiac performance. J Appl Physiol 1978;44:703–9

24. Robotham JL, Scharf SM. Effects of positive and negative pressure ventilation on cardiac performance. Clin Chest Med 1983;4:161–87

25. Rooke GA. Systolic pressure variation as an indicator of hypovolemia. Curr Opin Anaesthesiol 1995;8:511–5

26. Roy R, Powers SR, Feustel PJ, Dutton RE. Pulmonary wedge catheterization during positive end-expiratory pressure ventilation in the dog. Anesthesiology 1977;46:385–90

27. Teboul JL, Zapol WM, Brun-Buisson C, et al. A comparison of pulmonary artery occlusion pressure and left ventricular end-diastolic pressure during mechanical ventilation with PEEP in patients with severe ARDS. Anesthesiology 1989;70:261–6

28. Teplick RS. Measuring central vascular pressures: a surprisingly complex problem. Anesthesiology 1987;67:289–91

29. Tuman KJ, Carroll GC, Ivankovich AD. Pitfalls in interpretation of pulmonary artery catheter data. J Cardiothorac Anesth 1989;3:625–41

CHAPTER SEVENTEEN Patterns of Valvular Heart Disease

Advanced forms of valvular heart disease produce characteristic morphologic changes in monitored pressure waveforms. Although other diagnostic procedures such as echocardiography or cardiac catheterization are usually performed for definitive evaluation, hemodynamic monitoring and waveform interpretation may provide important ancillary diagnostic clues, especially in the critically ill patient. Keeping in mind the physiologic origins of normal central venous, pulmonary artery, pulmonary artery wedge, and systemic arterial pressure waveforms described in earlier chapters (Chs. 2 to 4, and 8), we can now proceed to review how these normal pressure waves are distorted in patients with cardiac valvular disease.

THE PROMINENT v WAVE: HALLMARK OF TRICUSPID AND MITRAL REGURGITATION

In patients with *tricuspid regurgitation,* tall systolic waves are inscribed in the central venous pressure (CVP) trace as blood leaks across the incompetent valve during systole (Fig. 17.1).[10,11] In contrast to the normal CVP v wave caused by venous filling of the right atrium from the vena cavae during late systole (see Figs. 2.3 and 2.4), this tall wave of tricuspid regurgitation begins earlier in systole and is most commonly termed a *regurgitant v wave.* Note that this wave begins with the onset of ventricular contraction, thereby eliminating the isovolumic phase of right ventricular systole, causing the c and v waves to merge, essentially obliterating the systolic x pressure descent (Figs. 17.1 and 17.2).[10,14] This prominent holosystolic v wave in the CVP trace is the hallmark of tricuspid regurgitation. Other terms applied to this pathologic waveform include *regurgitant c-v wave, giant v wave, r wave* (regurgitation), and *s wave* (systolic).[10]

As tricuspid regurgitation becomes more severe, the CVP trace comes to resemble that of the right ventricle, a condition termed ventricularization of the right atrial pressure (RAP) or CVP. Since the digital value displayed on the bedside monitor will display the mean CVP averaged over the cardiac cycle, this value will overestimate right ventricular end-diastolic pressure (RVEDP). This end-diastolic filling pressure is best estimated by measuring CVP at the time of the ECG R wave, prior to onset of the regurgitant v wave. Note that RVEDP will always be considerably lower than mean CVP in these patients (Figs. 17.1 to 17.3).

Several additional monitoring issues should be considered in patients with severe tricuspid regurgitation. It may be quite difficult to advance a balloon-tipped pulmonary artery catheter across the tricuspid valve, owing to the retrograde flow jet and right atrial enlargement that accompany this disease. Measurement of cardiac output by the thermodilution technique will be inaccurate because of the regurgitant flow across the tricuspid valve and the resulting recirculation and dilution of the intended bolus of cold indicator solution. This generally results in underestimation of the true cardiac output, although overestimation errors have also been reported.[2,5] Finally, the prominent systolic venous pulsations generated in the head and neck from tricuspid regurgitation may produce artifactual pulse oximeter readings when these are recorded from ear probes or other sites near the heart.[9] *Spurious arterial hemoglobin desaturation* apparently results from the superimposition of *systolic venous pulsations* on the normal *systolic arterial pulsations,* producing a pulse oximeter reading that is somewhere between venous and arterial hemoglobin saturation values (Fig. 17.4).

Inasmuch as tricuspid regurgitation inscribes a tall v wave in the CVP trace, the hemodynamic signature of *mitral regurgitation* should now be evident. In this condition, the left atrial pressure (LAP) trace will take on the same abnormalities just described for the RAP trace in patients with tricuspid valve regurgitation. Since we use pulmonary artery wedge pressure (PAWP) as a surrogate for LAP, we would expect the wedge pressure to display prominent regurgitant v waves in patients with mitral valve regurgitation (Fig. 17.5) (see also Figs. 4.4, 6.2, 6.16). Unlike normal wedge pressure v waves produced by late systolic pulmonary venous inflow, which fills the left atrium while the mitral valve is closed, the prominent v wave of mitral regurgitation begins in early systole and might be more precisely designated a regurgitant c-v wave. Mitral regurgitation produces fusion of the c and v waves and obliteration of the systolic x descent, as the isovolumic phase of left ventricular systole is eliminated owing to the retrograde ejection of blood into the left atrium.

Note that fusion of distinct c and v waves in the venous pressure trace is more evident in tricuspid regurgitation (Figs. 17.1 to 17.3) than in mitral regurgitation (Fig. 17.5), where the characteristic regurgitant wave appears to be more monophasic when observed in the PAWP trace. Direct LAP recordings in patients with severe mitral regurgitation may display distinct c and v waves that appear to fuse into one (Fig. 17.6), but recall that the PAWP trace is always a *delayed, damped* reflection of LAP (also see Ch. 4). As a result, a distinct PAWP c wave merging with a v wave is rarely evident in patients with mitral regurgitation. Nonetheless, the pathophysiologic basis of the regurgitant v wave is the same, whether it is recorded in the CVP trace in patients with tricuspid regurgitation or in the PAWP trace in patients with mitral regurgitation.

Since the prominent v wave of mitral regurgitation is generated during ventricular systole, measurement of mean PAWP will result in overestimation of left ventricular end-diastolic pressure (LVEDP). Instead, the latter should be estimated by measuring wedge pressure prior to onset of the regurgitant v wave (Figs. 17.5 and 17.7). (Remember that when a distinct a wave is evident in the wedge pressure tracing, measuring a wave peak pressure will provide an even closer estimate of LVEDP, since the hemodynamic impact of the atrial contraction is incorporated in this measurement. Also see Ch. 6.)

Although mean wedge pressure exceeds LVEDP in patients with mitral regurgitation, it remains a good approximation of mean LAP. Consequently, the regurgitant v wave contributes to left atrial hypertension and the subsequent risk of hydrostatic pulmonary edema. In patients with giant v waves, the mean wedge pressure and the v wave peak pressure should both be recorded. For example, in Figure 17.7, wedge pressure is 50 (v 90) mmHg.

When large v waves are present, it is important to recognize and distinguish the wedge pressure from the unwedged pulmonary artery pressure (PAP) trace. At first glance, a wedge trace with a tall systolic v wave has the same phasic characteristics as an unwedged PAP trace, namely, a prominent systolic pressure peak (Fig. 17.8). However, closer observation reveals a number of discriminating morphologic details. First, the PAP upstroke is steeper (more rapid) and slightly precedes the systemic arterial pressure upstroke, while the wedge pressure displaying a prominent v wave has a more gradual upstroke that begins after the radial artery pressure upstroke (Figs. 17.8 and 17.9). Second, the PAP peak occurs at about the same time or just before the systemic arterial pressure peak and the inscription of the ECG T wave (Fig. 17.9). In contrast, the wedge pressure v wave reaches its peak later in the cardiac cycle, after the ECG T wave (Figs. 17.5, 17.8, and 17.9).[13] This so-called *rightward shift* (Figs. 17.9 and 17.10) in the PAP waveform should be recognized by careful scrutiny and comparison of the ECG, systemic arterial, pulmonary artery, and wedge pressure traces. A third feature that distinguishes pulmonary artery and wedge pressure traces in patients with severe mitral regurgitation is the unusual morphology of the PAP waveform itself. The prominent regurgitant v wave distorts the pulmonary artery waveform, giving it a bifid appearance in systole and obscuring the normal end-systolic dicrotic notch (Figs. 17.5, 17.10 to 17.12). This is most evident in patients with the tallest wedge pressure v waves[6,12] (see also Fig. 4.10).

By recognizing these subtle but important diagnostic details, a clinician may monitor the wedge pressure v wave by observing the unwedged PAP trace, thus obviating the need for repeated balloon inflation. Of greater importance, one should hope to avoid the disastrous situation where a pulmonary artery catheter migrates distally, becomes wedged unintentionally without balloon inflation, and the clinician, not recognizing the wedge tracing, attempts to inflate the balloon and causes pulmonary artery rupture.

v WAVE HEIGHT AS A PREDICTOR OF MITRAL REGURGITATION SEVERITY

From the preceding discussion, one might think that the height of the PAWP v wave would provide a good guide to the severity of mitral valve regurgitation, but this has not proven to be the case.[1,7,8,15,17] For example, the giant v waves seen in Figure 17.11 (v wave 77 mmHg) and Figure 17.12 (v wave 44 mmHg) were oblitered when left ventricular afterload was reduced by lowering the systemic arterial blood pressure. However, in both examples, transesophageal Doppler echocardiography continued to demonstrate severe valvular regurgitation, despite the absence of tall v waves in the wedge pressure traces. Although pharmacologic afterload reduction with anesthetics or vasodilators will reduce the regurgitant fraction,[8] this will not totally eliminate the mitral regurgitation in patients with structural abnormalities of the mitral valve. Why then are the tall wedge pressure v waves no longer evident?

Since the wedge pressure is a damped reflection of true LAP, there may be some instances when a prominent v wave is present in the LAP trace but is obscured in the wedge pressure trace[16] (see Ch. 4, Fig. 4.4). In addition, one must keep in mind that the wedge pressure v wave is a *pressure surrogate for a volume event*—regurgitant flow across the mitral valve that increases atrial volume during systole. A closer look at left atrial pressure–volume relations helps to elucidate the apparently paradoxic coexistence of severe mitral regurgitation and a normal PAWP trace[4,7] (also see Ch. 15).

Three factors determine whether mitral regurgitation produces a prominent v wave in the left atrial or wedge pressure traces: *left atrial volume* (often termed the patient's volume status), *left atrial compliance*, and *volume of regurgitation* (Fig. 17.13). Since the left atrial pressure–volume relation is curvilinear, the same volume of regurgitation will result in a small increment in systolic pressure or a large increment in pressure, depending on the preexisting atrial volume at onset of systole (Fig. 17.13, top). Similarly, the shape of the left atrial pressure–volume curve, which reflects atrial stiffness or compliance, will determine the height of the pressure wave for any given regurgitant volume (Fig. 17.13, middle). This may explain why patients with acute mitral regurgitation tend to have prominent wedge pressure v waves, since they have smaller, stiffer left atria than patients with chronic valvular regurgitation.[4,8] Finally, the volume of blood entering the left atrium during systole will influence the height of the pressure wave (Fig. 17.13, bottom). However, since this is not the only determinant of v wave height, it is not surprising that wedge pressure v waves are neither sensitive nor specific indicators of severity of mitral regurgitation.[7,8,15,17]

Prominent PAWP v waves may exist in the absence of mitral regurgitation when LAP is elevated, as might occur when the left atrium is compressed,[18] and prominent v waves are seen commonly in patients with hypervolemia, congestive heart failure, and ventricular septal defect.[7] The last condition is instructive because the *giant v waves seen in patients with ventricular septal defect result from exaggerated antegrade systolic flow* into the left atrium, caused by the left to right shunt, which increases pulmonary blood flow, and thus increases systolic pulmonary venous return into the left atrium.[1] In this case, the prominent wedge pressure v wave is an exaggerated form of the normal antegrade systolic filling wave rather than a regurgitant systolic filling wave.

Thus, while tall v waves do not always predict severe mitral regurgitation, these prominent pressure waves contribute to raising mean wedge pressure or LAP, regardless of their origin. Consequently, tall v waves will result in left atrial hypertension and thereby increase the risk of pulmonary edema (Figs. 17.11 and 17.12). Perhaps the best way to interpret a prominent v wave is to recognize that it reveals the *hemodynamic impact rather than the volumetric severity* of mitral regurgitation (or any other cardiovascular abnormality that has produced the v wave).

In summary, it is impossible to assign a threshold value to the height of the PAWP v wave that predicts accurately the presence or absence of mitral valve regurgitation. Some investigators have suggested a rule of thumb in which a v wave peak pressure greater than twice mean wedge pressure *suggests* severe mitral regurgitation, and a v wave peak pressure greater than three times mean wedge pressure makes the diagnosis *virtually certain*.[8] Others have used the slope of the wedge pressure v wave as a discriminating factor. Pichard et al[15] demonstrated that wedge pressure v waves having flatter slopes (less than 100 mmHg/sec) were seen in patients with mitral regurgitation, while steeper v waves were present in patients without mitral regurgitation who had other reasons for the prominent v wave. However, this slope analysis has not found wide application in clinical practice. In the end, the clinician is best served by carefully observing the monitored waveforms, appreciating the underlying physiologic principles, and applying this information in the full light of all available clinical data.

TRICUSPID STENOSIS AND MITRAL STENOSIS

In contrast to atrioventricular valve regurgitation, which distorts the systolic portion of the venous pressure trace, atrioventricular valve stenosis alters the diastolic portion of these waveforms, including the y descent and the a wave.

Tricuspid stenosis is a diastolic defect in right atrial emptying and right ventricular filling. Mean CVP is elevated because of obstruction to flow at the level of the tricuspid valve, which produces a holodiastolic pressure gradient between the right atrium and right ventricle. As long as right atrial contractile function is preserved, the CVP trace displays an unusually prominent a wave and a slurred y descent, owing to the impaired diastolic flow across the stenotic tricuspid orifice (Figs. 17.14 and 17.15).[10,11] When atrial fibrillation is present (Fig. 17.16), the a wave will no longer be evident in the venous pressure waveform, but obstruction to flow across the tricuspid valve is still suggested by the elevated mean CVP and the slow y descent. (Compare the slope of the y descent in Figs. 17.14 to 17.16 with 17.1 to 17.3).

Right atrial myxoma may mimic the hemodynamic abnormalities of tricuspid stenosis when the tumor obstructs the tricuspid valve. On the other hand, diseases that increase right ventricular stiffness (e.g., right ventricular infarction, pericardial constriction, pulmonic stenosis, and pulmonary hypertension) may produce an elevated venous pressure and a prominent end-diastolic a wave in the CVP trace, but the y descent should be preserved or even exaggerated in these conditions, unlike the pattern seen in tricuspid stenosis.

Mitral stenosis produces abnormalities in the LAP and PAWP traces that resemble those just described on the right side of the heart in patients with tricuspid stenosis. Because of obstruction to flow across the stenotic mitral valve, a holodiastolic pressure gradient is present (see Fig. 6.15), mean LAP is elevated, the y pressure descent is obscured, and the end-diastolic a wave is prominent in patients who remain in sinus rhythm (Figs. 17.17 to 17.19). These hemodynamic abnormalities may be seen in other conditions that produce obstruction to blood flow across the mitral valve, like left atrial myxoma.

Diseases that increase left ventricular stiffness (e.g., left ventricular infarction, pericardial constriction, aortic stenosis, and systemic hypertension) produce changes in PAWP that resemble in part those seen in mitral stenosis. In these conditions, mean wedge pressure is increased and the trace displays a prominent a wave. However, the y descent remains steep, since there is no obstruction to flow across the mitral valve during diastole. The preservation of the y descent in the PAWP trace helps distinguish these conditions from mitral stenosis.

AORTIC STENOSIS AND REGURGITATION

The systemic arterial pressure waveform may show characteristic abnormalities when the aortic valve is diseased. **Aortic stenosis** produces a fixed obstruction to left ventricular ejection, resulting in a reduced stroke volume and an arterial pressure waveform that rises slowly *(pulsus tardus)*, peaks late, and is often of diminished amplitude *(pulsus parvus)*. In the examples in Figures 17.20 and 17.21, note the slow arterial pressure upstroke and delayed pressure peak. (Contrast with normal arterial pressure waveforms, Figs. 8.1 and 8.2.) In addition, the arterial pressure upstroke may reveal a shoulder or notch, termed the *anacrotic notch* (Fig. 17.22).[3]

In **aortic regurgitation,** the arterial pressure wave rises rapidly, pulse pressure is increased, and diastolic pressure is low, owing to the runoff of blood into the left ventricle as well as the periphery during diastole. Because of the large stroke volume ejected from the left ventricle in this condition, the arterial pressure pulse may have two systolic peaks *(bisferiens pulse)* (Figs. 17.23 and 17.24). These two peaks represent separate percussion and tidal waves, with the former resulting from left ventricular ejection and the latter arising from the periphery as a reflected wave[3] (see Ch. 8). The bisferiens pulse is also described in patients with mixed aortic regurgitation and stenosis and in patients with hypertrophic cardiomyopathy, although the physiologic basis is different in the latter condition. When advanced aortic stenosis and regurgitation coexist, the arterial pressure waveform may show features characteristic of both diseases (Fig. 17.25).

It is important to reemphasize the qualitative nature of all the pressure waveform abnormalities described in patients with valvular heart disease, particularly the abnormal arterial waveforms associated with aortic stenosis and regurgitation. Rarely is a single waveform abnormality pathognomonic. Instead, the waveforms displayed on the bedside monitor provide pieces to the puzzle and require the clinician's skills to integrate the information with other available history, physical findings, and laboratory data. Because one can never hope to gain all the information that may be available from the pressure waveforms without a detailed knowledge of normal and abnormal patterns, a wide range of hemodynamic waveform abnormalities from patients with valvular heart disease has been presented in this chapter.

Illustrations for Patterns of Valvular Heart Disease

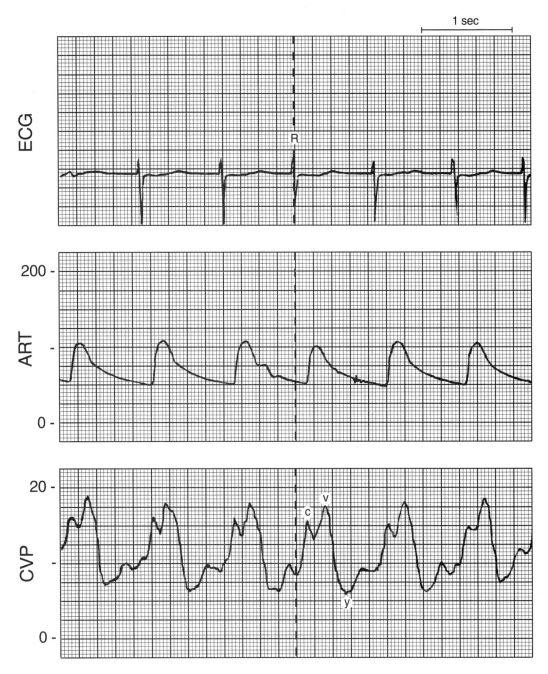

Figure 17.1 A tall regurgitant v wave and a steep y descent in the central venous pressure (CVP) trace are the hallmarks of tricuspid regurgitation. The holosystolic nature of the regurgitation is illustrated by the fusion of c and v waves, which essentially obliterates the normal systolic x descent in CVP. The arterial blood pressure (ART) waveform clarifies the timing of the abnormal CVP waveform components. Since the tall regurgitant v wave (18 mmHg) during *systole* increases mean CVP (11 mmHg), the best estimate for right ventricular *end-diastolic* filling pressure is recorded at the time of the ECG R wave (8.5 mmHg), prior to inscription of the CVP v wave. To appreciate fully the abnormalities of the CVP produced by tricuspid regurgitation, compare this recording with a normal CVP trace (Fig. 2.4). See text for more detail. (Modified from Mark,[11] with permission.)

Figure 17.2 Severe tricuspid regurgitation. A tall systolic c-v wave (greater than 24 mmHg) in the central venous pressure (CVP) exceeds the scale of the recorder, but the steep y descent remains evident. The CVP trace resembles a right ventricular pressure waveform, a condition termed ventricularization of the atrial pressure trace. Right ventricular end-diastolic pressure is estimated best by choosing venous pressure prior to inscription of the regurgitant systolic wave, approximately 19 mmHg in this example. Note the absence of the a wave in the CVP trace, because of atrial fibrillation. Compare with Fig. 17.1, which displays a small a wave in the CVP trace at end-diastole. The arterial blood pressure (ART) trace highlights the systolic timing of the abnormal CVP waveforms. (Modified from Mark,[9] with permission.)

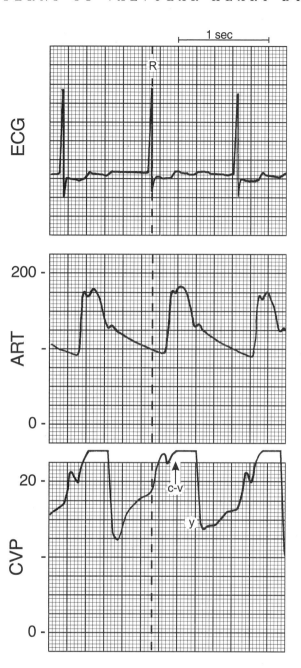

Figure 17.3 Severe tricuspid regurgitation. Tall systolic c-v waves exceed the scale of the recorder and raise mean central venous pressure (CVP). Because of atrial fibrillation, tachycardia (heart rate 115 beats/min), and the ventricularization of the venous pressure trace caused by tricuspid regurgitation, right ventricular end-diastolic pressure is hard to discern in the CVP trace, except in the last beat in the recording. In this case, right ventricular end-diastolic pressure is estimated best at the time of the ECG R wave (7 mmHg, *arrows*). These traces were recorded from a 56-year-old woman with severe pulmonary hypertension, scheduled to undergo repeat mitral and tricuspid valve replacement.

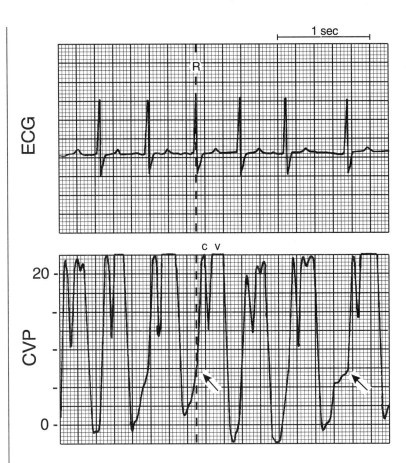

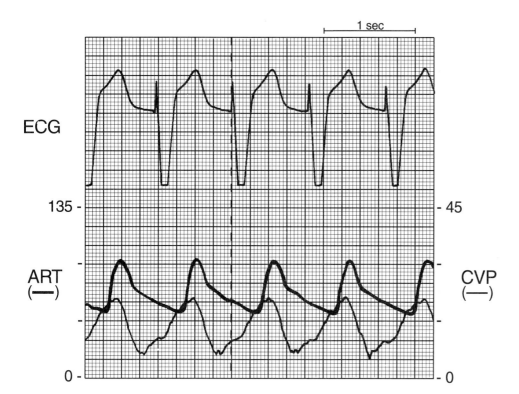

Figure 17.4 Artifactual arterial hemoglobin desaturation monitored by pulse oximetry in a patient with tall systolic v waves (21 mmHg) in the central venous pressure (CVP) trace caused by tricuspid regurgitation. The systolic timing of these huge venous pressure waves is highlighted by the arterial blood pressure (ART) trace and the ECG, which shows ventricular pacing. These traces were recorded from a 58-year-old man with severe tricuspid regurgitation, who had undergone two previous mitral valve replacements. Arterial hemoglobin saturation was 90 percent by ear pulse oximetry and 100 percent by finger pulse oximetry, when measured simultaneously at these two sites. The prominent systolic venous pulsations caused by tricuspid regurgitation resulted in an artifactual recording by the ear pulse oximeter, which apparently misinterpreted the systolic venous pulsations as systolic arterial pulsations.[9] See text for more detail.

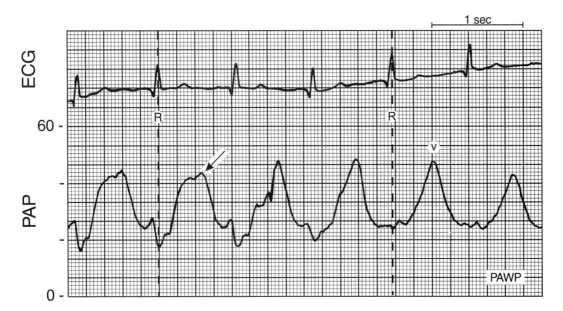

Figure 17.5 A tall regurgitant v wave in the pulmonary artery wedge pressure (PAWP) trace is the hallmark of mitral regurgitation. Unlike the normal small end-systolic PAWP v wave, the regurgitant v wave begins earlier in systole, represents fusion of both systolic c and v waves, and thus is often termed a regurgitant c-v wave. In contrast to the regurgitant c-v of tricuspid regurgitation, which usually displays fusion of distinct c and v waves in the central venous pressure trace (Figs. 17.1 to 17.3), the regurgitant c-v wave of mitral regurgitation generally inscribes a monophasic systolic pressure peak in the PAWP. In this example, this tall *systolic* v wave (48 mmHg) elevates mean PAWP (32 mmHg), so the best estimate of left ventricular *end-diastolic* filling pressure (24 mmHg) is recorded at the time of the ECG R wave, prior to inscription of the systolic v wave. Note that the regurgitant v wave distorts the unwedged pulmonary artery pressure (PAP) waveform, giving it a bifid appearance (*arrow*) which obscures the normal dicrotic notch. The regurgitant v wave pressure peak appears after the ECG T wave, later in the cardiac cycle than the normal systolic peak in PAP. To appreciate fully the abnormalities of the PAWP produced by mitral regurgitation, compare this recording with a normal PAWP trace (Fig. 4.7). See text for more detail.

Figure 17.6 Severe mitral regurgitation inscribes a tall systolic c-v wave in the left atrial pressure (LAP) waveform. In mitral regurgitation, fusion of distinct c and v waves may be noted in a direct LAP recording, while a monophasic regurgitant v wave is more common in the pulmonary artery wedge pressure waveform because of the damping effect of the interposed pulmonary vasculature (cf. Fig. 17.5). The systolic timing of this abnormal LAP c-v wave is highlighted by the arterial blood pressure (ART) waveform. These traces were recorded from a 74-year-old woman who had early postoperative failure of a mitral valvuloplasty. Despite ART hypotension (104/57 mmHg), severe mitral regurgitation caused left atrial hypertension (mean LAP 30 mmHg [v 60 mmHg]).

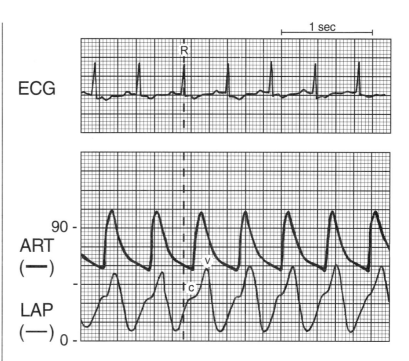

Figure 17.7 Mean pulmonary artery wedge pressure (PAWP) exceeds left ventricular end-diastolic pressure in patients with severe mitral regurgitation, because the regurgitant v wave during systole increases mean PAWP. The best estimate for left ventricular end-diastolic pressure is measured just prior to inscription of the systolic v wave (32 mmHg, *arrow*). Although the ECG R wave is highlighted to denote end-diastole (R, *dashed vertical line*), remember that the PAWP trace gives a delayed representation of left atrial pressure, and consequently, end-diastolic pressure is measured later in a PAWP trace than in a LAP trace (cf. Fig. 17.6) or a central venous pressure trace (compare Figs. 17.1 to 17.3). These PAWP waveforms were recorded from a 55-year-old woman who developed severe mitral regurgitation following acute myocardial infarction, resulting in a giant regurgitant c-v wave in her PAWP trace (mean PAWP 50 mmHg [v 90 mmHg]).

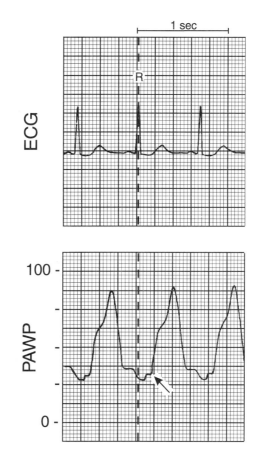

Figure 17.8 The tall systolic v wave of mitral regurgitation appears later in the cardiac cycle than the normal systolic pressure peak in the systemic arterial blood pressure (ART) trace. The regurgitant v wave inscribed in this pulmonary artery wedge pressure (PAWP) waveform has a more gradual upstroke than the systolic upstroke in the accompanying ART waveform, and it reaches its peak later, after the ECG T wave. These morphologic and timing characteristics help identify a PAWP waveform that displays a tall regurgitant v wave. A normal central venous pressure (CVP) waveform reinforces these details of waveform timing. See text for more detail.

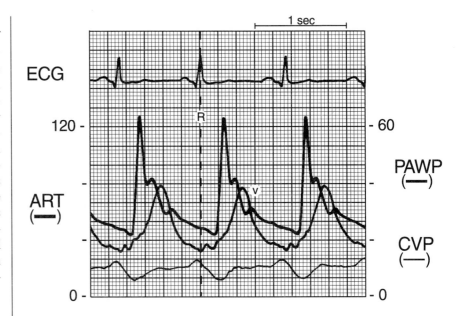

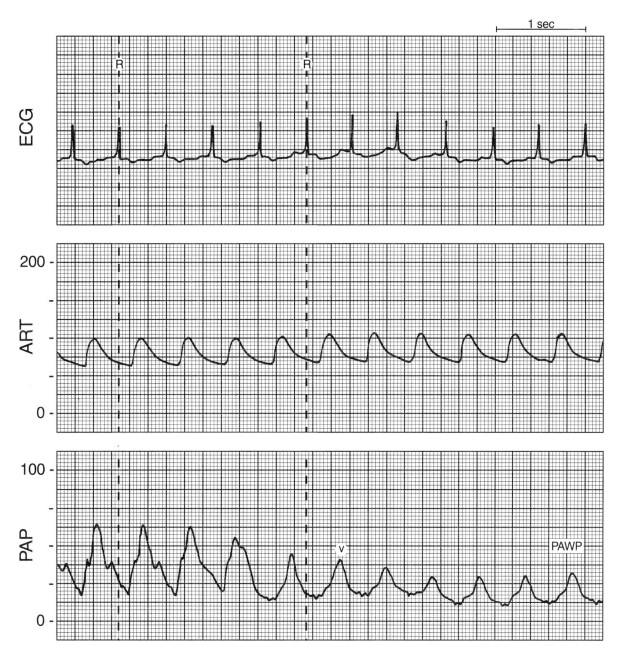

Figure 17.9 Temporal differences in the systolic pressure peaks recorded from the systemic arterial blood pressure (ART), pulmonary artery pressure (PAP), and pulmonary artery wedge pressure (PAWP, last seven heart beats) in a patient with mitral regurgitation. The PAP systolic upstroke is steeper than the PAWP systolic v wave upstroke and slightly precedes the systolic ART upstroke. The PAP systolic pressure peak coincides with the ART systolic pressure peak, while the PAWP v wave peak occurs later in the cardiac cycle. These traces were recorded from a 74-year-old woman with acute mitral regurgitation. She was tachycardic (heart rate 115 beats/min) and hypotensive (ART 105/65 mmHg), and the mitral regurgitation resulted in pulmonary hypertension (PAP 64/17 mmHg) and increased PAWP (mean 25 mmHg [v 40 mmHg]).

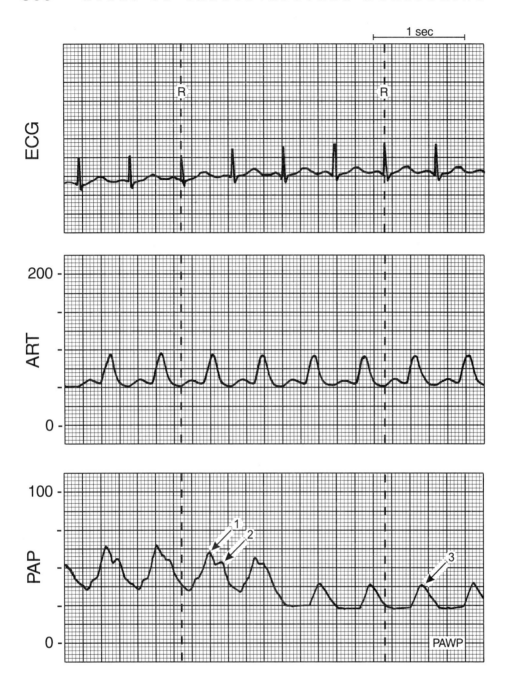

Figure 17.10 Temporal differences in the systolic pressure peaks recorded from the systemic arterial blood pressure (ART), pulmonary artery pressure (PAP), and pulmonary artery wedge pressure (PAWP, last four heart beats) in a patient with mitral regurgitation. The systolic PAP peak (*arrow 1*) slightly precedes the systolic ART peak, while the systolic peak in PAWP (*arrow 3*), which results from a regurgitant v wave, appears approximately 120 msec later in the cardiac cycle. The regurgitant v wave also distorts the unwedged PAP trace (*arrow 2*), giving it a bifid appearance, which obscures the dicrotic notch. This *rightward shift* in the location of the systolic pressure peak in the PAWP trace helps distinguish a PAWP that contains a tall regurgitant v wave from an unwedged PAP trace. These traces were recorded from a 31-year-old man who had staphylococcal endocarditis and severe mitral regurgitation. Note that the pulmonary artery diastolic pressure (35 mmHg) exceeds mean PAWP (28 mmHg), which suggests that pulmonary vascular resistance was increased in this case.

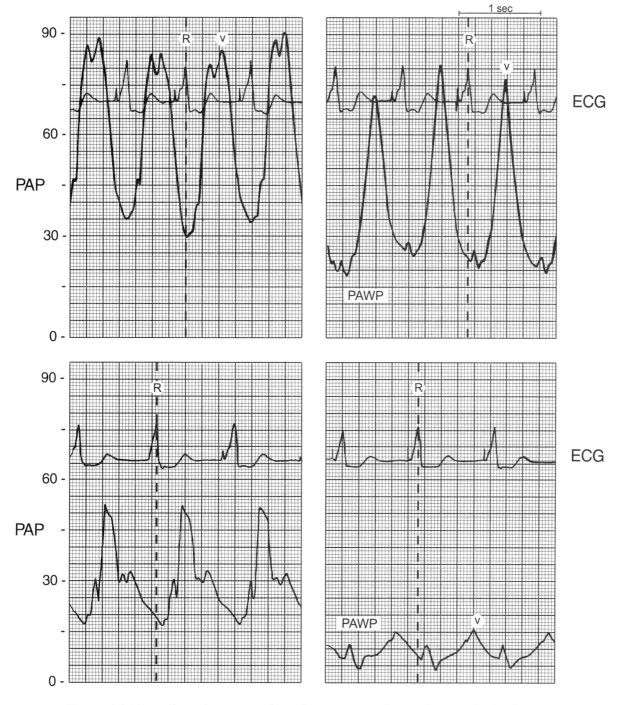

Figure 17.11 A tall systolic v wave of mitral regurgitation distorts the unwedged pulmonary artery pressure (PAP) trace, giving it a bifid appearance, which obscures the normal dicrotic notch. These traces were recorded from an 82-year-old man who had undergone coronary artery bypass graft surgery and subsequently developed severe mitral regurgitation. The ECG demonstrates ventricular pacing. The top panels show PAP and pulmonary artery wedge pressure (PAWP) recorded when mean arterial blood pressure was 85 mmHg. A giant regurgitant v wave (77 mmHg) is observed in the PAWP trace and can be observed in the unwedged PAP as well. The bottom panels were recorded after intravenous sodium nitroprusside was given to reduce mean arterial blood pressure to 70 mmHg, thereby decreasing left ventricular afterload and the regurgitant fraction. This treatment produced a dramatic decrease in PAWP, particularly the v wave magnitude (15 mmHg). The PAP waveform assumes a more normal morphology as well. Although transesophageal echocardiography showed that severe mitral regurgitation was still present following this therapy, the *hemodynamic impact* of the regurgitation was attenuated markedly by the afterload reduction. See text for more detail.

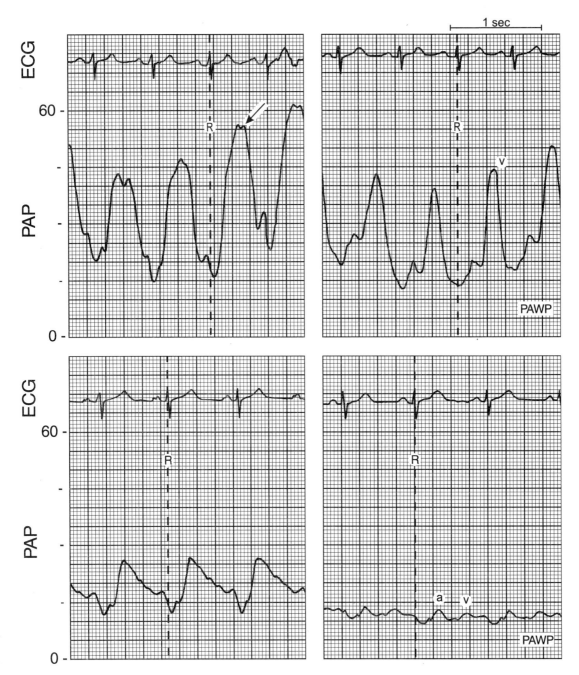

Figure 17.12 A tall systolic v wave of mitral regurgitation distorts the unwedged pulmonary artery pressure (PAP) trace, giving it a bifid appearance, which obscures the normal dicrotic notch. In the top panels, the PAP waveform has this abnormal morphology owing to the regurgitant v wave (*arrow*) that produces a double peak appearance. The pulmonary artery wedge pressure (PAWP) trace clearly reveals the v wave and its timing in the cardiac cycle. Following pharmacologic left ventricular afterload reduction, the bottom panels were recorded. This treatment obliterated the pathologic v wave in the PAWP trace. Mean wedge pressure is now normal (11 mmHg), and typical small a and v waves are evident. The PAP (26/12 mmHg) returns to normal as well. Although transesophageal echocardiography showed that severe mitral regurgitation was still present following treatment, the *hemodynamic impact* of the regurgitation was attenuated markedly by the afterload reduction. See text for more detail.

Figure 17.13 V wave height and severity of mitral regurgitation. Left atrial pressure–volume curves elucidate the three factors that determine v wave magnitude. (*Top*) Role of left atrial volume. For any given volume (x) of regurgitation, the left atrial volume at onset of systole will determine the height of the regurgitant v wave. In a hypovolemic patient (point A), regurgitant volume x will inscribe a small pressure v wave. In a normovolemic patient (point B), the identical regurgitant volume x results in a tall pressure **V** wave. (*Middle*) Role of left atrial compliance. For any given volume (x) of regurgitation, the shape of the left atrial pressure–volume curve will determine the height of the regurgitant v wave. In a patient with normal left atrial compliance (point A), regurgitant volume x will inscribe a small pressure v wave. In a patient with reduced left atrial compliance (point B), the identical regurgitant volume x results in a tall pressure **V** wave. (*Bottom*) Role of regurgitant volume. Assuming the same starting points for left atrial volume and pressure (points A and B), a small regurgitant volume (x) will produce a small v wave, while a large regurgitant volume (**X**) will produce a large **V** wave. However, owing to the confounding effects of left atrial volume and compliance, the volume of regurgitation is not the only predictor of v wave height. See text for more detail.

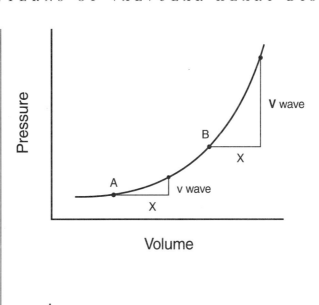

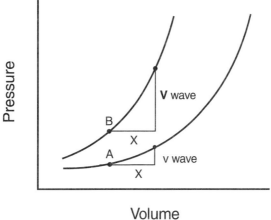

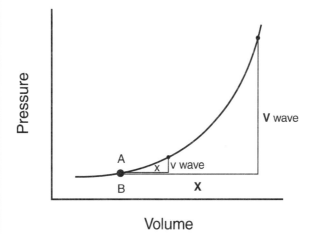

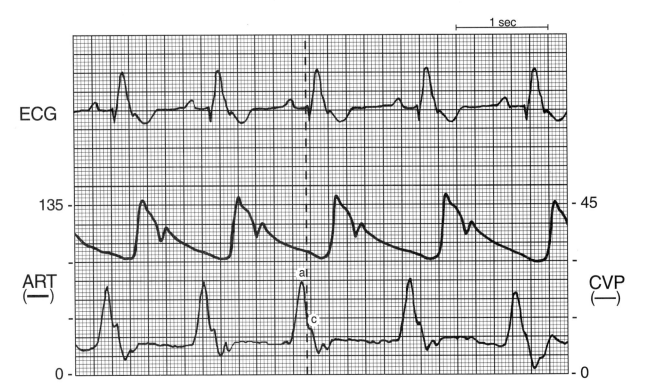

Figure 17.14 Tricuspid stenosis distorts the diastolic components of the central venous pressure (CVP) waveform. Because of obstruction to flow across the stenotic valve, the early diastolic y descent in CVP is obliterated, and atrial contraction at end-diastole inscribes a tall a wave (25 mmHg). The ECG and arterial blood pressure (ART) traces help identify the abnormal CVP waveform components. The ECG demonstrates first degree atrioventricular block and right bundle branch block. Onset of the ECG QRS complex is highlighted by the dashed line, which precedes the CVP c wave at onset of systole. See text for more detail. (Modified from Mark,[11] with permission.)

Figure   17.15 Tricuspid stenosis. Mean central venous pressure (CVP) is increased (14 mmHg), and the tracing demonstrates characteristic diastolic waveform abnormalities, including a slurred early diastolic y descent and prominent end-diastolic a wave (the peak of which exceeds the limits of the recorder). The normal CVP v wave and slow y descent seen in tricuspid stenosis should be compared to the tall regurgitant v wave and steep y descent characteristic of tricuspid regurgitation (Figs. 17.1 to 17.3). These traces were recorded from a 22-year-old man, born with Ebstein's anomaly of the tricuspid valve, who had undergone tricuspid valve replacement with a bioprosthesis that had become severely stenotic. The ECG demonstrates advanced conduction disease, including first degree atrioventricular block and right bundle branch block. (Modified from Mark,[10] with permission.)

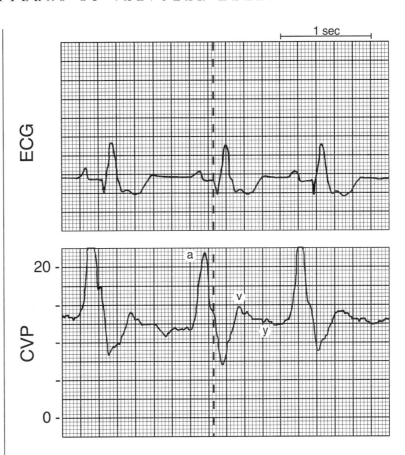

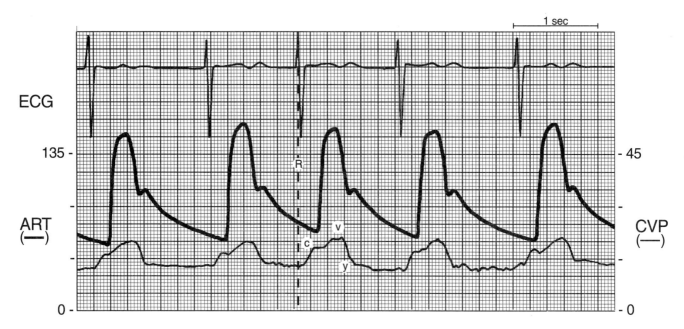

Figure 17.16 Moderate tricuspid stenosis. Because of atrial fibrillation, the a wave is not present in the central venous pressure (CVP) trace. However, characteristics of tricuspid stenosis include the increase in mean CVP (15 mmHg) and attenuation of the diastolic y descent. (Compare with Figs. 17.1 to 17.3.) The arterial blood pressure (ART) trace helps identify the c and v waves seen in the CVP trace and their timing in the cardiac cycle.

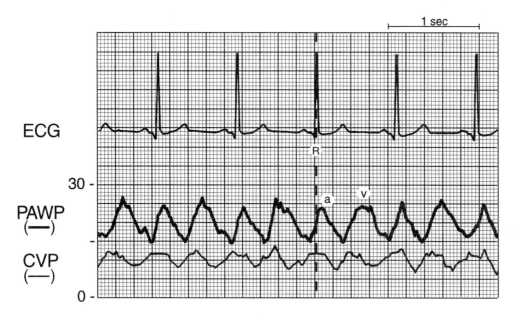

Figure 17.17 Mild mitral stenosis. Obstruction to flow across the mitral valve during diastole increases mean left atrial or pulmonary artery wedge pressure (PAWP, 20 mmHg). The PAWP waveform demonstrates a slurred early diastolic y pressure descent following the v wave and a prominent end-diastolic a wave. The wedge pressure waveform in mitral stenosis is different than that seen in mitral regurgitation (Figs. 17.5 and 17.7). The accompanying central venous pressure (CVP) waveform illustrates the temporal delay of a and v waves recorded in the PAWP trace.

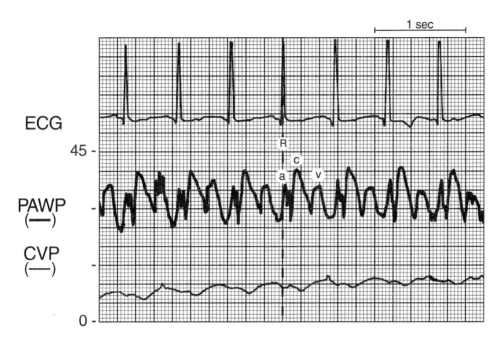

Figure 17.18 Moderate mitral stenosis. Mean pulmonary artery wedge pressure is significantly elevated (33 mmHg) and a, c, and v waves are identified. Although the increase in mean PAWP in mitral stenosis is similar to that seen in mitral regurgitation, the tall v wave and steep y descent characteristic of mitral regurgitation are not seen here (compare Figures 17.5, 17.11, and 17.12). Despite the increased PAWP, central venous pressure (CVP, 10 mmHg) morphology remains normal in this example.

Figure 17.19 Severe mitral stenosis and atrial fibrillation. Despite the marked increase in mean pulmonary artery wedge pressure (PAWP, 35 mmHg), the height of the v wave (43 mmHg) is comparatively small, and the diastolic y descent in pressure is markedly attenuated. Because of the arrhythmia, the a wave is not inscribed in either the PAWP or the central venous pressure (CVP) traces, although the c-v wave typical of atrial fibrillation is seen in the CVP waveform. This example clearly illustrates how obstruction to flow across the stenotic mitral valve distorts the normal early diastolic y descent in left atrial or wedge pressure. Compare the PAWP y descent with the CVP y descent. The arterial blood pressure (ART) waveform is included to aid waveform identification and timing.

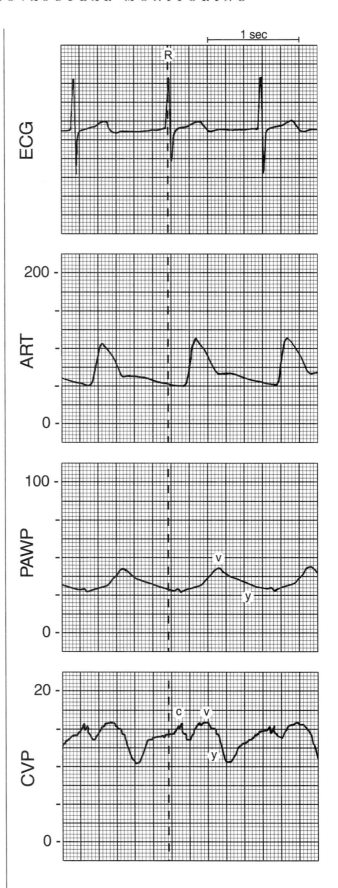

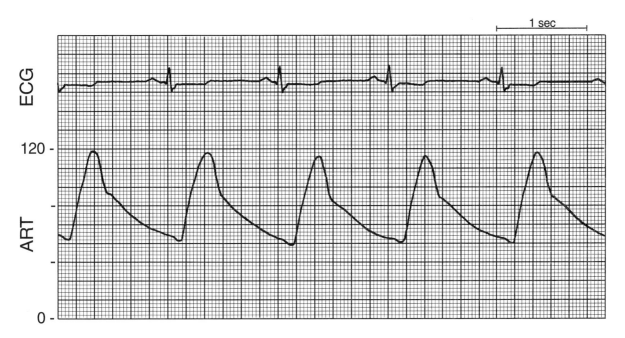

Figure 17.20 The arterial blood pressure (ART) waveform in aortic stenosis demonstrates a slow rise in pressure (*pulsus tardus*), a delayed pressure peak, and a diminished amplitude (*pulsus parvus*). Because of aortic stenosis, the radial ART systolic pressure peak is reached approximately 120 msec later than in a normal radial ART waveform (Figs. 8.1 and 8.2). Note that the dicrotic notch associated with aortic valve closure is not seen.

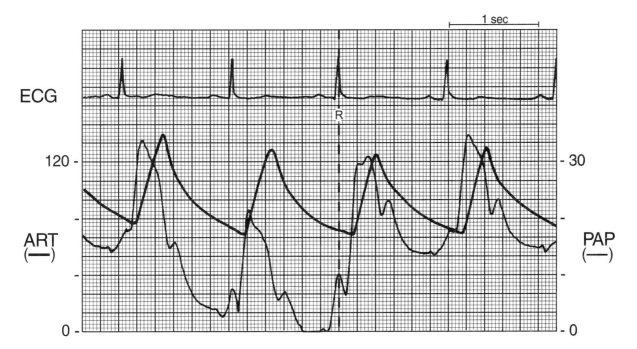

Figure 17.21 Aortic stenosis distorts the radial arterial blood pressure (ART) waveform. The slurred systolic pressure upstroke and delayed systolic ART peak are highlighted by comparing this waveform with a normal pulmonary artery pressure (PAP) waveform. Also note that forceful inspiration during spontaneous ventilation causes the PAP to decrease below zero (although the PAP waveform is clipped at the bottom of the recording grid).

Figure 17.22 Aortic stenosis. The characteristic slurred systolic pressure upstroke, delayed systolic pressure peak, and anacrotic notch (*arrow*) are evident in this radial arterial blood pressure (ART) waveform.

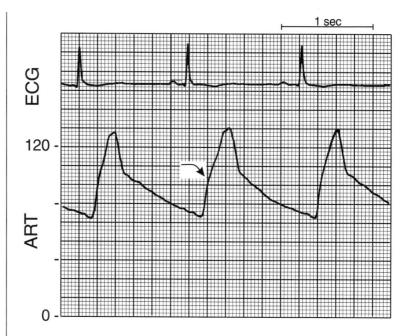

Figure 17.23 The arterial blood pressure (ART) waveform in aortic regurgitation demonstrates a steep systolic upstroke, wide pulse pressure (124/53 mmHg, pulse pressure 71 mmHg), and a double systolic peak (*bisferiens pulse*, white circle). Compare with the ART waveform seen in aortic stenosis (Figs. 17.20 to 17.22). See text for more detail.

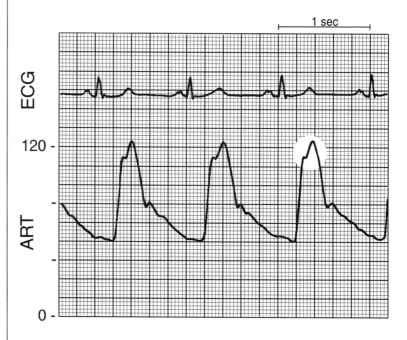

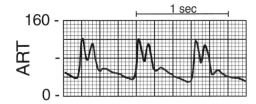

Figure 17.24 Aortic regurgitation. The radial arterial blood pressure (ART) waveform reveals a low diastolic pressure (32 mmHg), wide pulse pressure (120/32 mmHg, pulse pressure 88 mmHg), and double systolic peak. Compare with aortic stenosis (Figs. 17.20 to 17.22).

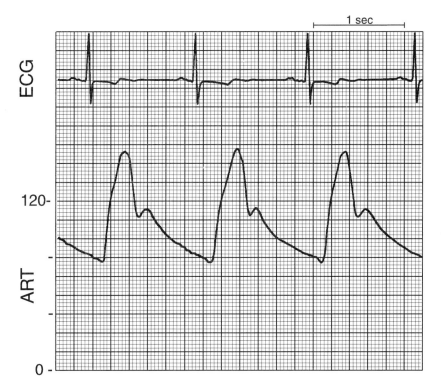

Figure 17.25 Moderate aortic stenosis and moderate aortic regurgitation. Features of both conditions are seen in the arterial blood pressure (ART) waveform. Characteristic of aortic stenosis, the waveform demonstrates a slurred systolic pressure upstroke and delayed systolic pressure peak. The widened pulse pressure and preserved dicrotic notch are more typical of aortic regurgitation.

References

1. Bethea CF, Peter RH, Behar VS, et al. The hemodynamic simulation of mitral regurgitation in ventricular septal defect after myocardial infarction. Cathet Cardiovasc Diagn 1976;2:97–104

2. Boerboom LE, Kinney TE, Olinger GN, Hoffmann RG. Validity of cardiac output measurement by the thermodilution method in the presence of acute tricuspid regurgitation. J Thorac Cardiovasc Surg 1993;106:636–42

3. Braunwald E. The physical examination. In: Braunwald E, ed. Heart Disease. A Textbook of Cardiovascular Medicine. Philadelphia: WB Saunders, 1992:13–42

4. Braunwald E, Awe WC. The syndrome of severe mitral regurgitation with normal left atrial pressure. Circulation 1963; 27:29–35

5. Cigarroa RG, Lange RA, Williams RH, et al. Underestimation of cardiac output by thermodilution in patients with tricuspid regurgitation. Am J Med 1989;86:417–20

6. Dobson GM, Horan BF, Bradburn NT. Significance of diastolic pulmonary artery pressure peaks. J Clin Monit 1992;8:62–5

7. Fuchs RM, Heuser RR, Yin FCP, Brinker JA. Limitations of pulmonary wedge V waves in diagnosing mitral regurgitation. Am J Cardiol 1982;49:849–54

8. Grossman W. Profiles in valvular heart disease. In: Grossman W, Baim DS, eds. Cardiac Catheterization, Angiography, and Intervention. Philadelphia: Lea & Febiger, 1991:557–81

9. Mark JB. Systolic venous waves cause spurious signs of arterial hemoglobin desaturation. Anesthesiology 1989;71:158–60

10. Mark JB. Central venous pressure monitoring: clinical insights beyond the numbers. J Cardiothorac Vasc Anesth 1991; 5:163–73

11. Mark JB. Getting the most from your central venous pressure catheter. In: Barash PG, ed. ASA Refresher Courses in Anesthesiology (vol 23). Philadelphia: Lippincott-Raven, 1995:157–75

12. Mark JB, Chetham PM. Ventricular pacing can induce hemodynamically significant mitral valve regurgitation. Anesthesiology 1991;74:375–7

13. Moore RA, Neary MJ, Gallagher JD, Clark DL. Determination of the pulmonary capillary wedge position in patients with giant left atrial V waves. J Cardiothorac Anesth 1987;1:108–13

14. O'Rourke RA, Silverman ME, Schlant RC. General examination of the patient. In: Schlant RC, Alexander RW, eds. The Heart Arteries and Veins. New York: McGraw-Hill, 1994:238–41

15. Pichard AD, Kay R, Smith H, et al. Large V waves in the pulmonary wedge pressure tracing in the absence of mitral regurgitation. Am J Cardiol 1982;50:1044–50

16. Royster RL, Johnson JC, Prough DS, et al. Differences in pulmonary artery wedge pressures obtained by balloon inflation versus impaction techniques. Anesthesiology 1984;61:339–41

17. Snyder RW, Glamann DB, Lange RA, et al. Predictive value of prominent pulmonary arterial wedge V waves in assessing the presence and severity of mitral regurgitation. Am J Cardiol 1994;73:568–70

18. Velky PJ, Harte FA. The appearance of large "V" waves in association with sternal retraction during coronary artery surgery. J Cardiothorac Vasc Anesth 1992;6:453–5

CHAPTER EIGHTEEN *Pericardial Constriction* and *Cardiac Tamponade*

THE VENOUS WAVEFORM IN CONSTRICTION AND TAMPONADE

While many pathologic conditions cause a marked increase in central venous pressure (CVP), cardiac compression by pericardial fluid or constrictive pericarditis deserves special mention because of certain characteristic hemodynamic features. **Pericardial constriction** (also termed constrictive pericarditis or pericardial restriction) limits cardiac filling because of the rigid, often calcified pericardial shell. Impaired venous return results in reduced end-diastolic volume, stroke volume, and cardiac output. Despite reduced cardiac volumes, cardiac filling pressures are markedly elevated and equal in all four chambers of the heart at end-diastole (Fig. 18.1).

Additional diagnostic clues are provided by the CVP waveform. Mean CVP is increased, and all of the normal phasic venous waveform components are exaggerated. Thus, the characteristic CVP waveform in pericardial constriction displays tall a and v waves and steep x and y descents, which give the waveform a sawtooth appearance described as an *M* or *W* configuration, depending on whether the heart rate is faster (M) or slower (W) (Figs. 18.1 and 18.2).[8,9,14,15] Venous return to the right atrium is biphasic in patients with pericardial constriction, with vena caval flow reaching velocity peaks during both the systolic x and diastolic y descents in atrial pressure.[23] Note that this biphasic pattern of venous return is similar to the pattern seen under normal conditions.

Another hemodynamic hallmark of pericardial constriction is observed in the right and left ventricular pressure traces. Owing to the restrictive pericardial shell, early diastolic ventricular filling is rapid but short-lived, resulting in a *diastolic dip and plateau* pattern,[9,23] also termed a *square root sign* (Fig. 18.3).[6] In some cases, particularly when heart rate is slow, a similar waveform pattern may be noted in the CVP trace: A steep y descent (the *diastolic dip*) results from rapid early diastolic flow from atrium to ventricle, and a mid-diastolic h wave (the *plateau*) reflects the interruption in flow imposed by the restrictive pericardial shell (Figs. 18.1 to 18.3). (See Ch. 2, Fig. 2.7, for more complete discussion of the mid-diastolic h or plateau wave and normal venous pressure waves.) Although the dip and plateau pattern of pericardial constriction is well seen in these examples (Figs. 18.1 to 18.3), it will be obscured during tachycardia because of the shortened duration of diastole.[9]

The CVP waveform in pericardial constriction shares many morphologic features with that recorded from patients with *restrictive cardiomyopathy* or *right ventricular infarction,* including elevated mean pressure, prominent a and v waves, and steep x and y descents[11,13] (compare Figs. 18.1 and 18.2

with 12.15 and 12.16). This underscores the fact that all three conditions share the pathophysiologic feature of reduced right ventricular diastolic compliance. In pericardial constriction, this results from the restraining effects of the diseased pericardium, while in restrictive cardiomyopathy and right ventricular infarction, diastolic dysfunction results from an intrinsic increase in right ventricular stiffness or an impairment in right ventricular relaxation.

Additional experimental and clinical observations highlight the shared pathophysiologic mechanisms in these three conditions. Extensive right ventricular infarction leads to right ventricular dilatation, which may increase intrapericardial pressure to the point where pericardial restraint also reduces left ventricular filling and stroke volume. This mechanism is supported by the observation that the hemodynamic abnormalities of experimentally induced right ventricular infarction can be ameliorated by opening the pericardium.[18] The diagnostic dilemma posed in differentiating restrictive cardiomyopathy from constrictive pericarditis is another example of just how similar the pathophysiologic features may be in these two conditions. Indeed, clinical improvement following pericardiectomy is often the only means of making this diagnostic distinction, since only patients with constrictive pericarditis will benefit from this surgical procedure.[11] Thus, it is not surprising that pericardial constriction, restrictive cardiomyopathy, and right ventricular infarction have many hemodynamic similarities, including the morphology of the CVP waveform. All represent examples of *restrictive physiology.*[11,13]

Like pericardial constriction, **cardiac tamponade** causes impaired cardiac filling, but in the case of tamponade, a compressive pericardial fluid collection produces this effect. This results in a marked increase in CVP and a reduced cardiac diastolic volume, stroke volume, and cardiac output. Despite many similar hemodynamic features, tamponade and constriction may be distinguished by the different CVP waveforms seen in these two conditions. *In tamponade, the venous pressure waveform appears more monophasic and is dominated by the systolic x pressure descent, while the diastolic y pressure descent is attenuated or absent,* because early diastolic flow from right atrium to right ventricle is impaired by the surrounding compressive pericardial fluid collection (Figs. 18.4 and 18.5).[1,8,12–15,23]

The distinctly different CVP waveforms observed in cardiac tamponade and pericardial constriction are accompanied by equally distinct patterns of venous return in these two conditions. Whereas caval blood flow is biphasic in patients with pericardial constriction, with flow peaks occurring during both the x and y CVP descents, *caval flow is monophasic in cardiac tamponade, with venous return to the right atrium limited to the period of the systolic x venous pressure descent.*[1,23] Why are the CVP waveforms and the patterns of venous return to the heart so strikingly different in cardiac tamponade as compared to pericardial constriction?

In cardiac tamponade, the liquid pericardial fluid collection produces a marked increase in pericardial pressure homogeneously surrounding all four cardiac chambers and thereby produces mechanical *coupling* of volume changes in the atrium with reciprocal volume changes in the ventricle.[1] As a result, caval blood flow or venous return is limited to the period of ventricular ejection during systole, when right and left ventricular volumes decrease and the x pressure descent is inscribed in the CVP trace. In patients with severe cardiac tamponade, this is the only time during the cardiac cycle when CVP falls to a level at which venous return to the right atrium can occur, thus accounting for the monophasic pattern of venous return seen in this condition.[1]

Thus, although elevation and equalization of diastolic pressures in all four cardiac chambers are seen in both cardiac tamponade and pericardial constriction, important but subtle differences in venous pressure waveform morphology help discriminate these conditions. Although supplemental diagnostic tests like echocardiography are used to distinguish cardiac tamponade from other causes of elevated CVP,[2] careful scrutiny of the venous waveform may provide important early or ancillary diagnostic clues.[4] As emphasized above, *predominance of the diastolic y descent in the CVP trace is an important observation that makes the diagnosis of tamponade unlikely.* In the example in Figure 18.6, CVP is very high, and the waveform is monophasic, a pattern expected in cardiac tamponade. However, closer scrutiny of the venous pressure waveform reveals that it is dominated by a steep y descent. This tracing was recorded from a patient with pericardial constriction and coexisting atrial fibrillation. In this case, the steep dominant y descent makes cardiac tamponade unlikely, and the presence of atrial fibrillation, which is common in pericardial constriction, accounts for the absence of the a wave and deep x descent.

Another example, recorded from a 38-year-old woman with mitral valve disease and pulmonary hypertension, further illustrates the subtle diagnostic clues provided by the hemodynamic traces (Fig. 18.7). This patient had just undergone mitral valve replacement, and postoperative cardiac tamponade was considered in this case because of a marked elevation in CVP, which coexisted with arterial hypotension and low cardiac output. Although the CVP demonstrates preservation of the diastolic y descent (Fig. 18.7), making cardiac tamponade unlikely, the diagnosis of tamponade after cardiac surgery is often difficult, and characteristic hemodynamic findings may not be present.[22] Consequently, this patient returned to the operating room for mediastinal exploration. At this time, pressures recorded at end-diastole from the pulmonary artery, right atrium,

and pulmonary wedge position were unequal (pulmonary artery diastolic pressure 21 mmHg, CVP 18 mmHg, pulmonary artery wedge pressure 16 mmHg) (Fig. 18.8). Instead of cardiac tamponade, these tracings suggest the diagnosis of right ventricular ischemia and failure, and elevated pulmonary vascular resistance from long-standing mitral stenosis leading to a gradient between the pulmonary artery diastolic and wedge pressures. (See Ch. 6, Figs. 6.11 and 6.13, for more detail regarding wedge pressure measurement in patients with pulmonary hypertension.) In this complex example, note also that the CVP a wave and x descent are not as prominent as normally seen in patients with right ventricular failure, because ineffective atrial contraction (atrial failure) coexists with ventricular failure in this case. All of these diagnostic observations were confirmed during mediastinal exploration, when no hemopericardium was encountered, but instead, a dilated, hypokinetic right ventricle and right atrium were observed.

In summary, CVP traces in pericardial constriction and cardiac tamponade have many similarities but important distinguishing features (Fig. 18.9).[12–15,23] As a general rule, the CVP waveform in pericardial constriction has prominent x and y descents or a predominant y descent, while in cardiac tamponade, the CVP waveform shows attenuation or obliteration of the y descent.[8] As illustrated above, coexisting abnormalities such as tachycardia, arrhythmias, and atrial contractile failure may complicate interpretation of these waveforms.[1,8–10] On occasion, localized pericardial constriction may simulate valvular stenosis,[23] and coexisting hypovolemia may lower cardiac filling pressures to within the normal range and confound the diagnosis.[9,10] In some instances, patients may show features of more than one condition, such as seen in patients with **effusive-constrictive pericarditis**[5] who have constriction of the heart by the visceral pericardium coexisting with a pericardial effusion that compresses the heart. In these cases, pericardiocentesis reduces the pericardial pressure and eliminates the features of tamponade, but the underlying restrictive physiology remains after pericardial fluid drainage.[5,9,10] As in other diagnostic situations, it is best not to consider the diagnosis of tamponade or constriction as an all or none phenomenon but rather in terms of degrees of severity.[8]

PULSUS PARADOXUS

Pulsus paradoxus is said to be present when spontaneous inspiration causes a decline in systolic arterial blood pressure of more than 10[23] or 12 mmHg.[8] This term remains a source of confusion because a slight inspiratory fall in blood pressure is a normal phenomenon, and *pulsus paradoxus is not paradoxic, but rather an exaggeration of this normal inspiratory decline in blood pressure.* Mild pulsus paradoxus is diagnosed using a standard blood pressure cuff and stethoscope or by observing a continuous arterial blood pressure tracing (Fig. 18.10), while more extreme inspiratory reductions in systolic blood pressure can be detected by simple palpation of a peripheral pulse and noting a reduced amplitude (palpable pulsus) or obliteration of the pulse (total paradox) during inspiration. It should be emphasized that pulsus paradoxus is a phenomenon described during spontaneous ventilation, not during positive pressure mechanical ventilation.[3] Dramatic cyclic changes in systolic blood pressure occur in many patients receiving positive pressure ventilation, and these pressure changes arise from hypovolemia and a variety of other causes more common than cardiac tamponade.[3,7,16,20,21] (See Ch. 16, Figs. 16.16 to 16-18, for more complete discussion of respiratory–circulatory interaction and changes in arterial blood pressure during positive pressure ventilation.)

Whenever the diagnosis of cardiac tamponade is entertained, the patient should be examined for the presence of pulsus paradoxus. Although *Beck's triad* of systemic arterial hypotension, elevated CVP, and a small, quiet heart is characteristic of cardiac tamponade resulting from sudden intrapericardial hemorrhage, it is seen less often in cases where tamponade develops slowly. In the latter situation, new onset of pulsus paradoxus is an important clinical clue that may lead to further diagnostic studies.

The mechanism of pulsus paradoxus in cardiac tamponade has been extensively studied and is described in detail elsewhere.[12,17,23] In brief, CVP is elevated in cardiac tamponade and the decrease in pleural pressure during spontaneous inspiration augments vena caval return to the right atrium and ventricle more than normal. Owing to the restraining effects of the tense, fluid-filled pericardium, the increased right-heart filling causes leftward shift of the intraventricular septum and reduced left ventricular diastolic compliance, resulting in decreased left ventricular filling, left ventricular stroke volume, and systemic arterial blood pressure. A second, perhaps less important mechanism contributing to pulsus paradoxus is the inspiratory increase in transmural left ventricular pressure that occurs as pleural pressure decreases during inspiration. The increased left ventricular transmural pressure results in increased left ventricular afterload, which further reduces left ventricular stroke volume and systemic arterial blood pressure. Thus, both of these mechanisms lead to the important observation that *pulsus paradoxus in cardiac tamponade is associated with a diminished pulse pressure and left ventricular stroke volume during early inspiration*, and this distinguishes it from the inspiratory decline in systolic blood pressure seen in patients with airway obstruction, bronchospasm, chronic lung disease, or dyspnea of any origin.[17,23] In these patients, respiratory variation in arterial blood pressure may be unusually large, but pulse pressure remains normal. These respiratory fluctuations in blood pressure result from exaggerated changes in intrathoracic and juxtacardiac pressure that accompany these other conditions. (See Ch. 16 for more detail about respiratory-circulatory interaction.)

In pericardial constriction, pulsus paradoxus is observed less frequently, since the pericardial space is obliterated by the disease process and inspiration does not produce a fall in pericardial pressure or CVP or any accompanying augmentation in venous return to the right atrium. Pulsus paradoxus may be seen in patients with pericardial constriction at a stage in the disease when the pericardium has not yet become totally inelastic, but the mechanism by which it occurs in advanced pericardial constriction remains less clear.[23] One additional clinical observation commonly seen in patients with pericardial constriction but not cardiac tamponade is Kussmaul's sign, an inspiratory increase in CVP.[9] In pericardial constriction, the rigid pericardial shell prevents transmission of normal phasic changes in intrathoracic pressure that occur during the respiratory cycle. Consequently, inspiration does not result in a fall in CVP, but instead, venous pressure paradoxically increases because the descent of the diaphragm increases intraabdominal pressure and presumably translocates blood from the engorged splanchnic visceral bed into the thorax.[19]

Illustrations for Pericardial Constriction and Cardiac Tamponade

Figure 18.1 Pericardial constriction. Inspection of the pulmonary artery pressure (PAP), pulmonary artery wedge pressure (PAWP), and central venous pressure (CVP) traces reveals equalization of end-diastolic filling pressures (22 mmHg). The tall a and v waves and steep x and y descents in the CVP waveform create the sawtooth *M* or *W* configuration characteristic of this condition. The CVP trace also displays a prominent mid-diastolic plateau wave or h wave (°), which follows the steep early diastolic y descent inscribed after the v wave. The arterial blood pressure (ART) waveform is shown to highlight waveform timing. See text for more detail. (Modified from Mark,[14] with permission.)

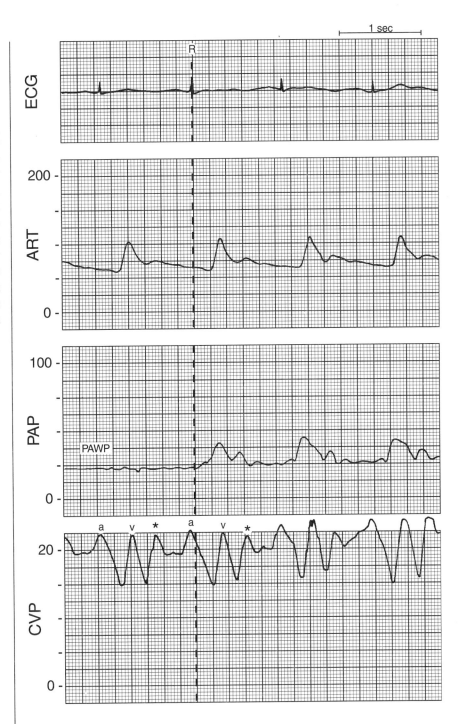

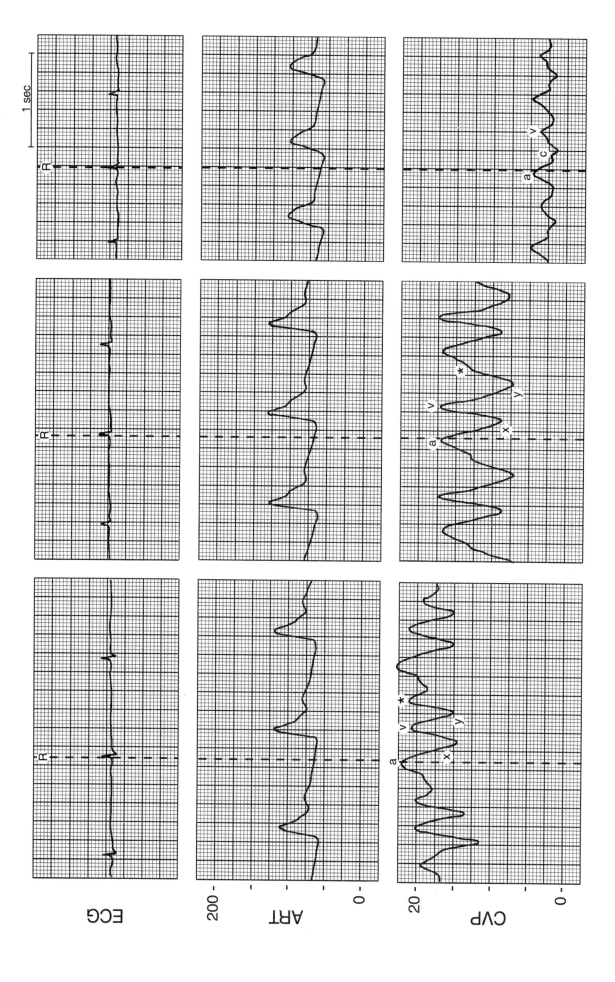

Figure 18.2 Pericardial constriction and its resolution following pericardiectomy. Striking changes in central venous pressure (CVP) are seen by comparing waveforms before (*left panels*), during (*middle panels*), and after (*right panels*) pericardial stripping. The characteristic CVP waveform of pericardial constriction seen preoperatively reveals tall a and v waves, steep x and y descents, and an unusual mid-diastolic plateau wave or h wave (°) (*left panels*). The steep early diastolic y descent followed by the mid-diastolic pressure plateau is analogous to the *dip and plateau* or *square root sign* described in the ventricular pressure trace in patients with this condition. This dominant y descent in the CVP trace distinguishes pericardial constriction from cardiac tamponade. Compare with Figs. 18.4 and 18.5. An increased mean CVP is still present intraoperatively after partial excision of the pericardium, although the diastolic dip and plateau pattern is less prominent (*middle panels*). Postoperatively, a normal CVP is recorded (3 mmHg), and normal venous a, c, and v waves can be identified (*right panels*). The arterial blood pressure (ART) waveform is shown to highlight waveform timing. See text for more detail. (Modified from Mark,[14] with permission.)

Figure 18.3 The diastolic filling abnormality of pericardial constriction produces a characteristic *dip and plateau pattern* or *square root* sign in both the ventricular and atrial pressure traces. Although this pattern may be seen on both the left and right sides of the heart, it is illustrated here for the right side with right ventricular (RV) and central venous pressure (CVP) wave-forms. The prominent a and v waves, steep x and y descents, and mid-dia-stolic pressure plateau wave (*) in the CVP are highlighted, and their temporal relationship to the ECG P, R, and T waves is noted. See text for more detail.

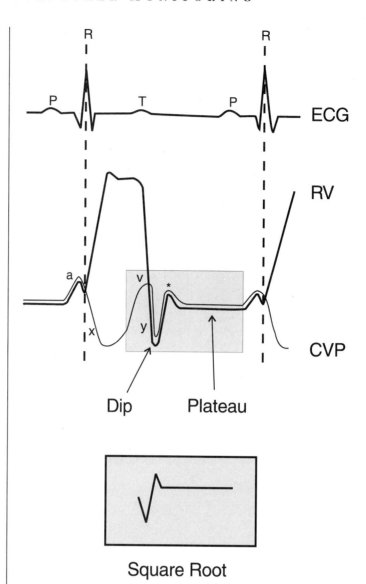

Figure 18.4 Cardiac tamponade. This central venous pressure (CVP) waveform was recorded from a 45-year-old woman following major thoracic trauma. Mean CVP is increased (16 mmHg), and the waveform shows marked attenuation of the diastolic y descent, unlike the pattern seen in pericardial constriction. Compare with Figs. 18.1 and 18.2. Other CVP waveform components (a, c, and v waves, x descent) are identified here. See text for more detail.

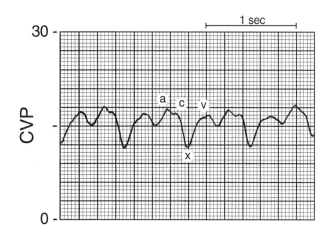

Figure 18.5 Cardiac tamponade. The arterial blood pressure (ART) is low (84/55 mmHg), and the central venous pressure (CVP) is increased. Furthermore, the CVP waveform appears monophasic, with a dominant systolic x descent and a markedly attenuated diastolic y descent. Although the ECG is not available here to aid waveform interpretation, the venous waveform components (a, c, x, v) may be identified by comparison with the ART waveform. See text for more detail. (Modified from Mark,[15] with permission.)

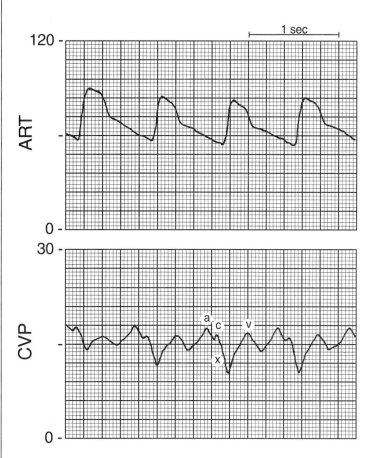

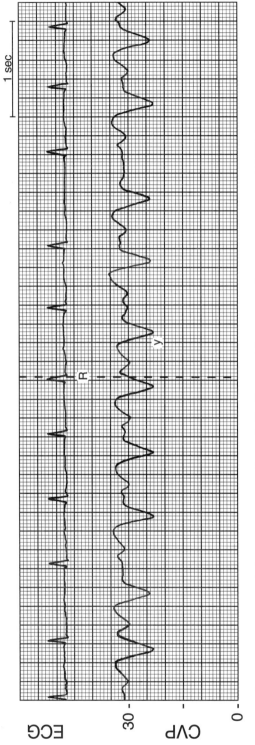

Figure 18.6 Pericardial constriction and atrial fibrillation. Mean central venous pressure (CVP) is extremely high (31 mmHg). Although the venous waveform is monophasic, the predominant pressure descent is the diastolic y descent, a pattern not seen in cardiac tamponade. In this instance, coexisting atrial fibrillation and constrictive pericarditis produce a monophasic CVP waveform with a dominant y descent preceded by small c and v waves. Compare with Figs. 18.1, 18.2, and 18.5.

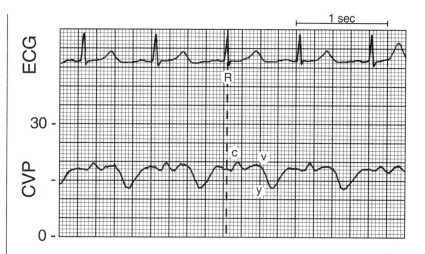

Figure 18.7 Pseudotamponade. This central venous pressure (CVP) waveform was recorded from a 38-year-old woman following mitral valve replacement. Postoperative cardiac tamponade was diagnosed because of persistent arterial hypotension and elevated cardiac filling pressures, including this CVP of 18 mmHg. Note, however, that the venous waveform is not typical for tamponade, because it shows a predominant diastolic y descent, which is normally obliterated or attenuated in patients with this diagnosis. In this instance, the abnormal CVP waveform resulted from right ventricular failure. Additional hemodynamic recordings (Fig. 18.8) clarify this diagnosis. See text for more detail.

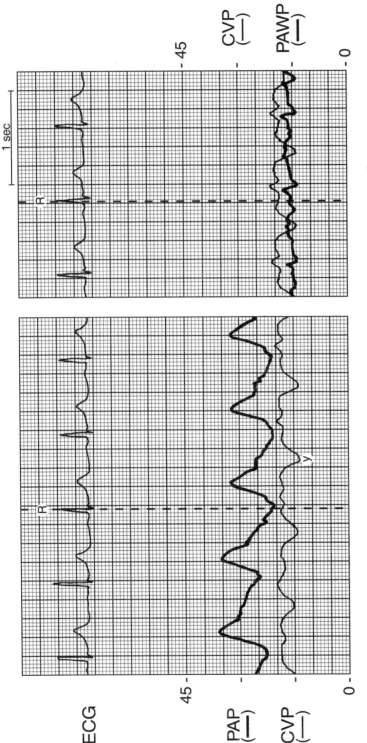

Figure 18.8 Pseudotamponade. Pulmonary artery pressure (PAP), pulmonary artery wedge pressure (PAWP), and central venous pressure (CVP) waveforms were recorded from a 38-year-old woman following mitral valve replacement. Postoperative cardiac tamponade was diagnosed based on persistent arterial hypotension, low cardiac output (2.3 L/min), and elevated cardiac filling pressures. Closer scrutiny of the hemodynamic waveforms reveals a number of features that are not typical for cardiac tamponade. Although the filling pressures are all abnormally high, there is no end-diastolic pressure equalization (pulmonary artery diastolic pressure 21 mmHg, CVP 18 mmHg, PAWP 16 mmHg). Furthermore, the morphology of the CVP waveform is very unusual for cardiac tamponade because the diastolic y pressure descent is preserved as the dominant pressure descent. In this case, these hemodynamic recordings result from right ventricular failure, which accounts for the disproportionate increase in CVP compared to the mild elevation in PAWP. The gradient between pulmonary artery diastolic pressure and PAWP (21 – 16 = 5 mmHg) reflects an increased pulmonary vascular resistance that accompanies long-standing pulmonary hypertension. Finally, the small CVP a wave and attenuated x descent following the ECG P and R waves result from impaired right atrial contractility. At the time of mediastinal exploration, cardiac tamponade was not present, and instead, the alternative diagnoses of right atrial and right ventricular failure were confirmed by direct cardiac inspection. Intravenous dobutamine ameliorated these abnormalities and produced a significant increase in cardiac output. Compare these traces with those seen in pericardial constriction (Figs. 18.1 and 18.2) and cardiac tamponade (Figs. 18.4 and 18.5). (Modified from Mark,[15] with permission.)

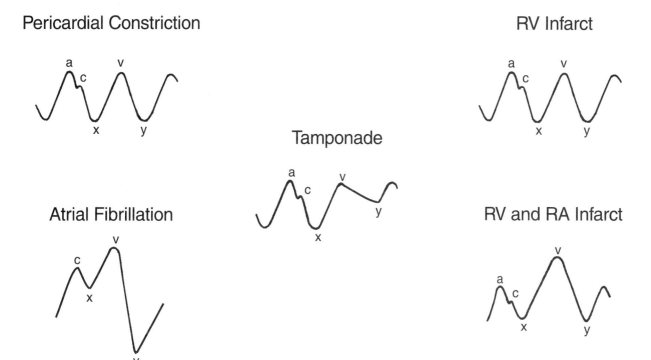

Figure 18.9 Central venous pressure morphologies in different forms of restrictive physiology. Pericardial constriction results in exaggeration of all phasic waveform components, with tall a-c and v waves and steep x and y descents. The venous waveform in right ventricular (RV) infarction mimics pericardial constriction, unless there is coexisting right atrial (RA) infarction, which reduces the amplitude of the a-c wave and systolic x descent. Cardiac tamponade is distinguished by the attenuation or obliteration of the early diastolic y descent. When atrial fibrillation accompanies pericardial constriction (or right ventricular infarction), the a wave is no longer present and the ensuing systolic x descent will be attenuated, leaving a dominant y descent.

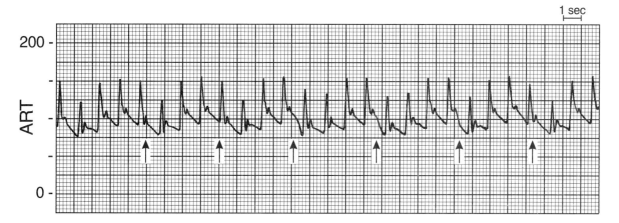

Figure 18.10 Pulsus paradoxus. Each spontaneous inspiratory effort (*arrows*, respiratory rate 15/min) produces a marked decline in arterial blood pressure (ART), with the systolic pressure falling as much as 25 mmHg. Note that there is a concomitant reduction in ART pulse pressure during inspiration. See text for more detail.

References

1. Beloucif S, Takata M, Shimada M, Robotham JL. Influence of pericardial constraint on atrioventricular interactions. Am J Physiol 1992;263:H125–34

2. Fowler NO. Cardiac tamponade. A clinical or an echocardiographic diagnosis? Circulation 1993;87:1738–41

3. Fowler NO. Clinical problem-solving. A broken heart. N Engl J Med 1996;334:1474–6

4. Greenberg MA, Gitler B. Left ventricular rupture in a patient with coexisting right ventricular infarction. N Engl J Med 1983; 309:539–42

5. Hancock EW. Subacute effusive-constrictive pericarditis. Circulation 1971;43:183–92

6. Hirschmann JV. Pericardial constriction. Am Heart J 1978; 96:110–22

7. Jardin F, Farcot J-C, Gueret P, et al. Cyclic changes in arterial pulse during respiratory support. Circulation 1983;68:266–74

8. Kern MJ, Aguirre F. Interpretation of cardiac pathophysiology from pressure waveform analysis: pericardial compressive hemodynamics, part I. Cathet Cardiovasc Diagn 1992;25:336–42

9. Kern MJ, Aguirre F. Interpretation of cardiac pathophysiology from pressure waveform analysis: pericardial compressive hemodynamics, part II. Cathet Cardiovasc Diagn 1992;26:34–40

10. Kern MJ, Aguirre F. Interpretation of cardiac pathophysiology from pressure waveform analysis: pericardial compressive hemodynamics, part III. Cathet Cardiovasc Diagn 1992;26:152–8

11. Kushwaha SS, Fallon JT, Fuster V. Restrictive cardiomyopathy. N Engl J Med 1997;336:267–76

12. Lorell BH, Braunwald E. Pericardial disease. In: Braunwald E, ed. Heart Disease. A Textbook of Cardiovascular Medicine. Philadelphia: WB Saunders, 1992:1465–1516

13. Lorell BH, Leinbach RC, Pohost GM, et al. Right ventricular infarction. Clinical diagnosis and differentiation from cardiac tamponade and pericardial constriction. Am J Cardiol 1979; 43:465–71

14. Mark JB. Central venous pressure monitoring: clinical insights beyond the numbers. J Cardiothorac Vasc Anesth 1991; 5:163–73

15. Mark JB. Getting the most from your central venous pressure catheter. In: Barash PG, ed. ASA Refresher Courses in Anesthesiology (vol 23). Philadelphia: Lippincott-Raven, 1995:157–75

16. Massumi RA, Mason DT, Vera Z, et al. Reversed pulsus paradoxus. N Engl J Med 1973;289:1272–5

17. McGregor M. Pulsus paradoxus. N Engl J Med 1979;301: 480–2

18. Pantely GA, Bristow JD. Ischemic cardiomyopathy. Prog Cardiovasc Dis 1984;27:95–114

19. Pauker SG, Kopelman RI, Lechan RM. Clinical problem-solving. Diverted by the chief complaint. N Engl J Med 1995; 333:45–8

20. Perel A, Pizov R. Cardiovascular effects of mechanical ventilation. In: Perel A, Stock MC, eds. Handbook of Mechanical Ventilatory Support. Baltimore: Williams & Wilkins, 1992:51–65

21. Robotham JL, Scharf SM. Effects of positive and negative pressure ventilation on cardiac performance. Clin Chest Med 1983;4:161–87

22. Russo AM, O'Connor WH, Waxman HL. Atypical presentations and echocardiographic findings in patients with cardiac tamponade occurring early and late after cardiac surgery. Chest 1993;104:71–8

23. Shabetai R, Fowler NO, Guntheroth WG. The hemodynamics of cardiac tamponade and constrictive pericarditis. Am J Cardiol 1970;26:480–9

CHAPTER NINETEEN

Hemodynamic Observations During Cardiopulmonary Bypass

Although cardiopulmonary bypass is often considered to be a relatively quiet or inactive time for hemodynamic monitoring, a number of unique diagnostic waveform patterns may be observed during the bypass period. Some have considerable physiologic importance and, if left untreated, could result in substantial morbidity, while others remain physiologic curiosities. One of these, atrioventricular dysynchrony during cardiopulmonary bypass, has been highlighted earlier (Ch. 14, Fig. 14.21). A number of additional waveform patterns are presented in this chapter, including several that are observed only during the period of cardiopulmonary bypass.

HYPOTHERMIA: OSBORNE WAVES AND OTHER ECG MANIFESTATIONS

As temperature falls, heart rate slows and PR, QRS, and QT intervals lengthen. As temperatures approach 28°C, atrial arrhythmias and ventricular arrhythmias are observed, and below this temperature, ventricular fibrillation is common.[5] This sequence of events can be observed daily during cardiac surgery when cardiopulmonary bypass is initiated and the core temperature is lowered progressively through active cooling of the arterial blood (Fig. 19.1). One particularly notable observation in the ECG trace is a unique wave that rises steeply at the termination of the QRS, giving the appearance of ST-segment or J-point elevation (Figs. 19.1 and 19.2). This wave, termed an *Osborn wave*, *J wave*, or *camel-hump sign*, is virtually pathognomonic for hypothermia.[2,5,9]

Although the Osborn wave usually appears when myocardial temperatures fall below 30°C, there is considerable variation between patients. Appearance of this wave provides an important diagnostic clue, since it may herald more catastrophic arrhythmias like ventricular fibrillation (Fig. 19.1),[5,8] and myocardial hypothermia may be recognized before onset of cardiac arrest. An example in Figure 19.3, recorded during noncardiac surgery, shows the dramatic effect of cardiac hypothermia on the ECG. Irrigation of the surgical field with room temperature saline during extrapleural pneumonectomy caused transient unintentional myocardial cooling, which was not accompanied by any reduction in the core temperature measured with a nasopharyngeal thermistor (Fig. 19.3). Although these ECG changes might suggest transmural myocardial ischemia, the diffuse nature of the ST-segment elevation is a pattern more typical for pericarditis or pericardial/epicardial irritation from the irrigating fluid. Regardless of the precise etiology of these ST-segment elevations, recognition of the unusual sudden ECG changes helps avoid further myocardial hypothermia and other associated deleterious cardiac effects.

RECOGNIZING LEFT VENTRICULAR DISTENTION

Patients with aortic valve regurgitation present unique problems during cardiopulmonary bypass. Antegrade delivery of cardioplegia may be ineffective owing to the incompetent aortic valve, and alternative techniques of myocardial preservation may be needed, like retrograde cardioplegia delivered through the coronary sinus.

An additional concern in these patients is that ventricular fibrillation prior to aortic cross clamping results in severe left ventricular distention. This occurs because the incompetent aortic valve now allows continuous regurgitation of blood from aorta to left ventricle. The fibrillating ventricle can no longer eject this regurgitant volume, and progressive ventricular distention results. Although precautions may be taken to avoid this problem in patients known to have aortic valve regurgitation, functional aortic insufficiency may develop in any patient during bypass when the aortic valve is distorted by surgical retraction.

Fortunately, this problem may be diagnosed by careful observation of the hemodynamic traces on the bedside monitor. Normally, when cardiopulmonary bypass is initiated, venous drainage will empty the heart, leading to central venous pressure (CVP) and pulmonary artery pressure (PAP) approaching 0 mmHg and a nonpulsatile systemic arterial pressure trace (Fig. 19.4). Although the left ventricle continues to beat, it is empty and does not eject a stroke volume. Thus, the arterial pressure trace shows only the nonpulsatile flow pattern generated by the extracorporeal pump (Fig. 19.4).

In contrast, when the arterial pressure waveform is pulsatile despite adequate venous drainage (as evidenced by CVP and PAP near 0 mmHg), left ventricular ejection must be occurring (Fig. 19.5). In this situation, an incompetent aortic valve allows abnormal retrograde filling of the left ventricle and thus explains the pulsatile arterial blood pressure trace observed (Fig. 19.5). Under these conditions, if ventricular fibrillation develops prior to aortic cross clamping, the left ventricle can no longer empty itself and left ventricular distention occurs (Fig. 19.5). This problem can be recognized by noting the *progressive rise in pulmonary artery pressure*, which reflects the regurgitant filling of the left ventricle from the aorta. If aortic regurgitation continues untreated, left ventricular filling pressure (estimated by PAP) rises toward the level of systemic arterial blood pressure, resulting in a diminished pressure gradient for coronary perfusion, which may approach 0 mmHg (Figs. 19.5 and 19.6). Careful observation of the PAP trace will allow rapid detection of these events and help direct prompt treatment, including manual decompression of the left ventricle, left ventricular venting, and aortic cross clamping to prevent further aortic valve regurgitation (Figs. 19.5 to 19.7). It is important to recognize that while left ventricular venting prevents ventricular distention, it does not ensure adequate systemic blood flow in patients with severe aortic regurgitation. Under these circumstances, net forward flow rate equals the measured pump flow rate minus the return flow from the left ventricular vent, since the vent return represents a functional left to right shunt, which does not contribute to effective perfusion of the patient. Thus, if there is a 5 L/min pump flow rate and a 3 L/min vent return rate, the effective net flow rate to the patient is only 2 L/min.

BLOOD PRESSURE WAVES

During cardiopulmonary bypass, the arterial blood pressure trace may appear to be nonpulsatile at first glance (Fig. 19.4), but in some patients, a low-amplitude, 2- to 5-mmHg, pulsatile component can be discerned when a standard roller pump is used to generate arterial inflow. This subtle pulsatile waveform is termed *roller head artifact* (Fig. 19.8) and results from the pumping action of the roller head as it revolves in the pump raceway or housing. Since roller pumps consist of two rotating arms, each complete revolution of the pump arms will produce *two bumps* in the arterial pressure trace. Consequently, by counting the number of these bumps generated during a given time interval in the arterial pressure recording, and knowing the effective stroke volume displaced by the roller head for a given size tubing, one can calculate the extracorporeal pump flow rate. In the example in Figure 19.8, there are 19 bumps in a 3-second time interval, generated from a pump fitted with 3/8-inch diameter tubing, which produces an effective stroke volume of 27 ml with each revolution of the pump roller head. Proceeding through this calculation: (19 bumps/3 sec) × (1 revolution/2 bumps) × (27 ml/revolution) × (60 sec/min) = 5,130 ml/min. This calculated flow rate agrees closely with the cardiopulmonary bypass pump flow rate displayed on the pump console, which was 5.2 L/min in this example. The important message is that small, regular pressure waves produced by the extracorporeal pump are commonly seen in the arterial blood pressure trace. By observing these waves, the clinician has a means to calculate the blood flow rate to the patient and confirm that the flow rate displayed on the pump console is correct.

Another more unusual cyclic oscillation in arterial blood pressure may be observed on occasion, which has a larger amplitude, but a much lower frequency of approximately 4 waves/min (Fig. 19.9). These curious blood pressure waves are more pronounced when the mean arterial pressure is higher[6] and are more easily recognized when their amplitude exceeds 10 or 15 mmHg (Figs. 19.10 and 19.11). Despite receiving little attention in the anesthesiology, medicine, and critical care literature, these waves may be observed in many patients during cardiopulmonary bypass.[1,6,7] These *vasomotor waves* have received various appellations including *Traube-Hering waves*,[1] *Mayer waves*,[4] and *second-order* and *third-order waves*.[1] Not only is their nomenclature confusing, but their physiologic basis in patients undergoing cardiopulmonary bypass remains unclear. Proposed etiologies include linked oscillation in the respiratory and vasomotor center output from the brain, which can be produced experimentally by a variety of central nervous system ischemic and hypoxemic insults.[1,3,4,6,7] However, despite a substantial experimental animal literature, little is known of the meaning of these pressure waves in patients undergoing cardiac surgery, other than the suggestion that the vasomotor waves reflect a baroreceptor reflex, which is frequently observed in this setting[7] and not known to be associated with any adverse central nervous system outcome after these surgical procedures. Since these cyclic variations in arterial blood pressure occur when pump flow rate remains constant, the pressure oscillations must result from phasic changes in arterial resistance. Numerous pharmacologic agents have been reported to ablate these waves, particularly drugs that lower the blood pressure such as phentolamine,[4] chlorpromazine, droperidol, and thiopental (Fig. 19.12),[6,7] but it is not clear whether or not treatment is necessary. One practical point is that hypercarbia may be suspected as a cause of these vasomotor waves in some cases, because experimental evidence suggests a linked stimulation of both the respiratory and vasomotor centers by the elevated partial pressure of carbon dioxide in the blood (Fig. 19.11). The reader is referred elsewhere for a more complete discussion of this topic.[3]

Illustrations for Hemodynamic Observations During Cardiopulmonary Bypass

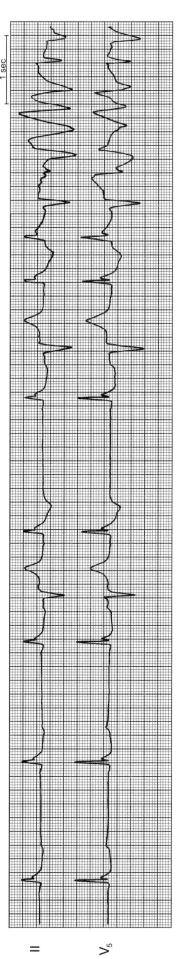

Figure 19.1 ECG changes during hypothermia. Bradycardia, ventricular ectopic beats, and ventricular fibrillation appear in rapid succession during onset of cooling associated with initiation of cardiopulmonary bypass. One additional ECG feature of hypothermia is the Osborn wave, which is seen in the initial supraventricular beats as a slowly inscribed positive deflection at the J point. At the time these traces were recorded, bladder temperature was 35.8°C and nasopharyngeal temperature was 31.4°C, a reflection of the temperature gradients created during the cooling phase of cardiopulmonary bypass. Presumably, aortic blood and myocardial temperatures were even lower than the nasopharyngeal temperature reading, as a result of rapid core cooling produced by the bypass pump through the arterial inflow cannula placed in the ascending aorta.

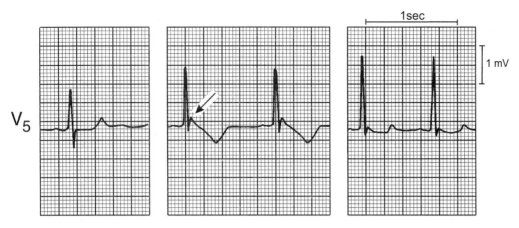

Figure 19.2 The characteristic ECG change during hypothermia is the Osborn wave (*arrow*), also termed J wave or camel-hump sign. This wave appears as a positive deflection at the junction of the QRS complex and the initial portion of the ST-segment and is most prominent in the mid-precordial and inferior leads. These traces were recorded before (*left panel*), during (*middle panel*), and after (*right panel*) hypothermic cardiopulmonary bypass.

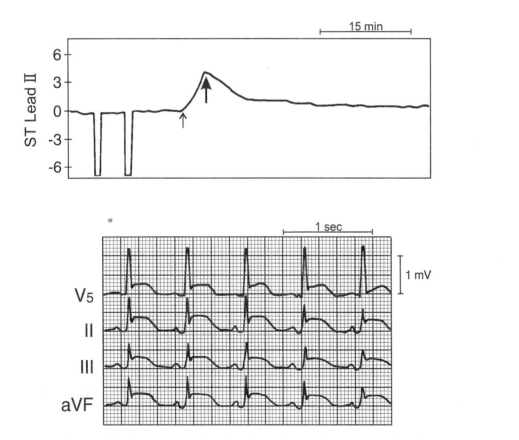

Figure 19.3 Unintentional cardiac hypothermia during extrapleural pneumonectomy. A 1-hour trend recording of ST-segment deviations, displayed as millimeters of ST displacement in lead II, illustrates the ECG changes during this event (*top panel*). Irrigation of the surgical field with room temperature saline (*thin arrow*) causes sudden cooling of the heart and results in transient, but striking 4-mm ST-segment elevation in lead II (*thick arrow*), which improves over 10 minutes. The ST-segment abnormalities during this episode are seen in virtually every lead, including the four shown here (*bottom panel*). The diffuse nature of these ST-segment elevations and their temporal association with the cold pericardial irrigation suggest that they more likely result from pericardial/epicardial irritation from the fluid than from transmural myocardial ischemia. (Also note the two brief periods in the ST-segment trend recording [*top panel*] where artifacts interrupt the recording and appear as sudden 6-mm ST depression.)

Figure 19.4 Normal hemodynamic pattern during cardiopulmonary bypass. Although the heart still beats in normal sinus rhythm, effective venous drainage to the pump empties the cardiac chambers. Consequently, the right- and left-sided filling pressures are nearly zero, as illustrated here by the central venous pressure (CVP) and pulmonary artery pressure (PAP) traces, which hover close to 0 mmHg. The beating left ventricle is empty and does not generate a stroke volume, thus accounting for the nonpulsatile arterial blood pressure (ART, 66 mmHg) trace.

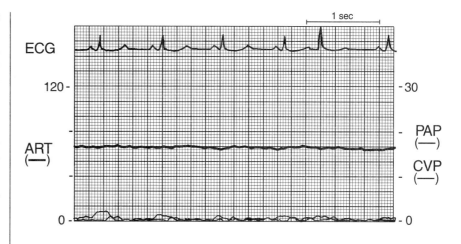

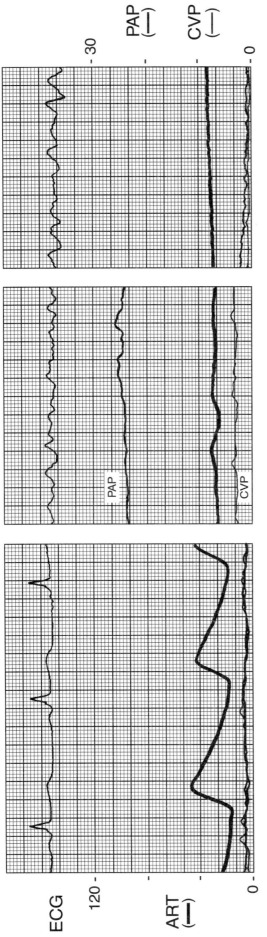

Figure 19.5 Left ventricular distention from aortic regurgitation during cardiopulmonary bypass. These traces were recorded from a patient with severe regurgitation of a porcine aortic valve prosthesis. In contrast to the hemodynamic pattern normally seen during initiation of cardiopulmonary bypass (Fig. 19.4), the arterial blood pressure (ART) trace remains pulsatile while the patient is in sinus rhythm, despite the fact that good venous drainage to the pump has been achieved, as indicated by the pulmonary artery pressure (PAP) and central venous pressure (CVP) traces, which approach 0 mmHg (*left panel*). This hemodynamic pattern is seen typically in patients with significant aortic value regurgitation and reflects the continued left ventricular filling through the incompetent aortic valve and its subsequent ejection with each heart beat. A serious problem arises when this situation is not recognized, and the heart stops beating, either in asystole or in ventricular fibrillation (*middle panel*). Aortic regurgitation continues, but the fibrillating left ventricle no longer ejects the regurgitant volume, and left ventricular distention results. This pattern is recognized by the progressive rise in PAP caused by back-filling of the left ventricle from the aorta. Note that PAP can rise to equal systemic pressure, as shown here where PAP (24 mmHg) and ART (27 mmHg) are nearly identical (*middle panel*). Under these circumstances, the coronary perfusion pressure gradient, estimated as ART – PAP, approaches 0 mmHg, and severe myocardial ischemia will occur if corrective action is not taken. Left ventricular venting will relieve left ventricular distention and restore a pressure gradient for coronary perfusion (*right panel*). This hemodynamic pattern now resembles the normal one during cardiopulmonary bypass, where the ART trace is nonpulsatile and the CVP and PAP are approximately 0 mmHg. Note that effective venting ameliorates left ventricular distention but does not guarantee adequate systemic blood flow in patients with severe aortic valve regurgitation. See text for more detail.

Figure 19.6 Left ventricular distention during cardiopulmonary bypass detected by pulmonary artery pressure (PAP) monitoring. This slow speed recording shows the hemodynamic pattern during the initial 9 minutes of bypass, when the rhythm is atrial fibrillation (AF). Aortic regurgitation can be suspected from the observation that the arterial blood pressure (ART) remains pulsatile (approximately 100/65 mmHg), despite good venous drainage to the pump, as indicated by the low PAP (approximately 7 mmHg). With onset of ventricular fibrillation (VF, dashed line), left ventricular ejection ceases, the ART waveform becomes nonpulsatile, and PAP increases progressively over 2 minutes to reach systemic ART values. *By continuously monitoring PAP during cardiopulmonary bypass, this potentially dangerous situation of left ventricular distention and inadequate myocardial perfusion can be recognized promptly.* Left ventricular venting (LV Vent) corrects the problem by draining the regurgitant volume from the left ventricle, causing PAP to fall, and thus restoring an acceptable pressure gradient for coronary perfusion. In the face of severe aortic regurgitation and left ventricular venting, the adequacy of systemic blood flow during bypass should be determined. See text for more detail.

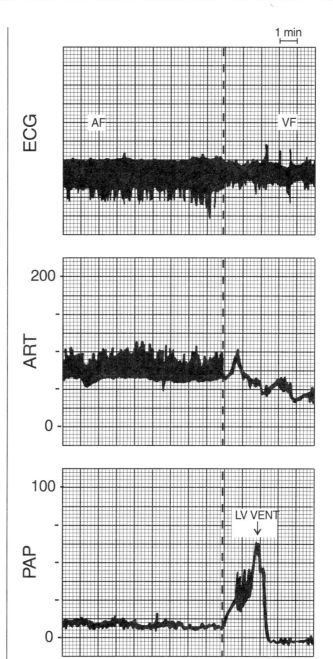

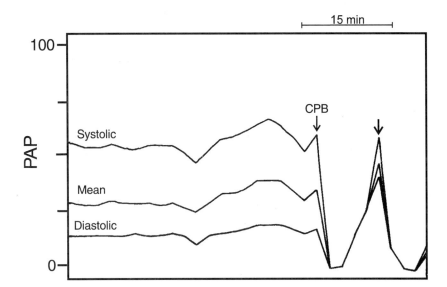

Figure 19.7 Left ventricular distention during cardiopulmonary bypass (CPB) detected by pulmonary artery pressure (PAP) monitoring. A trend recording for systolic, mean, and diastolic PAP is shown. With onset of CPB (*light arrow*), PAP falls to 0 mmHg, as anticipated with effective venous drainage to the pump. However, PAP begins to rise during CPB, and approximately 10 minutes later (*dark arrow*) reaches high levels suggesting left ventricular distention. A left ventricular vent (*dark arrow*) relieves the ventricular distention and returns PAP to 0 mmHg. These PAP values were recorded from an 84-year-old man with severe aortic stenosis and coronary artery disease who was scheduled to undergo aortic valve replacement and coronary artery bypass grafting. The significance of the aortic regurgitation was not appreciated preoperatively, but it was detected easily intraoperatively by continuous PAP monitoring during bypass.

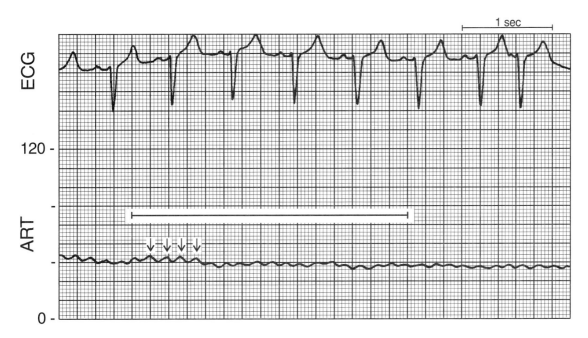

Figure 19.8 Roller head artifact seen in the arterial blood pressure (ART) trace during cardiopulmonary bypass. Small phasic pulsations often noted in the ART trace (*arrows*) result from the mechanical action of the roller pump arms as they revolve in the bypass pump raceway. When visible, these small pulsations allow an estimate of the cardiopulmonary bypass pump flow rate to be calculated. In this example, there are 19 bumps in a 3-second time interval (horizontal line on grid), generated from a bypass pump fitted with 3/8-inch diameter tubing, which produces an effective stroke volume of 27 ml with each revolution of the pump roller head. Pump flow rate is calculated as follows: (19 bumps/3 sec) × (1 revolution/2 bumps) × (27 ml/revolution) × (60 sec/min) = 5,130 ml/min. This calculated flow rate should agree closely with the cardiopulmonary bypass pump flow rate displayed on the pump console, which was 5.2 L/min in this example. See text for more detail.

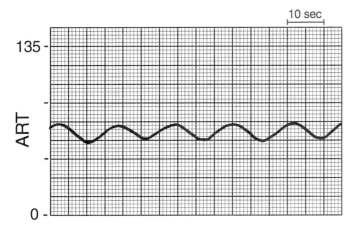

Figure 19.9 Vasomotor waves (also termed Traube-Hering waves, Mayer waves, second-order waves, and third-order waves) during cardiopulmonary bypass may be seen in the arterial blood pressure (ART) trace. These waves have a frequency of approximately 4 waves/min and an amplitude of 15 mmHg. The etiology and significance of these waves are uncertain. See text for more detail.

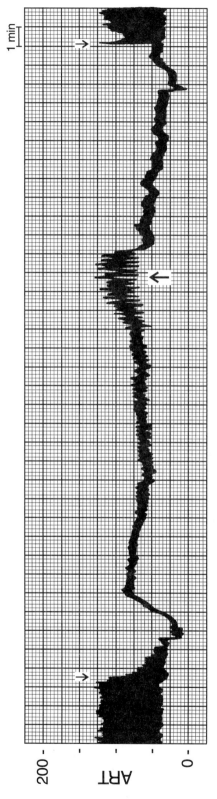

Figure 19.10 Large vasomotor waves recorded during cardiopulmonary bypass in a 26-year-old patient with staphylococcal endocarditis who underwent tricuspid valvectomy. A slow speed recording of arterial blood pressure (ART) shows progressive development of these vasomotor waves during the first 20 minutes of bypass. At their peak (*bold, up arrow*), these waves have a frequency of 4 waves/min and an amplitude of nearly 50 mmHg. Intravenous sodium thiopental given at this time attenuates these vasomotor waves for the remaining 13 minutes of bypass. The 33-minute bypass period is highlighted (*down arrows*). See text for more detail.

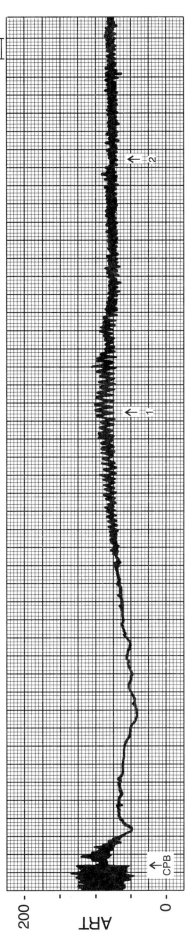

Figure 19.11 Vasomotor waves associated with hypercarbia during cardiopulmonary bypass (CPB). Approximately 25 minutes after initiation of CPB (*arrow CPB*), the arterial blood pressure (ART) trace shows prominent cyclic variations in pressure, which have a frequency of 3 waves/min and a peak amplitude of 25 mmHg (*arrow 1*). An arterial blood gas measured at this time shows an elevated partial pressure of carbon dioxide (pCO_2) of 49 mmHg. When this is treated by increasing the sweep gas flow to the pump oxygenator, the ART vasomotor waves are attenuated, and a repeat arterial blood gas measurement reveals a normal pCO_2 of 39 mmHg (*arrow 2*). See text for more detail.

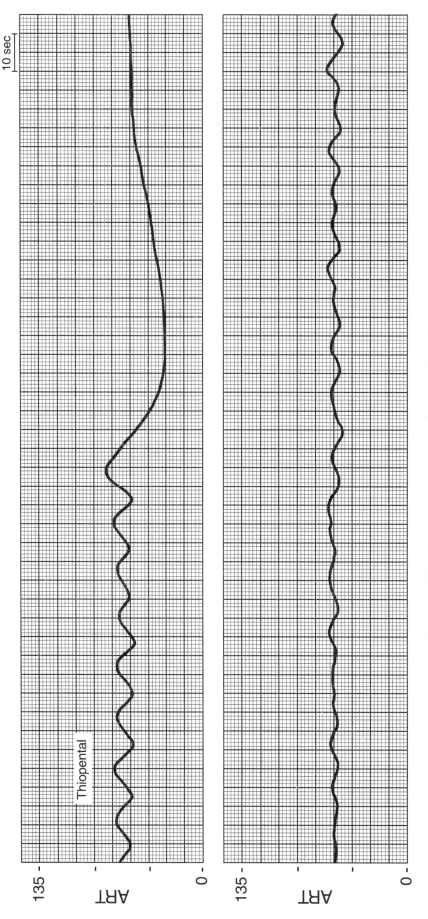

Figure 19.12 Vasomotor waves seen in the arterial blood pressure (ART) trace during cardiopulmonary bypass may be attenuated by a number of drugs that reduce blood pressure. In the top panel, ART vasomotor waves (frequency 4 waves/min, amplitude 15 mmHg) are obliterated following intravenous administration of thiopental 150 mg. The hypotensive effect that reduces ART to 30 mmHg is transient, and ART rises to 60 mmHg within 1 minute. The bottom panel is recorded 2.5 minutes later and shows that the ART vasomotor waves have returned but are less regular and have a reduced magnitude. See text for more detail.

References

1. Carroll GC. Fourth-order blood pressure waves. JAMA 1990; 263:856–7

2. Chou T-C, Knilans TK. Diseases of the central nervous system; hypothermia. In: Chou T-C, Knilans TK, eds. Electrocardiography in Clinical Practice. Adult and Pediatric. Philadelphia: WB Saunders, 1996:547–52

3. Miyakawa K, Koepchen HP, Polosa C. Mechanisms of Blood Pressure Waves. New York: Springer-Verlag, 1984

4. Preiss G, Iscoe S, Polosa C. Analysis of a periodic breathing pattern associated with Mayer waves. Am J Physiol 1975;228: 768–74

5. Reuler JB. Hypothermia: pathophysiology, clinical settings, and management. Ann Intern Med 1978;89:519–27

6. Suwa K, Asahara H. Vasomotor waves during cardiopulmonary bypass. Tohoku J Exp Med 1978;125:45–51

7. Suwa K, Yamamura H. Analysis of the vasomotor waves observed during cardiopulmonary bypass. Tohoku J Exp Med 1980;132:323–8

8. Towne WD, Geiss WP, Yanes HO, Rahimtoola SH. Intractable ventricular fibrillation associated with profound accidental hypothermia—successful treatment with partial cardiopulmonary bypass. N Engl J Med 1972;287:1135–6

9. Vandam LD, Burnap TK. Hypothermia. N Engl J Med 1959; 261:546–53

CHAPTER TWENTY *Intraaortic Balloon Counterpulsation*

The most common form of mechanical circulatory support is provided by counterpulsation using an intraaortic balloon pump (IABP). Three general methods are used to trigger the cycling period of the IABP. The most common triggering source is the ECG waveform. With ECG triggering, the balloon inflates on the T wave (onset of diastole) and deflates on the R wave (end of diastole, onset of systole). If the ECG signal is inconsistent, for example, because of electrical artifacts produced by the electrosurgical unit in the operating room, the arterial pressure waveform can be used as the trigger, with balloon inflation set at the dicrotic notch and deflation set just prior to the systolic pressure upstroke. Finally, the IABP can be set to cycle independently at a fixed rate in the absence of intrinsic cardiac electrical (ECG) or mechanical (arterial pressure) activity. This manual or internal mode of IABP triggering might be selected to provide some degree of pulsatile flow during nonpulsatile cardiopulmonary bypass.

The physiologic benefits of IABP counterpulsation are ascribed to both an increase in diastolic coronary perfusion and decrease in systolic left ventricular afterload. By inflating during diastole, the balloon augments diastolic aortic pressure and coronary perfusion pressure, thereby helping to relieve myocardial ischemia. Balloon deflation immediately prior to onset of systole reduces left ventricular afterload, thereby aiding ventricular ejection and increasing stroke volume and cardiac output.[3,4,7] Finally, counterpulsation reduces left atrial pressure and causes a reflex slowing of the heart rate, which may further improve myocardial oxygen balance.[4] Thus, counterpulsation should ameliorate myocardial ischemia, both through an increase in oxygen supply during diastole and a decrease in oxygen demand during systole.

Recent physiologic investigations have questioned the precise mechanism by which the IABP exerts its beneficial clinical effects. Kimura et al[2] have shown that the increased diastolic aortic pressure generated by the IABP is not transmitted effectively beyond a severe coronary stenosis and consequently does not lead to an increase in distal flow in diseased coronary vessels. Using transesophageal echocardiography in patients undergoing cardiac surgery, Cheung et al[1] have shown that the predominant acute effect of counterpulsation is a reduction in left ventricular systolic wall stress. Both of these studies point to the important role of afterload reduction as the mechanism by which the beneficial effects of the IABP are realized. Since optimal timing of the IABP is required in order to provide successful afterload reduction, this chapter provides a detailed consideration of IABP timing guided by arterial blood pressure monitoring.

IABP TIMING

Timing of balloon inflation and deflation becomes critically important if the beneficial effects of counterpulsation are to be achieved and detrimental circulatory effects are to be avoided. Although triggering of balloon inflation and deflation is often provided by the ECG, optimal timing of the balloon cycle requires an arterial pressure trace, since the precise duration of the mechanical cardiac events of interest (systole and diastole) cannot be determined accurately from the electrical ECG signal alone. Balloon inflation should occur with closure of the aortic valve, which is marked by the dicrotic notch on the arterial pressure waveform (also see Ch. 8). Balloon deflation should occur just prior to aortic valve opening and the systolic pressure upstroke (Fig. 20.1). When timed properly, balloon inflation during diastole will raise mean diastolic pressure, and balloon deflation prior to systole will lower peak systolic pressure as well as reduce the pressure at onset of systolic ejection. In most patients, the increment in diastolic pressure will exceed the decrement in systolic pressure, and as a result, mean arterial pressure will increase (Fig. 20.1).

The arterial blood pressure waveform thus assumes a characteristic morphology when the IABP is in place and properly timed during the cardiac cycle (Figs. 20.1 and 20.2; compare Fig. 8.1). The most notable feature of the arterial waveform is the double pressure peak that occurs with each cardiac cycle. The first peak corresponds to the normal systolic pressure peak, and the second results from balloon inflation during diastole. In most instances, the diastolic pressure peak, termed the *augmented diastolic pressure*, exceeds the systolic pressure peak. Note that balloon inflation occurs at the dicrotic notch, producing a sharp V shape, while balloon deflation occurs at end-diastole, creating an end-diastolic or *presystolic dip* and a reduced peak systolic pressure following balloon deflation (Fig. 20.2). Both the presystolic dip and the reduced peak systolic pressure are the hallmarks of successful afterload reduction.

It should now be evident that accurate IABP timing requires the clinician to examine both balloon-assisted beats as well as unassisted beats, in order to recognize all of the pertinent morphologic changes introduced in the arterial pressure waveform. *Consequently, balloon timing always should be adjusted with every other beat assisted by the balloon, generally termed a balloon-assist ratio of 1:2.* In the examples in Figures 20.1 and 20.2, this pattern of a 1:2 balloon-assist ratio is readily apparent. Note all of the important arterial pressure waveform changes described above: a steep rise in diastolic pressure beginning at the dicrotic notch, an augmented diastolic pressure peak exceeding systolic pressure, a presystolic pressure dip, and an ensuing peak systolic pressure that is lower than the systolic pressure generated following an unassisted beat (Fig. 20.2). After balloon timing has been adjusted to achieve these goals, the IABP-assist interval can be increased to 1:1, thereby providing maximal hemodynamic support to the patient.

The digital display of arterial blood pressure values on the bedside monitor may be confusing when a patient is receiving IABP support. First, the pressure displayed as "systolic" arterial pressure may be the diastolic augmented pressure peak rather than the true blood pressure during systole. This occurs when the algorithm in the bedside monitor inappropriately identifies the diastolic pressure peak as the systolic pressure peak, owing to its being the highest pressure during the cardiac cycle. In addition, the pressure displayed as "diastolic" pressure may be the presystolic dip or nadir pressure produced by IABP deflation. This extremely low "diastolic" pressure value belies the fact that mean diastolic pressure is actually very high because of balloon inflation during this portion of the cardiac cycle. In the example in Figure 20.2, the bedside monitor displays a blood pressure of 126/18 mmHg and erroneously records the diastolic augmented pressure as the "systolic" pressure and the presystolic nadir pressure as the "diastolic" pressure.

Although some monitors have a "smart" IABP pressure monitoring mode, the digital values for systolic and diastolic pressure may be misleading, and it is best to focus simply on mean arterial pressure. During intraaortic balloon counterpulsation, mean arterial pressure should remain accurate and continue to provide the most reliable estimate for overall systemic arterial perfusion pressure. As mentioned earlier, *properly timed IABP counterpulsation will augment mean diastolic pressure more than it reduces systolic pressure, resulting in a small increase in mean arterial pressure in most patients*.[3]

IABP TIMING PROBLEMS

By scrutinizing the arterial blood pressure trace, one should be able to determine whether balloon inflation and deflation are timed optimally during the cardiac cycle. Timing errors fall into four different categories: early inflation, late inflation, early deflation, and late deflation (Fig. 20.3). When the balloon is *inflated too early*, aortic pressure rises prematurely, before aortic valve closure and before inscription of the dicrotic notch in the arterial pressure trace. As a result, the left ventricle is forced to empty against an increased pressure or afterload, resulting in premature aortic valve closure, and consequently, reduced systolic ejection, stroke volume, and cardiac output. In contrast, *late balloon inflation* shortens the duration of diastolic augmentation in aortic pressure and diminishes the potential benefit provided by the balloon in augmenting coronary perfusion pressure. Late inflation of the IABP is recognized by the delayed rise in diastolic pressure, which occurs after the dicrotic notch and gives a U shape to the pressure rise rather than the ideal sharp V shape described above. Note that late inflation provides suboptimal IABP support, while early inflation may actually worsen the patient's condition because of the unintended increase in left ventricular afterload.

Like late balloon inflation, *early balloon deflation* diminishes the potential beneficial effects of balloon counterpul-

sation, because the duration of diastolic augmentation in aortic pressure is reduced. Early deflation may also cause a reduction in aortic pressure during diastole and thereby promote retrograde flow from the brachiocephalic and coronary arteries into the aorta.[3] Finally, early balloon deflation allows aortic pressure to rise to the normal unassisted end-diastolic value, prior to onset of systole. As a result, left ventricular afterload reduction does not occur. Inspection of the arterial pressure trace reveals this timing problem. The presystolic dip is no longer evident, and arterial pressure actually rises from its mid-diastolic nadir value to a higher pressure at end-diastole. Thus, the peak systolic pressure following a balloon-assisted beat is no lower than the peak systolic pressure generated after an unassisted beat, and afterload reduction is not realized.

The final timing problem is *late balloon deflation*. Like early inflation, late deflation may actually worsen the patient's condition by forcing the left ventricle to begin its ejection against an increased afterload imposed by the inflated balloon. When the balloon is not deflated appropriately at end-diastole, the arterial pressure trace will not display the normal presystolic dip in pressure, and instead, the arterial pressure at end-diastole is higher than that seen in an unassisted beat. Furthermore, the ensuing peak systolic pressure may be severely reduced, not because of afterload reduction, but resulting instead from failure of left ventricular ejection produced by excessive afterload imposed by the inflated aortic balloon.

In summary, proper timing of IABP inflation and deflation can be determined by careful observation of the arterial pressure waveform with a balloon-assist ratio of 1:2. Although late balloon inflation and early balloon deflation limit the therapeutic benefits of counterpulsation therapy, early balloon inflation or late balloon deflation are *unsafe* and may worsen the patient's medical condition because of increased left ventricular afterload resulting from balloon inflation during systole.

IABP TIMING: INFLUENCE OF PRESSURE MONITORING SITE

Current intraaortic balloons have a central lumen that permits direct arterial pressure monitoring from the balloon tip located in the proximal portion of the descending thoracic aorta (Fig. 20.4). Although the site of arterial pressure monitoring used for IABP timing has not been specified in the previous discussion, the central aortic pressure is the preferred site for optimal IABP timing. Alternatively, radial artery pressure monitoring should yield similar results. In both situations, the monitored pressures are recorded from sites above or proximal to the balloon and provide an estimate of aortic root pressure during diastole, when the balloon is fully inflated and nearly occluding the descending thoracic aorta (Fig. 20.4).[7] In most clinical situations, the central aortic pressure is displayed on the IABP console, and timing adjustments are guided by this pressure waveform. If the radial artery pressure is used for IABP timing, some authors have suggested that balloon inflation should appear approximately 50 msec earlier in this pressure waveform than it would in a central aortic pressure trace.[3,5] Presumably, this results from the IABP inflation pressure wave reaching the radial artery catheter slightly before the dicrotic notch would normally be inscribed. This small timing difference appears to be of minor importance in clinical practice. Consequently, radial artery pressure waveforms closely resemble central aortic pressure waveforms when the two are recorded simultaneously during IABP counterpulsation.

In contrast to radial artery pressure monitoring, femoral artery pressure monitoring presents unique problems in determining proper balloon timing. Unlike pressure monitoring from the IABP central lumen or radial artery, femoral artery pressure is recorded below or distal to the balloon, and the IABP pressure wave will arrive at the femoral recording site significantly earlier than the arterial pressure wave that originates from the heart (Fig. 20.4). As a result, the balloon inflation pressure wave arrives at a femoral artery recording site noticeably early, prior to the dicrotic notch, and gives the appearance of early balloon inflation. In the example in Figure 20.5, balloon inflation appears approximately 60 msec earlier than the apparent dicrotic notch. Although some authors have suggested that balloon inflation should be set to occur as much as 120 msec prior to the appearance of the dicrotic notch in the femoral artery pressure trace,[3,5,6] the safety of this timing method is not well established and introduces the theoretical risk that the balloon would be inflated prior to aortic valve closure. Thus, a more prudent approach to femoral artery timing of the IABP is to trigger balloon inflation approximately 40 to 80 msec prior to the position of the dicrotic notch in the femoral artery pressure trace.

Another consideration with femoral artery pressure monitoring is that balloon inflation produces occlusion or near-occlusion of the descending thoracic aorta, and consequently, the arterial vasculature is separated into two separate systems during diastole, one above and one below the balloon, each with different runoff characteristics. Although the pressures recorded above and below the balloon may be nearly identical when the IABP is in place but turned off, these pressures may be quite different when the IABP is on and the arterial vasculature is separated into these two distinct proximal and distal vascular beds. In the example in Figure 20.6, femoral artery pressure (102/48 mmHg, mean 66 mmHg) and radial artery pressure (108/48 mmHg, mean 68 mmHg) are essentially equal until 1:1 IABP counterpulsation begins. At this point, radial and femoral artery pressure traces take on different appearances, and the mean radial artery pressure (80 mmHg) exceeds the mean femoral artery pressure (70 mmHg) (Fig. 20.6). This highlights the functional separation of the arterial vasculature located above and below the balloon and underscores the fact that central aortic or radial artery pressure monitoring provides a better estimate of proximal aortic root pressure in these patients. Note also that balloon inflation appears 80 msec earlier in the femoral artery trace than in the radial artery trace in this example (Figs. 20.6 and 20.7), owing to the anatomic considerations related to these different monitoring sites described earlier.

Pressure monitoring from the femoral artery may also be subject to high-frequency artifacts, which distort the pressure signal and make IABP timing difficult. Owing to the proximity of the IABP drive line in the distal aorta, when the IABP is set in motion, the femoral artery pressure trace may display high-frequency artifacts associated with balloon movement during inflation and deflation (Figs. 20.6 and 20.7). These artifacts may distort the central aortic pressure trace as well (Fig. 20.8) but rarely compromise the fidelity of the radial artery pressure trace (Figs. 20.6 and 20.7). These artifacts arise from the motion of the IABP balloon and drive line during balloon inflation and deflation and are more readily transmitted to the central aortic pressure lumen or a nearby femoral or iliac artery catheter than the more remote radial artery catheter.

Illustrations for Intraaortic Balloon Counterpulsation

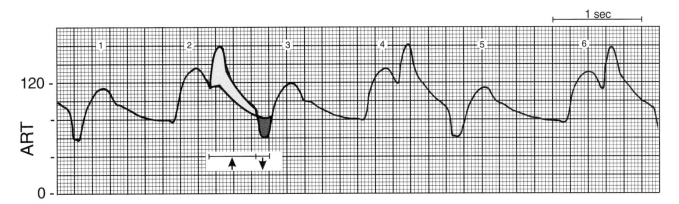

Figure 20.1 Intraaortic balloon counterpulsation produces a characteristic alteration in the arterial blood pressure (ART) waveform. With a balloon-assist ratio of 1:2, balloon inflation during every other heart beat creates a double peaked waveform (beats 2, 4, and 6). Properly timed balloon inflation beginning at the dicrotic notch causes an increase in diastolic pressure throughout most of diastole (*up arrow, light shading*). Prior to the systolic upstroke in ART, balloon deflation produces a transient decrease in aortic pressure, thereby reducing the pressure at onset of systolic ejection and the systolic pressure peak of the following beat (*down arrow, dark shading*). (Note that the balloon remains deflated beyond the down arrow and until the next balloon inflation at the dicrotic notch of beat 4.) This combination of effects results in an increased pressure gradient for coronary artery perfusion during diastole and left ventricular afterload reduction during systole. Note that the shaded areas of the diastolic portion of beat 2 illustrate the distortion in the ART waveform produced by the action of the intraaortic balloon pump, as well as the increase in mean arterial pressure resulting from counterpulsation. Compare beats 1, 3, and 5 with beats 2, 4, and 6. See text for more detail.

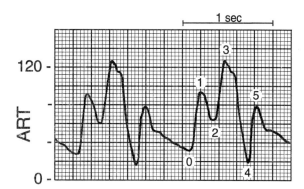

Figure 20.2 Characteristic arterial blood pressure (ART) waveform seen during intraaortic balloon counterpulsation with a 1:2 balloon-assist ratio. Four cardiac cycles are shown, two with balloon assistance and two without. Six points in the ART waveform are identified: (0) unassisted end-diastolic pressure (32 mmHg); (1) unassisted systolic pressure (92 mmHg); (2) dicrotic notch (64 mmHg); (3) assisted or augmented diastolic pressure (126 mmHg); (4) end-diastolic or presystolic dip (18 mmHg); and (5) assisted systolic pressure (78 mmHg). The actions of the intraaortic balloon create the augmented diastolic pressure and the presystolic dip and may cause the digital values displayed on the bedside monitor to be erroneous. Evidence for effective afterload reduction is provided by the observation that the presystolic dip (4) is lower than unassisted end-diastolic pressure (0), and the assisted systolic pressure peak (5) is lower than the unassisted systolic pressure peak (1). Compare these ART waveform components with those seen in a normal arterial pressure waveform (Fig. 8.1). See text for more detail.

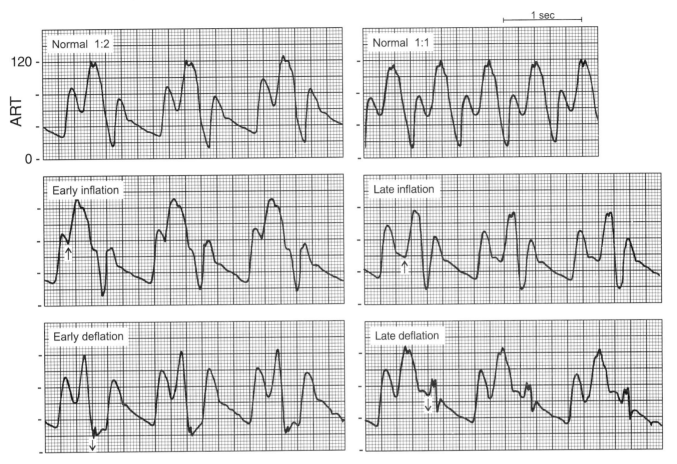

Figure 20.3 Intraaortic balloon counterpulsation timing problems. Arterial blood pressure (ART) wave-forms during normal 1:2 and 1:1 counterpulsation are shown in the top two panels. Timing errors are shown in the other four panels. *Early inflation* (*up arrow*), prior to the normal dicrotic notch, causes an increase in left ventricular afterload, premature aortic valve closure, and reduced systolic ejection. *Late inflation* (*up arrow*), after the dicrotic notch shortens the duration of diastolic augmentation and may be recognized by the U shape of the diastolic pressure rise, rather than the normal V shape. *Early deflation* (*down arrow*) prior to end-diastole reduces the duration of diastolic augmentation and does not provide effective afterload reduction, because the presystolic dip in pressure is lost, aortic pressure rises to the normal unassisted end-diastolic value, and the ensuing systolic pressure peak is no lower than peak systolic pressure generated following an unassisted beat. *Late deflation* (*down arrow*) after the onset of systolic ejection results in an increased left ventricular afterload and diminished systolic ejection. This may be recognized by the absence of the presystolic pressure dip and the distorted systolic pressure peak that follows. Although late inflation and early deflation reduce the potential therapeutic benefits of counterpulsation, early inflation and late deflation may actually worsen the patient's condition, because balloon inflation during systole increases left ventricular afterload. The ART pressure scale is identical in all six panels. See text for more detail.

Figure 20.4 Three common sites for arterial pressure monitoring during intraaortic balloon counterpulsation. The preferred site is the central aorta monitored from the central lumen of the balloon, which records the pressure at its tip located in the proximal descending thoracic aorta. Another acceptable alternative is the radial artery, which monitors arterial pressure above or proximal to the balloon and provides another estimate for aortic root pressure. Femoral artery pressure monitoring is less desirable because it monitors pressure below or distal to the balloon. Proper balloon timing from a femoral artery pressure trace is more difficult because pressure waves resulting from balloon inflation will arrive at the femoral recording site earlier than pressure waves originating from the actions of the heart, making it difficult to identify optimal timing patterns. See text for more detail.

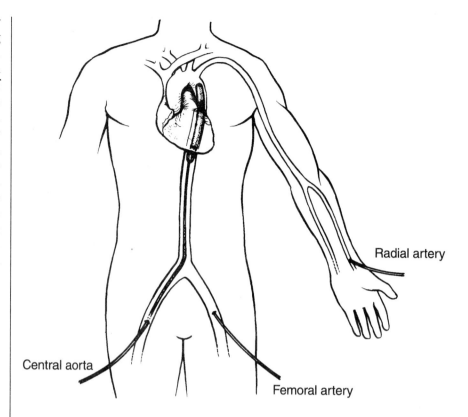

Radial artery

Central aorta

Femoral artery

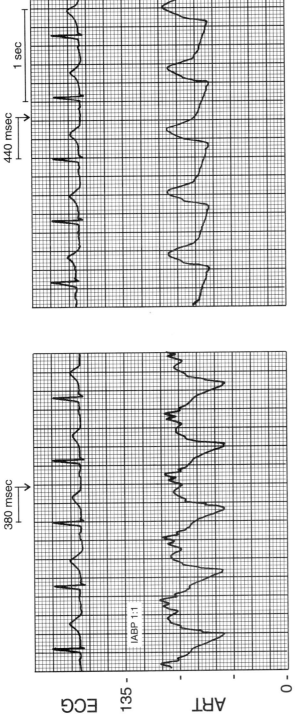

Figure 20.5 Femoral arterial blood pressure (ART) monitoring during 1:1 intraaortic balloon counterpulsation (IABP 1:1). Because the femoral ART is measured below or distal to the balloon, the balloon pressure wave arrives at this recording site significantly earlier than arterial pressure waves originating from the heart. Consequently, the femoral ART trace gives the appearance of early balloon inflation prior to the dicrotic notch during 1:1 counterpulsation (*left panel*). Although the precise location of the dicrotic notch in the femoral ART trace is hard to discern even with the balloon off (*right panel*), it appears that the balloon is inflating approximately 60 msec earlier than the dicrotic notch would normally appear. Balloon inflation occurs 380 msec after the ECG R wave in the left panel, and the position of the dicrotic notch appears closer to 440 msec after the ECG R wave in the right panel with the balloon pump off.

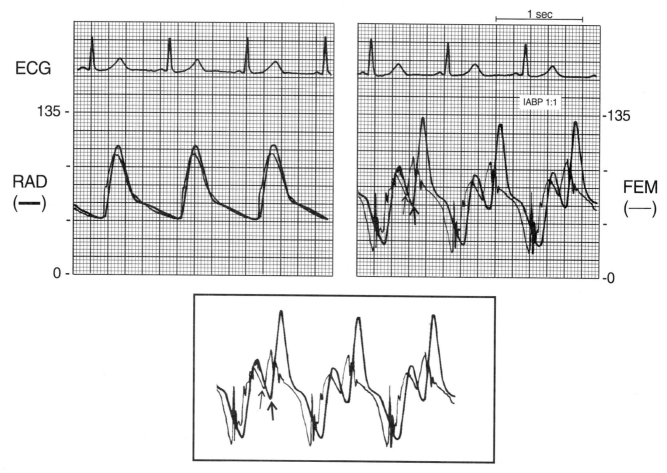

Figure 20.6 Arterial blood pressure monitoring from the radial artery (RAD) and the femoral artery (FEM) reveal important differences during intraaortic balloon counterpulsation. With the balloon off, RAD (108/48 mmHg, mean 68 mmHg) and FEM (102/48 mmHg, mean 66 mmHg) waveforms are nearly identical (*left panel*). In contrast, with 1:1 counterpulsation (IABP 1:1), RAD and FEM waveforms assume different appearances (*right panel*, also shown in *bottom panel* without grid). Because balloon inflation produces near occlusion of the descending thoracic aorta during diastole, this functionally separates the vasculature above the balloon from the vasculature below the balloon, creating two segments of the arterial system with distinct runoff characteristics. As a result, during 1:1 counterpulsation, mean RAD (80 mmHg) is higher than mean FEM (70 mmHg). Note that balloon inflation also appears 80 msec earlier in the FEM trace (*thin arrow*) than in the RAD trace (*thick arrow*), and that the FEM trace is distorted by a high-frequency motion artifact during counterpulsation (*right panel, bottom panel*). These traces were recorded from a 72-year-old woman undergoing coronary artery bypass grafting.

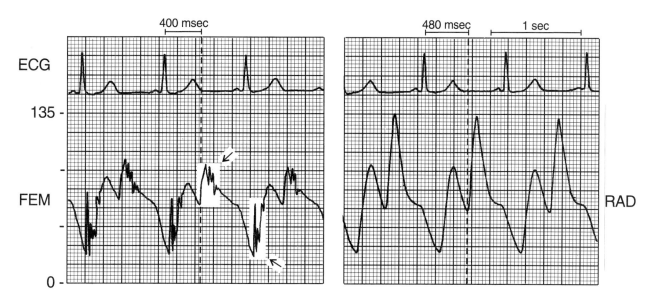

Figure 20.7 Arterial blood pressure monitoring from the femoral artery (FEM) and the radial artery (RAD) reveal important differences during intraaortic balloon counterpulsation. Balloon inflation appears 80 msec earlier in the FEM waveform (400 msec after the ECG R wave, *left panel*) than in the RAD waveform (480 msec after the ECG R wave, *right panel*). Mean arterial pressure during 1:1 counterpulsation is lower in the FEM (70 mmHg) than in the RAD (80 mmHg). A high-frequency artifact resulting from balloon movement during inflation and deflation distorts the FEM waveform (*white boxes, arrows, left panel*) but not the RAD waveform.

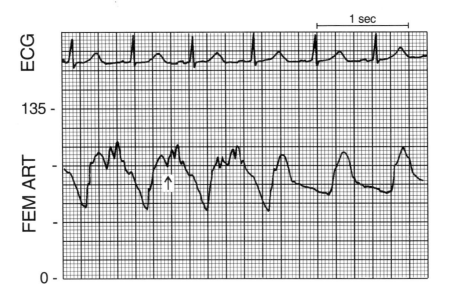

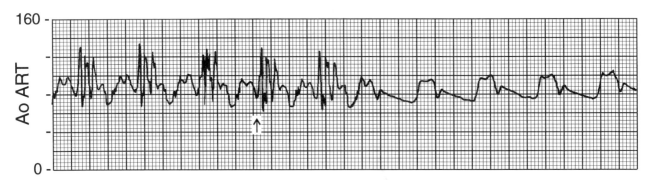

Figure 20.8 High-frequency motion artifacts caused by movement of the intraaortic balloon and its pneumatic drive line may distort femoral arterial blood pressure (FEM ART) and central aortic blood pressure (Ao ART) waveforms during counterpulsation. This waveform distortion is evident only when the balloon is turned on (first 3 beats, *top panel*; first 5 beats, *bottom panel*). Also note that balloon inflation appears early in the FEM ART trace (*arrow*, 240 msec after systolic pressure upstroke, *top panel*) compared to the Ao ART trace (*arrow*, 280 msec after systolic pressure upstroke, *bottom panel*).

References

1. Cheung AT, Savino JS, Weiss SJ. Beat-to-beat augmentation of left ventricular function by intraaortic counterpulsation. Anesthesiology 1996;84:45–54

2. Kimura A, Toyota E, Songfang L, et al. Effects of intraaortic balloon pumping on septal arterial blood flow velocity waveform during severe left main coronary artery stenosis. J Am Coll Cardiol 1996;27:810–6

3. Maccioli GA, Lucas WJ, Norfleet EA. The intra-aortic balloon pump: a review. J Cardiothorac Anesth 1988;2:365–73

4. Philips PA, Bregman D. Intraoperative application of intraaortic balloon counterpulsation determined by clinical monitoring of the endocardial viability ratio. Ann Thorac Surg 1977;23:45–51

5. Purcell JA, Pippin L, Mitchell M. Intra-aortic balloon pump therapy. Am J Nursing 1983;83:775–90

6. Quaal SJ. Counterpulsation timing: arterial pressure waveform. In: Comprehensive Intra-aortic Balloon Pumping. St. Louis: CV Mosby, 1984:130–45

7. Weber KT, Janicki JS. Intraaortic balloon counterpulsation. Ann Thorac Surg 1974;17:602–36

Index

Page numbers followed by *f* indicate figures; those followed by *t* indicate tables.

357

E

Electrical-mechanical dissociation, 207, 220
Electrocardiography, 127–143
  analog paper trace, importance of checking, 206–207
  aortic regurgitation and, 290, 310f
  aortic stenosis and, 290, 309f–310f
  artifacts, 4f–5f, 206, 212f
    during cardiopulmonary bypass, 206, 212f
    recognition of, 221–222, 228f–229f, 233f–235f
  atrial fibrillation and, 220, 224f–226f
  atrioventricular dissociation and, 220–221, 227f–228f, 230f–231f
  autogain, 130
  baseline, ST-segment abnormalities on, 147, 153f
  bedside monitoring, accuracy of, 128
  camel-hump sign. See Osborne wave
  displays, 2, 6f–9f
  electrical artifacts, 130, 139f, 206, 210f–211f
  filtering
    diagnostic mode, 130, 138f–139f
    filter mode, 130, 139f
    monitor mode, 130, 138f–139f
  filters
    bandpass, 130, 139f, 206
    high-frequency (low-pass), 130
    low-frequency (high-pass), 130
    moving average, 206
    selection of, 130, 138f–139f
  free-waveform display, 2, 7f
  gain adjustment, 130–131, 140f–142f
  for heart rate monitoring, 205–217
    artifacts on, 206, 212f
    digital display of, 206, 209f
    pacing and, 207, 213f–214f
  and hemodynamic monitoring, integrated approach for arrhythmia detection, 219–245
  hypothermia and, 148, 162f–164f, 328, 331f–332f
  J wave. See Osborne wave
  leads
    alternative systems for, 129, 135f
    atrial epicardial, 129, 137f
    color coding for, 128, 128t
    endotracheal, 129
    esophageal, 129, 136f
    intracardiac, 129, 136f
    invasive, 129, 136f–137f
    selection and display of, 129–130
    standard placement of, 128–129, 132f–134f
  limb leads
    modified bipolar, 129, 135f
    placement of, 128, 132f–133f
  mechanical influences on, 149
  with mitral regurgitation, 288, 296f–297f, 299f
  mitral stenosis and, 290, 306f–308f
  in myocardial ischemia, 145–179. See also Myocardial ischemia, electrocardiography in
  notch filter, 130, 139f

Osborne wave on, 148, 162f–163f, 328, 331f–332f
  during pacing, 222, 235f–243f
  patient positioning and, 148, 165f–166f
  precordial lead
    placement, 128, 134f
    and myocardial ischemia, 148, 160f–161f
    right-sided, 128, 134f
  P wave, 16, 19f–20f
  Q wave, 19f–20f
  recording, 3, 9f–10f
  respiratory cycle and, 149, 167f–168f
  right ventricular ischemia and, 185, 200f, 202f
  R wave, 16–17, 19f–20f, 28, 30f
    amplitude, gain adjustment and, 131, 141f–142f
    and central venous pressure, temporal relation of, 17, 22f
    detection, for heart rate monitoring, 206, 208f
  ST segment
    abnormalities on baseline recording, 147, 153f
    artifacts, with computer-aided monitoring, 149, 170f–171f
    changes in myocardial ischemia, 146–147, 151f–152f
    computer-aided monitoring, 149–150, 169f–177f
    depression, pseudonormalization, during computer-aided monitoring, 150, 177f
    display, with computer-aided monitoring, 149, 170f
    effects of filter selection on, 130, 138f–139f
    and limitations of individual lead monitoring, 148–149, 156f, 166f
    shift, gain adjustment and, 131, 141f–142f
    superimposition display format, with computer-aided monitoring, 149, 172f–173f
    trend displays, with computer-aided monitoring, 150, 173f–176f
    trend line, with computer-aided monitoring, 149, 169f
  surgical retraction and, 148–149, 166f
  S wave, 19f–20f
  temporal relations
    to central venous pressure recording, 18, 24f
    to left atrial pressure recording, 18, 24f
  tricuspid stenosis and, 290, 304f–306f
  T wave, 16–17, 19f–20f
EMD. See Electrical-mechanical dissociation

F

Fast flush method, for assessment of dynamic response of arterial blood pressure monitoring system, 101–102, 112f, 116f–118f
Fluid challenge, 250
Frank-Starling principle, 248

H

Heart rate
  definition of, 207
  versus pulse rate, 207
Heart rate monitoring, 205–217
Hemodynamic monitoring, electrocardiography and, integrated approach for arrhythmia detection, 219–245
Hemodynamic trends, 3
History, and interpretation of monitoring, 3
Hypercarbia, and vasomotor waves during cardiopulmonary bypass, 329, 339f
Hypertension. See also Pulmonary arterial hypertension
  systolic arterial, clinical interpretation of, 86f, 102–103, 107f–108f
Hypertrophic cardiomyopathy, 61
Hypothermia, electrocardiographic changes due to, 148, 162f–164f, 328, 331f–332f

I

IABP. See Intraaortic balloon pump
Incisura, 93
Integrated monitoring, 3, 12f, 220
  with aortic valve regurgitation, 290–291, 310f–311f
  with aortic valve stenosis, 290, 309f–310f
  for arrhythmia detection, 219–245
  and artifact recognition, 221–222, 234f–235f
  with mitral valve regurgitation, 288–289, 296f–299f
  with mitral valve stenosis, 290, 306f–308f
  during pacing, 222, 235f–243f
  with tricuspid valve stenosis, 290, 304f–306f
  with valvular heart disease, 287–312
Intraaortic balloon counterpulsation, 343–355
  and arterial blood pressure, 344, 347f–348f
    artifacts, 346, 352f–354f
    displays, 344–345
  augmented diastolic pressure with, 344–345
  beneficial effects of, 344
  pulse rate measurement during, 207, 216f
  timing, 344–345, 347f–348f
    arterial blood pressure artifacts and, 346, 352f–354f
    pressure monitoring site and, 345–346, 350f–354f
    problems with, 345, 348f–349f
Intraaortic balloon pump, cycling
  ECG triggering of, 344
  independent, 344
  mechanical (arterial pressure) triggering of, 344

J

Jugular venous pressure, 17
Junctional rhythm, 220, 227f, 230f. See also Atrioventricular dissociation
J wave. See Osborne wave